Statistics *for* Nursing Research

A Workbook for Evidence-Based Practice

THIRD EDITION

SUSAN K. GROVE, PhD, RN, ANP-BC, GNP-BC
Professor Emerita
College of Nursing and Health Innovation
The University of Texas at Arlington
Arlington, Texas;
Adult and Gerontological NP Consultant
Arlington, Texas

DAISHA J. CIPHER, PhD
Associate Professor
College of Nursing and Health Innovation
The University of Texas at Arlington
Arlington, Texas

ELSEVIER

Elsevier
3251 Riverport Lane
St. Louis, Missouri 63043

STATISTICS FOR NURSING RESEARCH:
A WORKBOOK FOR EVIDENCE-BASED PRACTICE
THIRD EDITION

ISBN: 978-0-323654111

Notice

Practitioners and researchers must always rely on their own experience and knowledge in evaluating
and using any information, methods, compounds or experiments described herein. Because of rapid
advances in the medical sciences, in particular, independent verification of diagnoses and drug dosages
should be made. To the fullest extent of the law, no responsibility is assumed by Elsevier, authors, editors
or contributors for any injury and/or damage to persons or property as a matter of products liability,
negligence or otherwise, or from any use or operation of any methods, products, instructions, or ideas
contained in the material herein.

Previous editions copyrighted 2017 and 2007

Library of Congress Control Number: 9780323654111

Executive Content Strategist: Lee Henderson
Content Development Specialist: Betsy McCormac
Publishing Services Manager: Shereen Jameel
Project Manager: Radhika Sivalingam
Design Direction: Amy Buxton

Printed in the United States of America.

Last digits the print number: 9   8   7   6   5   4   3   2   1

Susan K. Grove
In memory of my husband and sister:
Jay Suggs and Sheryl Grove: You both were the center of my world.

and

To our future:
Monece, Steve, Jack, Boone, and Cole Appleton
Nicole and Scott Horn

Daisha J. Cipher
To my husband and daughter:
Jason Moore and Gracie Alice Moore, for their love and support

and

To my parents:
John and Joyce Cipher, for their constant encouragement

Preface

With the emphasis in health care today on evidence-based practice, it is more important than ever for nurses to understand essential information about measurement, sampling, and statistical analysis techniques. Having this background enables students and practicing nurses to critically appraise the results of published studies and conduct data analyses to make evidence-based changes in practice.

The third edition of this workbook has been significantly revised to meet the needs of students and practicing nurses for basic and advanced statistical knowledge for practice. The revised workbook continues to focus on promoting understanding of statistical methods included in nursing studies and conducting selected statistical analyses for nursing data. This workbook was developed to meet the growing need for statistical knowledge by students in Doctor of Nursing Practice (DNP) programs, Master's in Nursing programs (e.g., Masters in Nursing Administration, Masters in Nursing Education), and RN-to-BSN and higher-level BSN programs. This workbook provides additional statistical content and practical application of that content to supplement what is provided in *Burns & Grove's The Practice of Nursing Research,* eighth edition, and *Understanding Nursing Research*, seventh edition. The content of this workbook is sufficient to enable graduate and undergraduate nursing students and practicing nurses to do the following:

- Critically appraise the sampling methods and measurement methods in nursing studies.
- Critically appraise the results sections of research articles.
- Understand power analysis and apply it in determining sample size and power of a study to determine relationships among variables and differences between groups.
- Select the most appropriate statistical procedures for analysis of data.
- Calculate selected statistical procedures using the computer and manually.
- Interpret statistical software output of the results of selected statistical procedures (mean, standard deviation, Pearson *r*, regression analysis, *t*-test, analysis of variance [ANOVA], chi-square, sensitivity, specificity, and odds ratio).
- Determine statistical significance and clinical importance of analysis results.

The exercises in this third edition of *Statistics for Nursing Research* are organized into two parts, to help differentiate basic content from more advanced content: Part 1 (Understanding Statistical Methods) and Part 2 (Conducting and Interpreting Statistical Analyses). The exercises in Part 1 were developed to promote understanding of measurement and sampling methods and to critically appraise the results sections of current, published studies.

Each exercise in Part 1 includes the following sections:

- Statistical Technique in Review
- Research Article
- Introduction

- Relevant Study results
- Study Questions
- Answers to Study Questions
- Questions to Be Graded

The *Statistical Technique in Review* at the beginning of each exercise provides a brief summary of the featured technique. The *Research Article* section then provides a current bibliographic reference to a pertinent published study from the nursing research literature. An *Introduction* follows to provide the reader with a base from which to interpret the study. A section called *Relevant Study Results,* based on the cited article, provides a relevant example taken directly from a current, published nursing study. The *Study Questions* section guides the reader in examining the statistical technique in the research article. The *Answer Key* section provides immediate feedback to ensure content mastery or to identify areas needing further study. Finally, *Questions to Be Graded* can be submitted to the instructor as assigned for additional feedback. *Instructor Answer Guidelines* for the questions to be graded are provided for the faculty on the Evolve site.

Each exercise in Part 2 features the following content:

- Statistical Formula and Assumptions
- Research Designs Appropriate for the Statistical Application
- Step-by-Step Hand Calculations [for selected statistics]
- Step-by-Step SPSS Computations [with screen shots]
- Interpretation of SPSS Output
- Final Interpretation in APA Format
- Study Questions
- Answers to Study Questions
- Data for Additional Computational Practice
- Questions to Be Graded

The *Statistical Formula and Assumptions* section at the beginning of each exercise provides the formula and mathematical properties of the statistic. The *Research Designs Appropriate for the Statistical Application* section lists the potential research designs that might require the calculation of the given statistic. The *Step-by-Step Hand Calculations* section provides the reader with a data set along with a step-by-step guide to computing the components of the statistic, using the example data. The *Step-by-Step SPSS Computations* section provides instructions on how to compute the statistics using SPSS statistical software and includes screenshots of SPSS at each step. The *Interpretation of SPSS Output* identifies each portion of statistical output and provides detailed explanations. The *Final Interpretation in APA Format* section provides the reader with an example of how to write the results of the analysis. The *Study Questions* section guides the reader in examining the statistical technique in the exercise. The *Answers to Study Questions* section provides immediate feedback to ensure content mastery or to identify areas needing further study. The *Data for Additional Computational Practice* section provides a new dataset for the reader to practice computing the statistic. *Questions to Be Graded* query the reader on the data provided for additional computational practice. An *Answer Guidelines* for the questions to be graded is provided for faculty on the Evolve website.

We believe that the hands-on approach in this workbook provides students with essential application of statistical content and an ability to assess their understanding of that content. We hope that this revised, expanded statistical workbook provides students and practicing nurses with relevant statistical knowledge for understanding the results of studies and conducting relevant data analyses. We believe that an increased understanding of statistical content provides a stronger background for implementing evidence-based nursing practice.

EVOLVE LEARNING RESOURCES

Resources for both students and instructors are provided on an Evolve Learning Resources website at http://evolve.elsevier.com/Grove/statistics/. For students and instructors, *Questions to Be Graded*, data sets in Excel and SPSS formats, and an article library with selected research articles are available on the Evolve site. Here, students can submit answers to the *Questions to Be Graded* by their faculty. For instructors, *Answer Guidelines for the Questions to Be Graded* are provided to help ensure that students have mastered the content.

DISCLAIMER

Data examples used for hand computations present either actual published data (where the individual data values have been made publically available) or simulated data. In the case of the simulated data examples, the observations were slightly altered to protect the identities of the research participants, so that it would be impossible to identify any participant. However, the statistical results of the analyses of simulated data are wholly consistent with the actual published results. For example, a significant difference yielded by the simulated data mimic the significant differences actually reported in the published studies. No significant effects were manufactured in this textbook.

Acknowledgments

Special thanks are extended to our reviewers, whose statistical knowledge was invaluable in ensuring the quality and accuracy of the information in this workbook. We also appreciate the time and effort that they spent verifying that this text is as current, accurate, and relevant as possible for nursing students and practicing nurses. We also want to thank the students who have provided us comments that have improved the clarity and quality of this text. Any errors that remain are, of course, our own.

Finally, we would like to thank the people at Elsevier who worked tirelessly to produce this book: Lee Henderson, Executive Content Strategist; Betsy A. McCormac, Content Development Specialist; Amy Buxton, Designer; Shereen Jameel, Publishing Services Manager; Radhika Sivalingam, Project Manager; and Priyanka Pradhaban, Multimedia Producer.

Susan K. Grove
Daisha J. Cipher

Contents

Part 2: Conducting and Interpreting Statistical Analyses

PART 1

Understanding Statistical Methods

Identifying Levels of Measurement: Nominal, Ordinal, Interval, and Ratio

STATISTICAL TECHNIQUE IN REVIEW

The levels of measurement were identified in 1946 by Stevens, who organized the rules for assigning numbers to objects so that a hierarchy of measurement was established. The **levels of measurement**, from lowest to highest, are nominal, ordinal, interval, and ratio. Figure 1-1 summarizes the rules for the four levels of measurement that are described in the following sections.

Nominal and Ordinal Levels of Measurement

Variables measured at the **nominal level of measurement** are at the lowest level and must conform to the following two rules: (1) the data categories must be exclusive (each datum will fit into only one category) and (2) the data categories must be exhaustive (each datum will fit into at least one category). The data categories are developed for the purpose of naming or labeling the variables for a study (Gray, Grove, & Sutherland, 2017; Waltz, Strickland, & Lenz, 2017). For example, the variable medical diagnosis of heart failure (HF) is measured at the nominal level and includes two categories, *yes* has HF or *no* HF. Variables measured at the nominal level that are frequently described in studies include gender, race/ethnicity, marital status, and medical diagnoses. For some nominal variables, such as medical diagnoses, some study participants might check more than one category because they have more than one medical diagnosis.

Ordinal level of measurement includes categories that can be rank ordered and, like nominal-level measurement, the categories are exhaustive and mutually exclusive (see Figure 1-1). In ranking categories of a variable, each category must be recognized as higher or lower or better or worse than another category. However, with ordinal level of measurement, you do not know exactly how much higher or lower one subject's value on a variable is in relation to another subject's value. Thus, variables measured at the ordinal level do not have a continuum of values with equal distance between them like variables measured at the interval and ratio levels (Grove & Gray, 2019). For example, you could have subjects identify their levels of acute pain as no pain, mild pain, moderate pain, or severe pain. Pain is measured at the ordinal level in this example because the categories can be ranked from a low of no pain to a high of severe pain; however, even though the subjects' levels of pain can be ranked, you do not know the differences between the levels of pain. The difference between no pain and mild pain might be less than that between moderate and severe pain. Thus, ordinal-level data have unknown, unequal intervals between the categories, such as between the levels of pain (Waltz et al., 2017).

Nonparametric or distribution-free analysis techniques are conducted to analyze nominal and ordinal levels of data to describe variables, examine relationships among variables, and determine differences between groups in distribution-free or non-normally

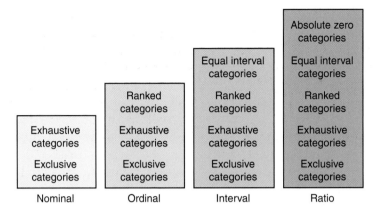

FIGURE 1-1 ▨ **SUMMARY OF THE RULES FOR THE LEVELS OF MEASUREMENT.**

distributed samples. The measure of central tendency, which is conducted to describe variables measured at the nominal level, is the mode or the most frequently occurring value in the data set. The median or middle value in a data set is calculated to describe variables measured at the ordinal level (see Exercise 8). Descriptive statistical analyses, such as frequencies and percentages, are often calculated to describe demographic variables measured at the nominal and ordinal levels in a study (see Exercise 6). Range is calculated to determine the dispersion or spread of values of a variable measured at the ordinal level (see Exercise 9).

Chi-square analysis is calculated to examine differences in variables measured at the nominal level (see Exercise 19). The Spearman Rank-Order Correlation Coefficient is calculated to examine relationships among variables measured at the ordinal level (see Exercise 20). The Mann-Whitney U and Wilcoxon Signed-Ranks tests can be conducted to determine differences among groups when study data are measured at the ordinal level (see Exercises 21 and 22). Nonparametric analyses are also conducted when interval- and ratio-level data are not normally distributed. The process for determining normality of a distribution is presented in Exercise 26. More details about conducting nonparametric analyses are presented in selected exercises of Part 2 of this text (Kim & Mallory, 2017; Pett, 2016).

Interval and Ratio Levels of Measurement

With **interval level of measurement**, the distances between intervals of the scale are numerically equal. However, there is no absolute zero, which means the score of zero does not indicate the property being measured is absent. Temperature is an example of a variable that is measured at the interval level, because the intervals between the different temperatures on either Fahrenheit or centigrade temperature scales are numerically equal. In addition, zero temperature is not the absence of temperature but only indicates it is very cold or freezing.

Subjects' scores obtained from multi-item scales are usually considered interval-level measurement. Likert scales are an example of multi-item scales commonly used to collect data about abstract concepts such as anxiety, perception of pain, quality of life, and depression. Each item on the scale has a response set for subjects to mark, which might include 1—strongly disagree to 4—strongly agree. The number and type of response options vary based on the scale. Usually the values obtained from each item in the scale are summed to obtain a single score for each subject. Although the values of each item are technically ordinal-level data, the summed score is often analyzed as interval-level data

(Gray et al., 2017; Waltz et al., 2017). The Center for Epidemiological Studies Depression Scale is an example of a 20-item, 4-point Likert scale that is used to measure depression in nursing studies, and the data from the scale is considered interval level for analysis.

Ratio level of measurement is the highest form of measurement; it adheres to the same rules as interval-level measurement, with numerically equal intervals on the scale (see Figure 1-1; Grove & Gray, 2019). In addition, ratio-level measurement has an absolute zero point, where at zero the property is absent, such as zero weight meaning absence of weight. In nursing, many physiological variables are measured at the ratio level, such as blood pressure, pulse, respiration, body mass index (BMI), and laboratory values (Stone & Frazier, 2017). Variables measured at the interval and ratio levels are also referred to as **continuous variables**. The data obtained from measuring continuous variables can usually be analyzed with parametric statistics.

Parametric statistics are powerful analysis techniques conducted on interval and ratio levels of data to describe variables, examine relationships among variables, and determine differences among groups (Kim & Mallory, 2017; Knapp, 2017). The assumptions of parametric statistics are introduced here and discussed in more detail for the parametric analysis techniques conducted in Part 2 of this text.

Assumptions:

1. The distribution of scores in a sample is expected to be normal or approximately normal.
2. The variables are continuous, measured at the interval or ratio level.
3. The data can be treated as though they were obtained from a random sample.
4. All observations within each sample are independent (Gray et al., 2017; Plichta & Kelvin, 2013).

Parametric analysis techniques are the same for variables measured at either the interval or the ratio level of measurement. For example, means and standard deviations can be calculated to describe study variables measured at the interval or the ratio level (see Exercises 8 and 9). Pearson correlational coefficient (Pearson r; see Exercise 13) is computed to determine relationships between variables, and the t-test (see Exercises 16 and 17) or analysis of variance (ANOVA; see Exercise 18) are calculated to determine significant differences among groups. **Significant results** are those in keeping with the outcomes predicted by the researcher, where the *null hypothesis is rejected*. Significant results are usually identified by * or p values less than or equal to alpha (α), which is often set at 0.05 in nursing research (Grove & Gray, 2019; Heavey, 2019). The symbol ≤ 0.05 means less than or equal to 0.05, so any p values ≤ 0.05 are considered significant. Because the analysis techniques are similar for variables measured at the interval and ratio levels, these levels of measurement are sometimes referred to as interval/ratio level; these variables are identified as continuous in this text.

RESEARCH ARTICLE

Source

Ha, F. J., Toukhsati, S. R., Cameron, J. D., Yates, R., & Hare, D. L. (2018). Association between the 6-minute walk test and exercise confidence in patients with heart failure: A prospective observational study. *Heart & Lung, 47*(1), 54–60.

Introduction

Ha and colleagues (2018, p. 54) conducted a descriptive correlational study to examine "the association between a single 6-min walk test (6MWT) and exercise confidence in HF [heart failure] patients." The sample included 106 HF patients from an outpatient clinic, who completed the Cardiac Depression Scale (CDS) and an Exercise Confidence Survey before and following the 6MWT. The CDS was a 26-item Likert scale developed to measure depressive symptoms in cardiac patients. The scale included response sets that ranged from "1 = not at all tearful" to "7 = very easily tearful," with higher numbers indicating increased severity of symptoms. The Exercise Confidence Scale is a self-reported measure of confidence of cardiac patients to perform a range of physical activities on a scale of 0 to 100 (where 0 = "Quite uncertain," 50 = "Moderately certain," and 100 = "Completely certain"). The Exercise Confidence Scale is a multi-item rating scale, and the values obtained from this scale are analyzed as interval-level data (Gray et al., 2017; Waltz et al., 2017).

"The 6MWT was associated with a significant improvement in exercise confidence in HF patients. Exercise confidence is associated with age, gender, duration of HF, New York Heart Association (NYHA) class, and severity of depressive symptoms" (Ha et al., 2018, p. 59). The researchers recommended further controlled studies to determine if the 6MWT and exercise confidence translate into improved exercise adherence and physical functioning in HF patients.

Relevant Study Results

"There were 106 participants, most of whom were male (82%) with a mean age of 64 ± 12 years (Table 1). Almost three-quarters (72%) had a history of reduced EF [ejection fraction] (<40%) and one-quarter (25%) had preserved EF (≥40%)... Approximately one-third of patients (36/106; 34%) were depressed (CDS ≥95) and the prevalence of depression increased with greater NYHA class (NYHA class I, 11%; NYHA class II, 44%; NYHA class III, 64%) ... There were no significant differences detected in any clinical characteristics between patients with HFrEF [heart failure with reduced ejection fraction] or HFpEF [heart failure with preserved ejection fraction].

One hundred two patients (96%) had complete data for Baseline Exercise Confidence. Participant mean scores indicated higher Baseline Exercise Confidence for Walking (70 ± 25), Climbing (75 ± 30), and Lifting objects of graded weight (71 ± 29) than for Running (35 ± 30). Total Exercise Confidence exceeded the mid-point of the Exercise Confidence Scale, indicating greater than 'moderate certainty' to complete exercise activities overall (62 ± 24). Total exercise Confidence and all sub-scales were inversely associated with age, NYHA class, CDS score, and 6MWD ... Additionally, duration of HF was inversely associated with Climbing and Lifting Confidence, while BMI [body mass index] was inversely associated with Walking Confidence. Male participants had significantly higher scores compared with females for the Total Exercise Confidence" (Ha et al., 2018, pp. 56–57).

TABLE 1   PATIENT DEMOGRAPHIC AND CLINICAL CHARACTERISTICS

Patient Demographic and Clinical Characteristics	Total (%) $N = 106$
Age, mean years ±	64 ± 12
Sex, female	19 (18)
Aetiology, ischaemic	36 (34)
Type of HF	
HFrEF	76 (72)
HFpEF	27 (25)
Not documented	3 (3)
Duration of HF, years ± SD	3.8 ± 3.6
NYHA class	
I	35 (33)
II	58 (55)
III	11 (10)
Not specified	2 (2)
BMI, kg/m^2	31 ± 7
Comorbidities	
Hypertension	71 (67)
Diabetes mellitus	40 (38)
CAD	37 (35)
Previous stroke	8 (8)
COPD	9 (9)
CKD (stage 3–5)	37 (35)
Current Therapy	
ACE-I/ARB	90 (85)
β blocker	100 (94)
Aldosterone antagonist	55 (52)
Antidepressant	15 (14)
Device therapy	
ICD	16 (15)
Pacemaker	16 (15)
CDS score, mean ± SD	86 ± 27
Depressed (CDS ≥ 95)	36 (34)
6MWD	
Feet ± SD	1325 ± 384
metres ± SD	404 ± 117

6MWD, 6-min walk test distance; ACE-I, Angiotensin-converting enzyme inhibitor; ARB, Angiotensin-II receptor blocker; BMI, Body mass index; CAD, Coronary artery disease; CDS, Cardiac depression scale; CKD, Chronic kidney disease; COPD, Chronic obstructive pulmonary disease; eGFR, estimated glomerular filtration rate; HF, Heart failure; HFpEF, Heart failure with preserved ejection fraction; HFrEF, Heart failure with reduced ejection fraction; ICD, Implantable cardioverter defibrillator; NYHA, New York Heart Association; SD, Standard deviation.

From Ha, F. J., Toukhsati, S. R., Cameron, J. D., Yates, R., & Hare, D. L. (2018). Association between the 6-minute walk test and exercise confidence in patients with heart failure: A prospective observational study. *Heart & Lung, 47*(1), p. 57.

STUDY QUESTIONS

1. Identify the level of measurement for the sex or gender demographic variable. Also identify the level of measurement for the BMI physiological variable in this study.

2. Identify the level of measurement for the type of HF variable in this study. Provide a rationale for your answer.

3. Identify the level of measurement for the NYHA class variable. Provide a rationale for your answer.

4. Identify the mode for the comorbidities variable. What is the meaning of these results?

5. Identify the level of measurement for the demographic variable of age. Provide a rationale for your answer.

6. What are the frequency and percent for the male sex or gender variable? Discuss the representativeness of this sample for males and females.

7. Identify the level of measurement for the duration of HF variables. What statistics were used to describe this variable in the study? Provide a rationale for your answer.

8. How many cardiac patients participated in this study? Determine the frequency and percent of these patients who did not have a pacemaker. Round your answer to the nearest whole percent (%).

9. Are parametric or nonparametric statistical analysis techniques used to analyze nominal-level data in Table 1? Provide a rationale for your answer.

10. How many cardiac patients in this study were depressed? Discuss the clinical importance of this result.

Answers to Study Questions

1. The Sex or gender demographic variable was measured at the nominal level and included two categories, male and female, that cannot be rank ordered (see Table 1). BMI was measured at the ratio level because it is a continuous physiological variable with an absolute zero (Grove & Gray, 2019; Stone & Frazier, 2017).

2. The type of HF variable was measured at the nominal level. The types of HF categories (HFrEF, HFpEF, and not documented) in this study were exclusive (each cardiac patient fit into only one category) and exhaustive (all cardiac patients fit into a category). The two common types of HF (HFrEF and HFpEF) included most of the study participants ($n = 103$), and the three other HF patients fit into the open category of "not documented," which ensures the categories are exhaustive (see Figure 1-1; Grove & Gray, 2019). The types of HF cannot be rank ordered, since one category is not clearly higher or lower than another category, resulting in a nominal level of measurement rather than an ordinal one.

3. The level of measurement for the NYHA class variable was ordinal. The NYHA class was measured with categories that are exclusive, exhaustive, and can be rank ordered (see Figure 1-1). The categories were exhaustive, since most of the cardiac patients ($n = 104$) fit into NYHA classes of I, II, or III and the two other patients fit into the open category "not specified." The categories were exclusive, since each patient with HF fit into only one category. The NYHA classes can be rank ordered because class I includes cardiac patients with the least severe heart disease and class III those with the most severe heart disease (Gray et al., 2017; Waltz et al., 2017).

4. The mode for the comorbidities variable for this sample of cardiac patients was hypertension, 71 (67%). The mode is the most frequently occurring category of a variable (Grove & Gray, 2019). These results indicate that the majority of the patients with HF have hypertension and should be closely monitored and managed for this comorbidity.

5. The level of measurement for the subjects' age was ratio, because age has an underlying continuum of years in this study. Each year includes the same equal intervals of 12 months or 365 days. Age has an absolute zero, since zero indicates the absences of age for a person. Age might also be called a continuous variable, since it has a continuum of values (Gray et al., 2017).

6. The sample was composed of 82% males (see the study narrative) and the frequency of males in the study was $n = 87$ (106 [sample size] − 19 [number of females] = 87). The sample was predominately males, making the results representative of the male gender; however, the study included only 19 females (18% of the sample), which limits the representativeness of the study results for females.

7. The duration of HF in this sample was measured in years, resulting in ratio-level data. Each year includes the same equal intervals of 12 months or 365 days. Duration of HF has an absolute zero, since zero indicates the absence of HF for a person. Duration of HF might also be called a continuous variable, since it has a continuum of values (Gray et al., 2017).

8. A total of 106 cardiac patients participated in this study. The sample included 16 patients with a pacemaker (see Table 1). The number of cardiac patients without a pacemaker was 90 (106 – 16 = 90). The group percent is calculated by the following formula: (group frequency ÷ total sample size) × 100%. For this study, (90 patients ÷ 106 sample size) × 100% = 0.849 × 100% = 84.9% = 85%. The final answer is rounded to the nearest whole percent as directed in the question. You could have also subtracted the 15% of patients with pacemakers from 100% and identified that 85% did not have pacemakers.

9. Nonparametric statistics, frequencies and percentages, were used to analyze the nominal-level data in Table 1. Nominal data can only be sorted into categories that are mutually exclusive and exhaustive, and only nonparametric or distribution-free analysis techniques can be conducted on this level of data (Kim & Mallory, 2017; Pett, 2016). Parametric analyses are usually conducted on variables measured at the interval or ratio level (Gray et al., 2017; Plichta & Kelvin, 2013).

10. The study narrative stated that "approximately one-third of patients (36/106; 34%) were depressed (CDC ≥95)" (Ha et al., 2018, p. 56). The researchers also found that the prevalence of depression increased with the greater NYHA class. Depression was a common problem for the cardiac patients in this study. As a nurse, you need to assess patients with HF for depression, especially those with higher NYHA classes (II and III). It is important to ensure patients with depression get diagnosed and receive adequate treatment.

Questions to Be Graded

Name: _____ Class: _____

Date: _____

Follow your instructor's directions to submit your answers to the following questions for grading. Your instructor may ask you to write your answers below and submit them as a hard copy for grading. Alternatively, your instructor may ask you to submit your answers online.

1. In Table 1, identify the level of measurement for the current therapy variable. Provide a rationale for your answer.

2. What is the mode for the current therapy variable in this study? Provide a rationale for your answer.

3. What statistics were conducted to describe the BMI of the cardiac patients in this sample? Discuss whether these analysis techniques were appropriate or inappropriate.

4. Researchers used the following item to measure registered nurses' (RNs) income in a study: What category identifies your current income as an RN?
   a. Less than $50,000
   b. $50,000 to 59,999
   c. $60,000 to 69,999
   d. $70,000 to 80,000
   e. $80,000 or greater

   What level of measurement is this income variable? Does the income variable follow the rules outlined in Figure 1-1? Provide a rationale for your answer.

5. What level of measurement is the CDS score? Provide a rationale for your answer.

6. Were nonparametric or parametric analysis techniques used to analyze the CDS scores for the cardiac patients in this study? Provide a rationale for your answer.

7. Is the prevalence of depression linked to the NYHA class? Discuss the clinical importance of this result.

8. What frequency and percent of cardiac patients in this study were not being treated with an antidepressant? Show your calculations and round your answer to the nearest whole percent (%).

9. What was the purpose of the 6-minute walk test (6MWT)? Would the 6MWT be useful in clinical practice?

10. How was exercise confidence measured in this study? What was the level of measurement for the exercise confidence variable in this study? Provide a rationale for your answer.

Identifying Probability and Nonprobability Sampling Methods in Studies

STATISTICAL TECHNIQUE IN REVIEW

A **sampling method** is a process of selecting people, events, behaviors, or other elements that are representative of the population being studied (Gray, Grove, & Sutherland, 2017). The sampling methods implemented in research are usually categorized as either probability (random) or nonprobability (nonrandom). Table 2-1 identifies the common probability and nonprobability sampling methods applied in quantitative, qualitative, and mixed methods studies in nursing (Heavey, 2019; Thompson, 2002). **Quantitative research** is an objective research methodology used to describe variables, examine relationships or associations among variables, and determine cause-and-effect interactions between independent and dependent variables (Grove & Gray, 2019; Shadish, Cook, & Campbell, 2002). **Qualitative studies** are scholarly, rigorous approaches used to describe life experiences, cultures, and social processes from the perspective of the persons involved (Creswell & Poth, 2018; Gray et al., 2017; Marshall & Rossman, 2016). **Mixed methods studies** include methodologies from both quantitative and qualitative research to better understand the area of study (Creswell & Clark, 2018). The sampling method used in a study is based on the type of research, the study problem and purpose, population studied, and the expertise and experiences of the researchers.

Probability Sampling Methods

Probability sampling, also known as random sampling, requires that every member of the study population have an equal and independent opportunity to be chosen for inclusion in a study. Probability sampling involves identifying the **sampling frame** or each person or element in a study target population and then randomly selecting a sample from that population (see Exercise 3; Grove & Gray, 2019). Thus, probability sampling allows every person or element of the study population to be represented without researcher bias and minimizes sampling error. The purpose of sampling in quantitative research is to obtain study participants who are as representative of the target population as possible. The sample's representativeness of the study population is increased by probability sampling. A large sample with limited attrition also increases the representativeness of the sample (Cohen, 1988; Gray et al., 2017). Four common probability sampling designs used to select random samples in quantitative studies include simple random sampling, stratified random sampling, cluster sampling, and systematic sampling (Grove & Gray, 2019; Heavey, 2019; Kandola, Banner, O'Keefe-McCarthy, & Jassal, 2014; Kazdin, 2017). Table 2-1 identifies these probability sampling methods, their common application in studies, and the sample's representativeness of the study population.

Simple random sampling is achieved by random selection of members from the sampling frame. The random selection can be accomplished many different ways, the

TABLE 2-1	PROBABILITY AND NONPROBABILITY SAMPLING METHODS	
Sampling Method	Common Application(s)	Representativeness of Sample or In-depth, Richness of Findings to Promote Understanding
Probability		
Simple random sampling	Quantitative research	Strong representativeness of the target population that increases with sample size.
Stratified random sampling	Quantitative research	Strong representativeness of the target population that increases with control of stratified variable(s).
Cluster sampling	Quantitative research	Less representative of the target population than simple random sampling and stratified random sampling, but representativeness increases with sample size.
Systematic sampling	Quantitative research	Less representative of the target population than simple random sampling and stratified random sampling methods, but representativeness increases with sample size.
Nonprobability		
Convenience sampling	Quantitative, qualitative, and mixed methods research	Questionable representativeness of the target population that improves with increasing sample size. Used in qualitative and mixed methods research so adequate participants might be found to promote understanding of the study area.
Quota sampling	Quantitative research and rarely qualitative and mixed methods research	Use of stratification for selected variables in quantitative research makes the sample more representative than convenience sampling. In qualitative and mixed methods research, participants of different ages or ethnic groups might be selected to increase the depth and richness of the study findings.
Purposeful or purposive sampling	Qualitative and mixed methods research and sometimes quantitative research	Focus is on insight, description, and understanding of a phenomenon, situation, process, or cultural element with specially selected study participants who have the potential to provide in-depth, rich data.
Network or snowball sampling	Qualitative and mixed methods research and sometimes quantitative research	Focus is on insight, description, and understanding of a phenomenon, situation, process, or cultural element in a difficult-to-access population.
Theoretical sampling	Qualitative research	Focus is on developing a theory in a selected area with specially selected study participants.

most common being a computer program to randomly select the sample from the sampling frame. Another example would be to assign each potential subject a number and then randomly select numbers from a random numbers table to fulfill the required number of participants needed for the sample. Random sampling helps ensure the sample is representative of the study population and that the study has adequate power to detect a difference or identify relationships if they are present (see Exercise 24). This sampling method is strongly representative of the target population, and the representativeness increases with sample size (Gray et al., 2017).

Random sampling is not to be confused with **random assignment of study participants to groups**, which is a design strategy to promote more equivalent groups (i.e., intervention and control groups) at the beginning of a study and to reduce the potential for error (Gray et al., 2017; Kazdin, 2017; Shadish et al., 2002). Researchers should clearly indicate if study participants are randomly assigned to groups because this makes the groups independent (see Exercise 16).

Stratified random sampling is used when the researcher knows some of the variables within a population that will affect the representativeness of the sample. Some examples of these variables include age, gender, race/ethnicity, medical diagnosis, and severity of illness. The study participants are selected randomly on the basis of their classification into the selected stratum of a variable. The strata identified ensure that all levels of the variable(s) are represented in the sample. For example, age could be the variable, and, after stratification, the sample might include equal numbers of subjects in the established age ranges of 20–39, 40–59, 60–79, and 80 years of age or older. Stratified random sampling is a strong sampling method that is representative of the target population, and the representativeness increases with control of the stratified variable(s) (Gray et al., 2017; Kandola et al., 2014).

Researchers use **cluster sampling** (also referred to as complex sampling) in two different situations: (1) when the time and travel necessary to use simple random sampling would be prohibitive; and (2) when the specific elements of a population are unknown, therefore making it impossible to develop a sampling frame. In either of these cases, a list of institutions or organizations associated with the elements of interest can often be obtained. To conduct cluster sampling, a list of all the states, cities, institutions, or organizations associated with the elements of the population is developed. The states, cities, institutions, or organizations are then randomly selected from the list to form the sample. However, the data collected from study participants from the same institution are likely to be correlated and thus not completely independent (Gray et al., 2017). Thus, cluster sampling produces a sample that is not as representative of the study population as with simple random sampling and stratified random sampling (see Table 2-1). Aday and Cornelius (2006) provide more details on the strengths and weaknesses of cluster sampling.

Systematic sampling requires an ordered list of all of the members of the population. Individuals are selected through a process that accepts every kth member on the list using a randomly selected starting point. k is calculated based on the size of population and the sample size desired. For example, if the population has 1000 potential participants and a sample size of 100 is desired, then $k = 1000 \div 100 = 10$, which means that every 10th person or unit on a list is invited to participate in the study. The initial starting point must be random for the sample to be considered a probability sample. Also, steps must be taken to ensure that the original list was not ordered in any way that could affect the study results. Probability sampling methods are more commonly used in quantitative studies and occasionally in mixed methods studies (Grove & Gray, 2019).

Nonprobability Sampling Methods

Nonprobability sampling is a nonrandom sampling technique that does not extend equal opportunity for selection to all members of the study population. Readers should never assume a probability sampling method was used in a study; rather, the researchers must identify the sampling method as probability or nonprobability for their study. In clinical research, nonprobability sampling methods are used much more frequently than probability sampling methods are due to the limited availability of potential subjects (Holmes, 2018). The common nonprobability sampling methods applied in nursing research include convenience, quota, network, purposive, and theoretical sampling (see Table 2-1). Convenience sampling is the most frequently used sampling method in quantitative, qualitative, and mixed methods nursing studies (Creswell & Clark, 2019; Creswell & Creswell, 2018; Creswell & Poth, 2018).

Researchers obtain a **convenience sample** by enrolling study participants who meet sample criteria, are accessible, and are willing to participate in a study (Grove & Gray, 2019; Kazdin, 2107). Subjects are enrolled in a study until the target sample size is obtained. Convenience sampling does not allow for the opportunity to control for sampling errors or biases. To counter the inability to control for biases, researchers must carefully examine the population being studied and adjust the sampling criteria to appropriately address the identified biases. For example, researchers might include only individuals with a new diagnosis of type 2 diabetes in their study of the effects of diet education on hemoglobin A1c values. This sampling criterion of newly diagnosed diabetic decreases the potential for errors or biases created by previous diabetic education and other management strategies patients might have experienced in the past to control their type 2 diabetes.

Researchers use **quota sampling** to ensure adequate representation of types of subjects who are likely to be underrepresented, such as women, minorities, the elderly, or the poor. A convenience sampling method is used in conjunction with quota sampling to help ensure the inclusion of the identified subject type. Quota sampling can be used to mimic the known characteristics of the population or to ensure adequate numbers of subjects in each stratum. This is similar to the strategy used for stratified random sampling and is more frequently applied in quantitative than in qualitative studies. Quota sampling is recognized as more representative of the target population than convenience sampling is because of the decreased opportunity for sampling error or bias (see Table 2-1; Grove & Gray, 2019; Heavey, 2019).

Purposive, network, and theoretical sampling methods are more commonly used in qualitative and mixed methods research rather than in quantitative research. **Purposive sampling** occurs when the researcher consciously selects participants, elements, events, or incidents to include in a study. Those selected by the researchers are information-rich cases or those from whom a lot of information can be obtained (see Table 2-1; Creswell & Clark, 2018; Creswell & Poth, 2018; Marshall & Rossman, 2016). Researchers usually make an effort to include typical and atypical cases in the sample. This type of sampling has been criticized because the researcher's judgments in the selection of cases cannot be evaluated. However, this sampling method can be a good way to explore new areas of study.

Network or snowball sampling makes use of social networks and the fact that friends often have common characteristics. The researcher identifies a few study participants who meet the sampling criteria and then asks them to assist in recruiting others with similar characteristics. Network sampling is useful for gathering samples that are difficult to obtain, have not been previously identified for study, or can help the researcher explore a particular area of interest or focus. Sampling errors or biases are inherent in networking samples because the study participants are not independent of one another (Grove & Gray, 2019).

Theoretical sampling is used in the research process to advance the development of a theory and is more commonly used in grounded theory studies. Data are gathered from individuals or groups who can provide relevant information for theory generation. For example, a researcher might interview family members and patients to develop a theory of surviving a near-death experience. The researcher continues to seek study participants and collect data until saturation of the theory concepts and relationships has occurred. **Saturation of data** occurs when collecting data from new study participants does not add new knowledge regarding the study purpose. Participant diversity in the sample is promoted to ensure that the developed theory is applicable to a wide range of behaviors and settings (Charmaz, 2014; Creswell & Poth, 2018).

STUDY QUESTIONS

Directions: Answer the following questions with a clear, appropriate response. For each question that includes an excerpt about sampling from a research article, provide the following information: (1) decide whether the sampling method presented is either a *probability* or *nonprobability sampling method*; (2) identify the *specific sampling method* used—that is, convenience, quota, purposive, network, or theoretical sampling for nonprobability samples or simple random, stratified random, cluster, or systematic sampling for probability samples (see Table 2-1); and (3) provide a *rationale for the sampling method* you selected. Some of the examples might include *more than one sampling method* to obtain the study sample.

1. Study excerpt: The purpose of the Buechel and Connelly (2018) study was to examine the knowledge of human papillomavirus (HPV) and immunization rate among U.S. Navy personnel. Participants ($N = 233$) were recruited from "both active duty and activated reservists, attached to Commander, Naval Surface Force, U.S. Pacific Fleet . . . located in Japan and the United States . . . Potential participants were contacted using three recruitment methods: (a) e-mail invitations; (b) advertisements via flyers, posters, Intranet, command newspapers, information cards, and command announcements; and (c) in-person recruitment at subordinate commands and military facilities. Interested participants were invited to complete and Internet-delivered survey."
Source: Buechel, J. J., & Connelly, C. D. (2018). Determinants of human papillomavirus vaccination among U.S. Navy personnel. *Nursing Research, 67*(4), 341–346. Excerpt from page 342.

2. Was the sample from the Buechel and Connelly (2018) study identified in Question 1 representative of the Navy personnel in the U.S. Pacific Fleet located in Japan and the United States? Provide a rationale for your answer.

3. Study excerpt: Mayer et al. (2013) conducted a qualitative study to examine family experiences after sudden cardiac death. "Multiple recruitment methods were used, including health professional referrals, advertising, and snowball sampling . . . where adult participants were asked to refer other families who might qualify. The purposive sample included seven families comprised of seventeen individual family members."
Source: Mayer, D. M., Rosenfeld, A. G., & Gilbert, K. (2013). Lives forever changed: Family bereavement experiences after sudden cardiac death. *Applied Nursing Research, 26*(4), 168-173. Excerpt from page 169.

4. Study excerpt: Han et al. (2018) conducted a pilot study to examine the effects of a tailored lifestyle intervention on body composition, obesity-related biomarkers, and lifestyle modification for women at high risk for breast cancer. "Seventy-three women were approached for the study. Of those, 30 were determined to be eligible, and 16 consenting participants completed the baseline study visit. These participants were then randomized through a computer-generated table with stratification based on menopausal status, with eight assigned to each groups."

   Source: Han, C. J., Korde, L. A., Reding, S., Allott, K., Doren, M. V. Schwarz, Y., Vaughan, C., & Reding, K. W. (2018). Investigation of a lifestyle intervention in women at high risk of breast cancer. *Western Journal of Nursing Research, 40*(7), 976–996. Excerpt from page 981.

5. Was the sample for the Han et al. (2018) study presented in Question 4 representative of the population of women at high risk for breast cancer? Provide a rationale for your answer.

6. Study excerpt: "A cross-sectional study stratified by age and sex [gender] was performed using computerized healthcare records belonging to Catalan health system between November and December 2007. . . . The sample size . . . was 317 participants. . . . The gender distribution of the randomly selected 317 patients of the study consisted of 157 women (49.5%) and 160 men (50.5%)."

   Source: Monteso-Curto, P., Ferre-Grau, C., Leixa-Fortuno, M., Albacar-Rioboo, N., & Lejeune, M. (2014). Diagnosed, identified, current, and complete depression among patients attending primary care in southern Catalonia: Different aspects of the same concept. *Achieves of Psychiatric Nursing, 28*(1), 50–54. Excerpt from page 51.

7. Study excerpt: "Healthcare providers in 206 Vaccine for Children (VFC) offices throughout this state [Indiana] were asked to participate in an assessment of their vaccine knowledge. A mailing list of the VFC offices was obtained from a local district health department. The estimated number of medical office personnel and providers who administer and handle immunizations in each office was determined by calling each VFC office. . . . Each office manager coordinated the completion and return of the informed consents and the Immunization Knowledge Assessment Tools." A total of 713 surveys were randomly distributed in 206 clinics and 344 surveys were returned, for a 48% response rate.

   Source: Strohfus, P. K., Collins, T., Phillips, V., & Remington, R. (2013). Healthcare providers' knowledge assessment of measles, mumps, and rubella vaccine. *Applied Nursing Research, 26*(4), 162–167. Excerpt from page 163.

8. Study excerpt: The Hurley et al. (2018) study examined the relationship between 804 registered nurses' personal health practices and their perceptions of themselves as role models for health promotion. "The population from which the study sample was drawn included all registered nurses in Tennessee ($n = 61,829$) listed in the Tennessee Board of Nursing 2015 database. After approval from East Tennessee State University's Institutional Review Board, a simple random sample was drawn from the databases. Inclusion criteria were active registered nurse licensed in the state of Tennessee, and a valid email in the database."

   Source: Hurley, S. Edwards, J., Cupp, J., & Phillips, M. (2018). Nurses' perceptions of self as a role models of health. *Western Journal of Nursing Research, 40*(8), 1131–1147.

9. "A cross-sectional study was conducted with a sample of qualified nurses recruited from two hospitals . . . The sample was representative of qualified nurses within the target population . . . A two-stage sampling approach was taken. The first stage involved the selection of different work areas within two teaching hospitals . . . The second stage involved the random selection of a sample of nurses from each of these work areas . . . Nurses were randomly selected from the nursing off-duty (work roster) using a random generator application . . . In total 300 nurses were invited to participate in the study . . . A response rate of 70% was obtained ($n = 210$); however, only $n = 203$ of the returned questionnaires were completed properly and thus included in these analyses."

   Source: McCarthy, V. J., Wills, T., & Crowley, S. (2018). Nurses, age, job demands and physical activity at work and at leisure: A cross-sectional study. *Applied Nursing Research, 40*, 116–121. Excerpt was from pages 117–118.

10. Study excerpt: Glaserian Grounded theory methodology was used in this qualitative study, with participants initially being selected purposefully for the first sets of interviews (Glaser, 2001). Using an additional sampling method, "[t]he final set of interviews was devoted to discussion of the emerging theory to confirm category saturation. Inherent within this process is the assessment by participants of the credibility or 'fit' . . . of the emerging theory" (Neill et al., 2013, p. 761). The final sample included 15 families with children aged 0 to 9 years who had experienced an acute childhood illness at home.

Source: Neill, S. J., Cowley, S., & Williams, C. (2013). The role of felt or enacted criticism in understanding parent's help seeking in acute childhood illness at home: A grounded theory study. *International Journal of Nursing Studies, 50*(6), 757–767. Excerpt from page 235.

Answers to Study Questions

1. Nonprobability, convenience sampling method. The researchers did not identify the sampling method in their study, but it was consistent with convenience sampling (see Table 2-1; Grove & Gray, 2019). Navy personnel in Japan and the United States were recruited using a variety of methods and invited to complete an online survey. With convenience sampling, participants are recruited because they are available, accessible, and willing to participate, as in this study.

2. Answers may vary. A nonprobability (nonrandom) convenience sample has reduced representativeness of the study population and an increased potential for sampling error or bias (see Table 2-1; Gray et al., 2017). However, the recruitment of participants by several methods, strong sample size ($N = 233$), and lack of participant attrition (online survey) strengthened the representativeness of the sample (Gray et al., 2017).

3. Nonprobability, purposive, and network or snowball sampling methods. You might have also identified convenience sampling because multiple recruitment methods were used, including advertising, which would result in convenience sampling. Mayer et al. (2013) clearly indicated that more than one sampling method was used and identified their main sampling method as purposive to gain an understanding of family bereavement. Network or snowball sampling was evident when health professionals were asked for referrals and study participants were asked to refer other families who might qualify for the study (Creswell & Poth, 2018).

4. Nonprobability, quota sampling method. A total of 30 women who met sample criteria and were available were asked to participate and only 16 consented. The women were randomized into groups with stratification by menopause status. The initial sample is one of convenience that was strengthened by stratification of menopause status, resulting in quota sampling. Remember that randomly assigning study participants to groups is a design strategy and not a sampling method (Gray et al., 2017; Shadish et al., 2002).

5. Answers may vary, but the best response is the sample has limited representativeness of the population of women at high risk for breast cancer. Nonprobability sampling decreases representativeness of the population; however, quota sampling is the strongest of nonprobability sampling method for promoting representativeness (see Table 2-1; Gray et al., 2017). The sample size for the pilot study was small at 16 because 14 (46.7%) of the women approached for the study refused to participate. The small sample size and high refusal rate reduce the representativeness of the sample.

6. Probability, stratified random sampling method. The sample of 317 patients was randomly selected and stratified by age and sex (gender) using health records of patients diagnosed with depression.

7. Probability, cluster sampling method. Strohfus et al. (2013) did not clearly identify their type of sampling method, but it is consistent with multilevel cluster sampling. Because the sampling frame for

the study could not be identified, the researchers identified study participants using the Vaccine for Children (VFC) offices throughout the state. Within these offices, managers were identified to collect data from the healthcare providers managing immunizations.

8. Probability, simple random sampling method. The sampling method was clearly identified by Hurley et al. (2018). The sampling frame was all RNs in the Tennessee Board of Nursing 2015 database. The researchers should have identified how the sample was randomly selected, but it was probably done by a computer program.

9. Probability, cluster sampling method. McCarthy et al. (2018) identified their sampling approach as having two stages. The first stage involved the selection of nursing units, which is done with cluster sample to identify the settings for the subjects. The second stage involved randomly selecting nurses from these units. This multistage process of sampling is consistent with cluster sampling when the sampling frame of potential subjects is not available, so the hospital units were identified and the nurses were randomly selected from the units.

10. Nonprobability, purposive and theoretical sampling methods. Neill et al. (2013) used purposive or purposeful sampling to select families with children who had experienced an acute childhood illness at home for the first sets of interviews. Theoretical sampling was used to identify participants for the final interviews to confirm category saturation and to determine the credibility of the emerging theory. Theoretical sampling is frequently used in grounded theory studies (Charmaz, 2014; Creswell & Poth, 2018).

Questions to Be Graded

Name: _____ Class: _____

Date: _____

Follow your instructor's directions to submit your answers to the following questions for grading. Your instructor may ask you to write your answers below and submit them as a hard copy for grading. Alternatively, your instructor may ask you to submit your answers online.

Directions: Answer the following questions with a clear, appropriate response. For each question that includes an excerpt about sampling from a research article, provide the following information: (1) decide whether the sampling method presented is either a *probability* or *nonprobability sampling method*; (2) identify the *specific sampling method* used—that is, convenience, quota, purposive, network, or theoretical sampling for nonprobability samples or simple random, stratified random, cluster, or systematic sampling for probability samples (see Table 2-1); and (3) provide a *rationale for the sampling method* you selected. Some of the examples might include *more than one sampling method* to obtain the study sample.

1. Study excerpt: "Participants in this study were all women who had had, or might have, sex with men; that is, women not in exclusively same-sex partnerships. All participants were 18 to 35 years old, English-speaking, and attended a large, public, Midwestern university. More than 2,000 women completed Phase 1 of the study, a survey; of these approximately 900 volunteered to participate in the Phase II interviews. Women were selected from this pool to be interviewed using a purposive maximum variation sampling strategy . . . Based on survey data, women were sampled based on variation in their knowledge and use of emergency contraception and on some aspects of sexual history . . . Theoretical sampling was used to select potential participants based on the data as they were collected, including women who had experienced a pregnancy termination or 'false alarm' pregnancy . . . This process yielded a sample of 35 women who represented a wide range of experiences. When saturation was reached, recruitment and data collection ended." The data for this study were obtained from a larger mixed methods study that included quantitative survey data and qualitative narrative interview data focused on collegiate women's sexual behavior.

   Source: Loew, N., Mackin, M. L., & Ayres, L. (2018). Collegiate women's definitions of responsible sexual behavior. *Western Journal of Nursing Research, 40*(8), 1148–1162. Excerpt from page 1151.

2. Study excerpt: "This study was a part of a multi-site prospective observational study of COPD [chronic obstructive pulmonary disease] patients to explore the relationship between depression, inflammation, and functional status . . . Participants were recruited from various sources including outpatient clinics from three medical centers, pulmonary rehabilitation programs, a research database maintained by the investigators, queries of medical records and pulmonary function tests, Better Breathers Club, community pulmonary practices, advertisements, study website, and other referrals." A total of 282 patients with COPD were included in the study. Source: Lee, J., Nguyen, H. Q., Jarrett, M. E., Mitchell, P. H., Pike, K. C., & Fan, V. S. (2018). Effect of symptoms on physical performance in COPD. *Heart & Lung, 47*(2), 149–156. Excerpt from page 150.

3. Study excerpt: The focus of this quasi-experimental study was to determine the effect of a three-stage nursing intervention to increase women's participation in Pap smear screening. Using "random sampling methodology, each apartment in the target area was identified by a number. Numbers were then drawn from a random numbers table. Women were contacted by home visits. . . . By the end of this stage, 237 participants had completed the pre-test." Source: Guvenc, G., Akyuz, A., & Yenen, M. C. (2013). Effectiveness of nursing interventions to increase Pap smear test screening. *Research in Nursing & Health, 36*(2), 146–157. Excerpt from page 148.

4. Was the sample identified in the Guvenc et al. (2013) study in Question 3 representative of the population of women requiring a Pap smear test in a target area? Provide a rationale for your answer.

5. "Participants were recruited from January 2003 through November 2007 during their initial evaluation at the Pediatric Pain Management Clinic at Children's Hospital Los Angeles . . . Ninety-six child-caregiver dyads were approached for study participant in order to obtain 65 sets of completed measures, resulting in a 68% participant rate. Nineteen sets were not returned, 7 sets did not have a complete child battery, 1 set did not have a complete caregiver battery, 2 child-caregiver dyads withdrew, and 2 families declined to participate . . . Children were considered eligible for the study if they were English speaking, between the ages of 8 and 18, had a diagnosis of chronic pain, and had a caregiver present."

   Source: Yetwin, A. K., Mahrer, N. E., John, C., & Gold, J. I. (2018). Does pain intensity matter? The relation between coping and quality of life in pediatric patients with chronic pain. *Journal of Pediatric Nursing, 40*(3), 7–13. Excerpt from page 8.

6. Study excerpt: "Participants were 559 substance users recruited from multiple sources (parks, streets, prisons, methadone maintenance therapy, and drop in centers) . . . a nonprobability sampling technique that is appropriate to use in research when the members of a population are difficult to locate. In this research, we collected data from substance abusers . . . and then asked those individuals to locate other substance abusers whom they knew."

   Source: Barati, M., Ahmadpanah, M., & Soltanian, A. R. (2014). Prevalence and factors associated with methamphetamine use among adult substance abusers. *Journal of Research in Health Sciences, 14*(3), 221–226. Excerpt from page 222.

7. Study excerpt: Mansfield et al. (2018) conducted a correlational study to examine the association between parental knowledge of human papillomavirus (HPV) and their intentions to have their daughters vaccinated. "This study used HINTS [Health Information National Trends Survey] 2006-2007 because it was the only data set that assessed the outcome variable, intention to vaccinate for HPV . . . HINTS's probability-based sample design used a random-digit dialing to conduct telephone surveys and a nationwide address list to administer surveys via mail. A sub-sampling screening tool, Westat's Telephone Research Center (TRC), was used to identify working residential numbers. A total of 3,767 telephone interviews were then completed, and 325 were partially completed ($n = 4,092$); 3,473 mail surveys were completed and 109 were partially completed ($n = 3,582$). The final total sample was 7,674 participants."

   Source: Mansfield, L. N., Onsomu, E. O., Merwin, E., Hall, N. M., & Harper-Harrison, A. (2018). Association between parental HPV knowledge and intentions to have their daughters vaccinated. *Western Journal of Nursing Research, 40*(4), 481–501. Excerpt from page 481.

8. Was the sample identified in the Mansfield et al. (2018) study in Question 7 representative of parents' intentions to have their daughters vaccinated? Provide a rationale for your answer.

9. Study excerpt: Initially, participants were selected in a purposeful manner "based on their familiarity with, interest in, and willingness to reflect and discuss their hope experience." Additional sampling was done to achieve "theoretical saturation that was defined as theoretical completeness in which no new properties of the categories were identified."
Source: Bally, J. M., Duggleby, W., Holtslander, L., Mpofu, C., Spurr, S., Thomas, R., & Wright, K. (2014). Keeping hope possible: A grounded theory study of the hope experience of parental caregivers who have children in treatment for cancer. *Cancer Nursing, 37*(5), 363–372. Excerpt from page 364.

10. Study excerpt: Macartney and colleagues (2018) studied the concussion symptoms in 136 adolescents, 74 female and 62 male. "A retrospective chart review was completed between 11/21/2014 to 11/20/2015. A purposive sample of all patients who visited the CHEO [Children's Hospital of Eastern Ontario] concussion clinic during the study period [was] included. Patients were excluded if symptoms records were not documented . . . CHEO's concussion clinic opened in the fall of 2014. The clinic provides care to patients less than nineteen years old who remain symptomatic at least four weeks post injury."
Source: Macartney, G., Simoncic, V., Goulet, K., & Aglipay, M. (2018). Concussion symptoms prevalence, severity and trajectory: Implications for nursing practice. *Journal of Pediatric Nursing, 40*(1), 58–62. Excerpt from page 59.

Understanding the Sampling Section of a Research Report: Population, Sampling Criteria, Sample Size, Refusal Rate, and Attrition Rate

STATISTICAL TECHNIQUE IN REVIEW

Sampling or eligibility criteria include a list of requirements or characteristics essential for membership in the target population. Sampling criteria include both inclusion and exclusion criteria. **Inclusion sampling criteria** are the requirements identified by the researcher that must be present for an element or participant to be included in a sample. **Sampling exclusion criteria** are the requirements identified by the researcher that eliminate or exclude participants from being in a sample. Researchers may identify from very broad sampling criteria to very specific criterion. Broad sampling criteria can promote a large, diverse, or heterogeneous population, while specific sampling criteria promote a smaller, more homogeneous population.

A **population** is the particular group of individuals who are being studied, such as adults with diabetes, women diagnosed with breast cancer, or overweight children. The sampling criteria determine the **target population**, and the sample is selected from the **accessible population** or the available potential study participants within the target population. The **sample** is the focus of a particular study. Figure 3-1 demonstrates the relationships among the concepts population, target population, accessible population, sample, and study elements (Gray, Grove, & Sutherland, 2017). The **study elements** are the participants, subjects, objects, or events that might be included in the sample for a study. When the study is completed, researchers determine the extent to which the findings can be generalized from the sample to the accessible population. If the findings from a study are significant and consistent with the findings from strong previous studies, the findings might be generalized to the target population.

An adequate sample size is essential for identifying significant relationships among variables or differences between groups. **Power** is the probability that a given statistic can detect relationships or differences that actually exist in the population studied (Gaskin & Happell, 2014). Put another way, statistical power refers to the probability of rejecting the null hypothesis when it is actually false. "Statistical power is indexed on a scale of 0.00 to 1.00, with zero indicating there is no chance of rejecting a false null hypothesis and 1.00 indicating the false null hypothesis will be rejected 100% of the time it is studied" (Taylor & Spurlock, 2018, p. 263). Large samples increase the power of the statistics conducted so that researchers might accurately accept or reject the null hypotheses for their

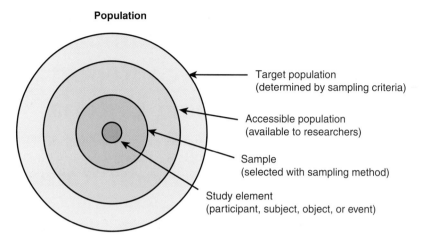

FIGURE 3-1 ▪ LINKING POPULATION, SAMPLE, AND ELEMENT IN A STUDY.

study. Power analysis includes the following four elements: (1) alpha or level of significance set by the researcher, usually at 0.05; (2) standard power for a study is usually 0.80 or 80%; (3) effect size (strength of relationships among variables or extent of group differences); and (4) sample size (Aberson, 2010; Cohen, 1988; Taylor & Spurlock, 2018). Power analysis is covered in more detail in Exercises 24 and 25 of Part 2 of this text.

Researchers need to identify a large enough accessible population to ensure an adequate sample is obtained after accounting for refusal and attrition rates. **Refusal rate** is the percentage of potential subjects who decide not to participate in a study. The refusal rate is calculated using the following formula:

Refusal rate = (Number refusing to participate ÷ Number of subjects approached) × 100%

Example: Refusal rate = (5 refuse to participate ÷ 50 approached) × 100% = 0.1 × 100% = 10%

Attrition rate is the percentage of subjects dropping out of a study after the sample size has been determined based on the sampling criteria. Attrition can occur actively when participants choose to drop out of a study for a variety of reasons or passively when participants are lost to follow-up. The attrition rate is calculated by dividing the number of subjects dropping out of the study by the total number of subjects in the study sample. Because subject attrition happens for a variety of reasons, researchers must anticipate this rate and increase the number of subjects recruited into a study to ensure an adequate sample size (Grove & Gray, 2019).

Attrition rate = (Number dropping out of a study ÷ Total sample size) × 100%

Example: Attrition rate = (4 dropped out of study ÷ 80 sample size) × 100% = 0.05 × 100% = 5%

The refusal and attrition rates decrease the sample's representativeness of the target population. Therefore refusal and attrition rates greater than 20% are of concern and researchers need to report the reasons people gave for refusing to take part in or for dropping out of a study. Researchers take these rates into consideration when determining the findings for their study. Sample attrition also reduces the final sample size and decreases the power of statistics to detect significant relationships among variables and differences between groups (Gaskin & Happell, 2014).

RESEARCH ARTICLE

Source

Ordway, M. R., Sadler, L. S., Dixon, J., Close, N., Mayes, L., & Slade, A. (2014). Lasting effects of an interdisciplinary home visiting program on child behavior: Preliminary follow-up results of a randomized trial. *Journal of Pediatric Nursing 29*(1), 3–13.

Introduction

Ordway et al. (2014) conducted a longitudinal follow-up study of a randomized controlled trial (RCT) to determine the effects of the Minding the Baby (MTB) home visiting program on parental reflective functioning (RF) and on child behavior. The study included intervention and control groups, and the women who participated in the MTB intervention described their children as having significantly fewer externalizing child behaviors post intervention. However, there was no significant difference between the intervention and control groups for parental RF. This study is clinically important because it adds support to the use of preventative home visitation programs, such as MTB, to reduce externalizing behavior problems in children. "The prevention of children's externalizing behaviors in the preschool years may help to reduce further effects later in their lives" (Ordway et al., 2014, p. 11). The sample section is presented as an example for this exercise. Data analyses were conducted with 24 mother–child dyads in the intervention group and 26 mother–child dyads in the control group.

Relevant Study Results

Ordway and colleagues (2014, p. 5) noted, "At the start of this follow-up study, there were 132 mother–child dyads that previously participated or were presently participating with the MTB program. Mother–child dyads were eligible for this study if they met the following criteria: (a) the targeted child was between the ages of 3 to 5 years at the time of data collection between March 2010 and March 2011, (b) the mother had primary custody or regular visitation with the child, (c) the dyad lived in state and/or was able to meet in state for the data collection, and (d) the mother participated in the MTB program or the control condition beyond the initial consent period. Among the 71 mother–child dyads with children 3–5 years old during the 1-year data collection period, 62 met all of the eligibility criteria. Fifty dyads (80.6%) were available for contact, and 12 dyads were unreachable. None of the mothers who were contacted refused to participate in the follow-up study (Figure 1).

Upon IRB approval from the university and local community health center where the women were originally recruited, subjects were consented and data were collected during two data collection visits with the mother–child dyads. The sample size was calculated using…significance level…$\alpha = 0.05$ and 80% power was selected for analyses of two outcomes, parental RF and child behavior. Accordingly, the required size for each group was determined to be 17 dyads. All of the eligible subjects were recruited thereby resulting in the enrollment of 29% more subjects from each group allowing for study attrition" (Ordway et al., 2014, p. 5).

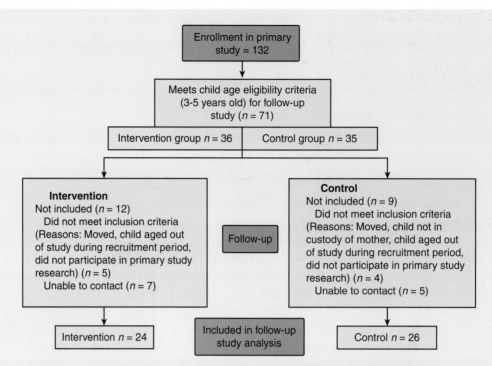

FIGURE 1 ■ **FLOW OF PARTICIPANTS FROM ORIGINAL STUDY THROUGH FOLLOW-UP.** Ordway, M. R., Sadler, L. S., Dixon, J., Close, N., Mayes, L., & Slade, A. (2014). Lasting effects of an interdisciplinary home visiting program on child behavior: Preliminary follow-up results of a randomized trial. *Journal of Pediatric Nursing 29*(1), p. 5.

STUDY QUESTIONS

1. What type of study was conducted? What dependent and independent variables were studied? What groups were included in the study?

2. What population was studied? Who were the study participants?

3. Did the study report sampling exclusion criteria? If so, what were these criteria?

4. How many mother–child dyads were included in the primary study? How many mother–child dyads met the child-age eligibility criteria of 3–5 years for the follow-up study?

5. Of the 35 mother–child dyads in the control group of the primary study, how many were included in the follow-up study reported in this article? How many mother–child dyads were lost from the primary study control group? Was a rationale provided for their not participating? If so, what were the reasons and did they seem appropriate or unusual?

6. What was the refusal rate for the mother–child dyads for participation in the follow-up study? Provide a rationale for your answer.

7. Calculate a refusal rate for a study where researchers approached 200 potential subjects and 179 consented to be in the study. Show your calculations and round your answer to the nearest tenth of a percent.

8. Was Figure 1 helpful in identifying the sample size of the original RCT and in determining the group sizes for the follow-up study? Discuss the importance of these diagrams in understanding the sampling process in quasi-experimental and experimental studies.

9. Define the term *power* as used in research. What is the usual power requirement set for a nursing study? What level of significance is often used for conducting a power analysis?

10. Where were the participants recruited for this study? Did they provide consent to participate in the study?

Answers to Study Questions

1. This study was a longitudinal follow-up to a randomized controlled trial (RCT) conducted to determine the effect of the Minding the Baby (MTB) home visiting program on child behavior problems and parental reflective functioning (RF). The MTB home visiting program was the intervention or independent variable implemented in this study. The child internalizing, externalizing, and total behavior problems and parental RF were the dependent variables measured in this study. Maternal depressive symptoms were also measured in this study but were not included in this exercise. The study included intervention and control groups (see Figure 1 of the sampling algorithm for the Ordway et al. (2014) study).

2. Women with children 3–5 years of age were the population for this study. Population was defined earlier in this exercise and identified in Figure 1. The study participants were mother–child dyads, where each mother and child pair was included as a participant.

3. No, the study report did not include sampling exclusion criteria. Only sampling or eligibility inclusion criteria were identified.

4. The primary study included 132 mother–child dyads (see study narrative and Figure 1). A total of 71 of the mother–child dyads (intervention group $n = 36$ and control group $n = 35$) met the eligibility criteria of child being 3–5 years old.

5. A total of 26 mother–child dyads were included in the control group of the follow-up study (see Figure 1). Thus, 9 dyads of the original 35 in the primary study were not included in the follow-up study. The researchers clearly identified the reasons for these 9 dyads not participating in the follow-up study: four of the mother–child dyads did not meet inclusion criteria since they had moved, the child was not in custody of mother, the child aged out of the study during the recruitment period, or the child did not participate in the primary study (see Figure 1). Researchers were unable to contact five of the mother–child dyads. These are common and appropriate reasons for participants not taking part in a follow-up study, and the study is strengthened by a discussion of what happened to these dyads (Gray et al., 2017).

6. The follow-up study had a 0% refusal rate. The mother–child dyads in the intervention group were $n = 24$ and in the control group were $n = 26$ for a total sample of 50 mother–child dyads. All mothers contacted who met the sampling criteria agreed to participate in the study and none refused.

7. Refusal rate = (number of subjects refusing to participate in a study ÷ by the number of potential subjects approached) × 100%. Number refusing = 200 − 179 = 21. Refusal rate = (21 refused to participate ÷ 200 potential subjects approached) × 100% = 0.105 × 100% = 10.5% or 11% (Grove & Gray, 2019).

8. Graphics, such as Figure 1, are strong additions to research reports for RCTs and quasi-experimental and experimental quantitative studies to document the sampling process. This type of figure can be used to identify the number of potential subjects, indicate those meeting or not meeting sampling or eligibility criteria, refusal numbers and rates, numbers in each group, attrition numbers and rates, and final size of study groups. When reporting RCTs or quasi-experimental and experimental studies, researchers need to consider including a sampling algorithm, such as Figure 1, that is recommended by the Consolidated Standards for Reporting Trials (CONSORT, 2010).

9. Power is the probability that a given statistic can detect differences or relationships that actually exist in the population studied. Put another way, statistical power refers to the probability of rejecting the null hypothesis when it is actually false (Taylor & Spurlock, 2018). With adequately powered statistical analyses, researchers are able to more accurately accept or reject the null hypotheses in their study. The minimum acceptable power is usually set at 0.80 or 80%, and the level of significance or alpha (α) is typically set at 0.05.

10. The researchers obtained institutional review board (IRB) approval from the university and the local health center to conduct their study. The women in this study were recruited from a community health center and invited to participate in the study, and those consenting were included in this follow-up study.

Questions to Be Graded

Name: _____ Class: _____

Date: _____

Follow your instructor's directions to submit your answers to the following questions for grading. Your instructor may ask you to write your answers below and submit them as a hard copy for grading. Alternatively, your instructor may ask you to submit your answers online.

1. Did the study include sampling inclusion criteria? What were those criteria? Were these criteria appropriate for this study?

2. Sampling inclusion and exclusion criteria are developed to determine what type of population? What is the accessible population? Document your answer.

3. How many of the mother–child dyads with children 3 to 5 years old were available for contact for the follow-up study? How many mother–child dyads were included in the initial intervention group for the follow-up study? What frequency and percent of the mother–child dyads were unable to be contacted in the intervention group?

4. Of the 36 mother–child dyads in the intervention group, how many were included in the follow-up study? How many mother–child dyads did not participate in the study? Was a rationale provided for their not participating? If so, what were the reasons and did they seem appropriate or unusual?

5. What was the attrition number and rate for this study? Provide a rationale for your answer.

6. Calculate the attrition rate for a study that included a sample size of 276 subjects and 10 subjects became too ill to continue in the study, 5 could not be contacted after hospital discharge, and 4 died. Round your answer to the nearest tenth of a percent.

7. What was the total sample for this study?

8. The intervention and control groups had unequal numbers. Is this a study strength or weakness? Provide a rationale for your answer.

9. Discuss the results of the power analysis conducted for this study. Was the sample size adequate for this study? Provide a rationale for your answers.

10. Are the findings from this study ready for use in practice? Provide a rationale for your answer.

Understanding Reliability of Measurement Methods

STATISTICAL TECHNIQUE IN REVIEW

The **reliability** of a measurement method or instrument denotes the consistency of the measures it obtains of an attribute, concept, or situation in a study or clinical practice. Broadly, reliability is concerned with the dependability, consistency, stability, precision, and reproducibility of a measurement method (Bartlett & Frost, 2008; Gray, Grove, & Sutherland, 2017). An instrument that demonstrates strong reliability in the measurement of a variable or concept has less random error (Bannigan & Watson, 2009; Bialocerkowski, Klupp, & Bragge, 2010). For example, the Center for Epidemiologic Studies Depression Scale (CES-D) was developed through research to diagnose depression in mental health patients (Radloff, 1977). Over the last 40 years, the CES-D has been expanded to different versions and has proven to be a quality measure of depression in clinical practice and in research for children, adolescents, adults, and elderly. If a scale like the CES-D consistently measures a concept, then it is considered to be reliable (Grove & Gray, 2019). However, a scale that produces inconsistent scores with repeat testing of study participants or has low reliability values is considered unreliable, resulting in increased measurement error (Waltz, Strickland, & Lenz, 2017).

Reliability testing examines the amount of random error in an instrument that is used in a study. Because all measurement methods contain some error, reliability exists in degrees and usually is expressed as a correlation coefficient. *Estimates of reliability are specific to the sample being tested.* High reliability values reported for an established instrument do not guarantee that reliability will be satisfactory in another sample or with a different population. Researchers need to perform reliability testing on each instrument used in a study to ensure that it is reliable for that study sample (Bialocerkowski et al., 2010; DeVon et al., 2007). The three most common types of reliability testing reported in health-care studies are stability reliability, equivalence reliability, and internal consistency or homogeneity. Table 4-1 summarizes these types of reliability testing (Grove & Gray, 2019; Waltz et al., 2017).

Stability reliability is concerned with the consistency of repeated measures of the same variable or attribute with the same scale or measurement method over time. Stability is commonly referred to as **test-retest reliability** due to the repeated measurement of a variable over time. Reliability testing examines the amount of random error in a measurement technique, and a quality measurement method should have acceptable reliability (Gray et al., 2017). For example, if a scale is being used to measure stress in a study, the study participants given this scale should mark the items similarly if they are given the same stress scale at a later time (e.g., 1–2 days later). If the participants complete the scale in a similar way from one time to the next, this indicates adequate test-retest reliability, which is designated by an intraclass correlation coefficient (ICC). The ICC values

TABLE 4-1	DETERMINING THE RELIABILITY AND READABILITY OF MEASUREMENT METHODS
Quality Indicator	**Description**
Reliability	**Stability reliability:** Is concerned with the reproducibility of scores with repeated measures of the same concept or attribute with an instrument or scale over time. Stability is usually examined with **test-retest reliability.**
	Equivalence reliability:
	Interrater or interobserver reliability: Comparison of judges or raters in determining their equivalence in rating variables or events in a study. Interobserver reliability is focused on the agreement between two or more observers in a study.
	Alternate forms reliability: Comparison of two paper-and-pencil instruments to determine their equivalence in measuring a concept.
	Internal consistency: Is also known as homogeneity reliability testing used primarily with multi-item scales where each item on the scale is correlated with all other items to determine the consistency of the scale in measuring a concept.
Precision	**Precision of physiological measure**: Degree of consistency or reproducibility of the measurements made with physiological instruments or equipment; comparable to reliability for multi-item scales.
Readability	**Readability level**: Conducted to determine the participants' ability to read and comprehend the items on an instrument. Researchers should report the level of education needed to read the instrument. Readability must be appropriate to promote reliability and validity of an instrument.

vary based on the test-retest reliability of the scale, the changes in the participants over time, and the changes in the administration of the scale. However, the higher the correlational coefficient obtained in a study, the stronger the test-retest reliability for the measurement method (Kim & Mallory, 2017). Koo and Li (2016, p. 161) recommend evaluating the ICC "level of reliability using the following general guideline: Values less than 0.50 are indicative of poor reliability, values between 0.50 and 0.75 indicate moderate reliability, values between 0.75 and 0.90 indicate good reliability, and values greater than 0.90 indicate excellent reliability."

Equivalence reliability compares two versions of the same scale or instrument or two observers measuring the same event. Comparison of two observers or judges scoring or evaluation of a behavior or situation in a study is referred to as **interrater or interobserver** reliability (Polit & Yang, 2016). There is no absolute value below which interrater reliability is unacceptable, because the behaviors or situations being judged vary in complexity and abstractness (Bialocerkowski et al., 2010). However, any Pearson r value below 0.70 should generate concern about the reliability of the data, data gatherer, or both. The interrater reliability value should be reported in the research report and is best to be 0.80 (80%) to 0.90 (90%) or higher, which means the raters or judges are equivalent during the study (Grove & Gray, 2019).

Studies that include two or more observers should report a statistic that measures the interobserver agreement. The kappa statistic or (kappa coefficient) is the most commonly used statistic to determine interobserver agreement in a study (Viera & Garrett, 2005). A kappa of 1 indicates perfect observer agreement that is never achieved due to measurement error, and a kappa of 0 indicates agreement equivalent to chance. Viera and Garrett (2005) recommended the following values be used when interpreting kappa: 0.01 to 0.20, slight agreement; 0.21 to 0.40, fair agreement; 0.41 to 0.60, moderate agreement; 0.61 to 0.80, substantial agreement; and 0.81 to 0.99, almost perfect agreement.

Comparison of two versions of a test or scale is referred to as **alternate-forms reliability** or **parallel-forms reliability** (see Table 4-1; Waltz et al., 2017). Alternative forms of tests are developed for normative knowledge testing such as the Scholastic Aptitude Test (SAT), which is used as a college entrance requirement. The SAT has been used for decades, and there are many forms of this test, with a variety of items included on each. These alternate forms of the SAT were developed to measure students' knowledge consistently and protect the integrity of the test. Multiple forms of the Graduate Record Exam (GRE) have been developed and used for entrance to graduate school. For most scales, the development of two comparable versions of a scale is difficult and not often done (Bannigan & Watson, 2009; Waltz et al., 2017).

Internal consistency, also known as homogeneity reliability testing, is used primarily with multi-item scales, where each item on a scale is correlated with all other items on the scale to determine consistency of measurement (see Table 4-1). The principle is that each item should be consistently measuring a concept such as depression and so should be correlated with the other items on the scale. The Cronbach's alpha coefficient is the most commonly used measure of internal reliability for scales with multiple items that are at least at the interval level of measurement. A Cronbach's alpha coefficients range from 0.00 to 1.00, where 1.00 indicates perfect reliability and a coefficient of 0.00 indicates no reliability or chance (Waltz et al., 2017).

A Cronbach's alpha coefficient ≥ 0.80 indicates a strong reliability for a scale that has been used in several studies. The stronger correlation coefficients, which are closer to 1.00, indicate less random error and a more reliable scale. For example, the CES-D has strong internal consistency reliability, with Cronbach's alphas ranging from 0.84 to 0.90 in field studies (Armenta, Hartshorn, Whitbeck, Crawford, & Hoyt, 2014). For relatively new scales, a reliability of 0.70 is considered acceptable because the scale is being refined and used with a variety of samples. Reliability coefficients of < 0.60 indicate limited instrument reliability or consistency in the measurement of a variable or concept with higher potential for error (Waltz et al., 2017).

The Cronbach's alpha coefficient can be used to calculate the error for a scale with a specific population. The Cronbach's alpha is squared and subtracted from 1.00 to determine the potential for error in the scores from a scale. The formula and example are presented as follows:

$1.00 - (\text{Cronbach alpha})^2 = \text{measurement error}$ $100\% \times \text{error} = \text{Percentage of error}$

$1.00 - (0.80)^2 = 1.00 - 0.64 = 0.36$ $100\% \times 0.36 = 36\%$

Many scales have subscales that comprise the concept measured, and the reliability of the subscales should also be included in a research report. The subscales of instruments usually have lower reliability coefficients (0.60 to 0.70) than the total scale. The number of items in the total scale provides a more stable measurement of a concept in a study than the subscales, with fewer items (Gray et al., 2017; Waltz et al., 2017). If the data are dichotomous (yes or no responses) the Kuder-Richardson formula (K-R 20) is used to estimate internal consistency (Waltz et al., 2017). A research report should include the results from stability, equivalence, and/or homogeneity reliability testing done on a measurement method from previous research and in the present study (Gray et al., 2017; Waltz et al., 2017).

Precision, similar to reliability, is the degree of consistency or reproducibility of measurements made with physiological equipment or devices. There should be close agreement in the replicated physiological measures of the same variable or element under specified conditions (Ryan-Wenger, 2017). The precision of most physiological equipment is determined by the manufacturer and is a part of the quality control testing done by the agency using the device. To promote precision in physiological measures or devices, researchers develop protocols to ensure consistent collection of physiological data, transfer of specimens, and analysis of physiological data or specimens. The physiological equipment used to collect and analyze physiological data should be recalibrated and maintained as indicated by the manufacturer (DeVon et al., 2007; Ryan-Wenger, 2017).

Test-retest reliability is appropriate for physiological variables that have minimal fluctuations, such as lipid levels, bone mineral density, or weight of adults (Ryan-Wenger, 2017). Test-retest reliability can be inappropriate if the variables' values frequently fluctuate with various activities, such as with pulse, respirations, and blood pressure (BP). However, test-retest is a good measure of precision if the measurements are taken in rapid succession. For example, the national BP guidelines encourage taking three BP readings 1 to 2 minutes apart and then averaging them to obtain the most precise and accurate measure of BP (Weber et al., 2014). Higher levels of precision (0.90 to 0.99) are important for physiological measures that are used to monitor critical physiological functions such as arterial pressure and oxygen saturation (Bialocerkowski et al., 2010).

Readability is an essential element of the reliability and validity of an instrument. Assessing the grade level for reading an instrument is simple and takes seconds with the use of a readability formula, of which there are more than 30. These formulas count language elements in the document and use this information to estimate the degree of difficulty a reader may have in comprehending the text. The formulas provide an overview of the readability of a document based on estimated grade level, ease of reading, and grammar in the document. Readability formulas are now a standard part of word-processing software. When researchers determine the readability level of their measurement methods are appropriate for a study population, this strengthens the reliability and validity of the instruments in the study. Often a scale needs to be at the sixth grade level for certain adults to be able to comprehend and complete it (Waltz et al., 2017). Study participants must be able to read and understand the items on a scale in order to complete the items consistently and accurately.

The concepts of reliability and validity (see Exercise 5) should be evaluated together to determine the quality of a measurement method. An instrument that has low reliability cannot be valid because it is inconsistent in its measurement of the study variable or concept. However, an instrument can be reliable but not necessarily valid. For example, a Likert scale that was developed to measure pain has a Cronbach's alpha of 0.84, but it is actually more focused on measuring stress and anxiety than pain, resulting in low validity for the scale. The measurement of study variables with reliable and valid measurement methods is essential for obtaining quality study results and findings. The questions in this exercise will help you critically appraise the reliability of scales and the precision of physiologic measures in published studies (Gray et al., 2017; Grove & Gray, 2019; Waltz et al., 2017). Some of the sources in this exercise are older because frequently used quality instruments are developed over years.

RESEARCH ARTICLE

Source

Williams, S. G., Turner-Henson, A., Langhinrichsen-Rohling, J., & Azuero, A. (2017). Depressive symptoms in 9th graders: Stress and physiological contributors. *Applied Nursing Research, 34*(1), 24–28.

Introduction

Williams, Turner-Henson, Langhinrichsen-Rohling, and Azuero (2017) conducted a predictive correlational study to determine if stressful life events, perceived stress, and bullying were predictive of depressive symptoms in ninth graders. In addition, cortisol values and diurnal rhythm were examined in these adolescents. "A non-probability, convenience sampling method was used; the resulting sample consisted of 143 9th graders recruited from two public suburban southeastern U.S. high schools" (Williams et al., 2017, p. 25). Nurses may encounter adolescents with depressive symptoms in many settings, but school is an optimal site to screen for these symptoms. The measurement methods for depressive symptoms, bullying, and cortisol values are presented in the following study excerpt.

Relevant Study Results

"Depressive symptoms were measured with The Center for Epidemiologic Studies Depression Survey (CESD-10) . . . The CESD-10 was chosen due to the applicability for adolescent populations and the length of the measure (10 questions). In a study of $n = 156$ adolescents, reliability of CESD-10 was found to be $\alpha = 0.85$ (Bradley, Bagnell, & Brannen, 2010). Reliability for the current study was $\alpha = 0.86$ . . .

Bullying was measured using The Personal Experiences Checklist (PECK), a 32-item Likert scale instrument that was previously used in adolescents' ages 8 to 15 years (Hunt, Peters, & Rapee, 2012). This self-report instrument is scored from 0 to 4: 0 (never), 1 (rarely), 2 (sometimes), 3 (most days), and 4 (every day). Bullying behaviors included the following number of items, internal consistency, and test-retest coefficients: verbal/relational bullying (11 items, $\alpha = 0.90$, $r = 0.75$); physical bullying (9 items, $\alpha = 0.91$, $r = 0.61$); cyberbullying (8 items, $\alpha = 0.90$, $r = 0.86$; and cultural bullying (4 items, $\alpha = 0.78$, $r = 0.77$). High scores indicate more bullying. Reliability for the overall scale was $\alpha = 0.94$ in the current study . . .

Cortisol diurnal rhythm (cortisol change from morning to afternoon) was assessed by collecting salivary specimens during an elective course in the morning school hours (8 am–11 am) and again in the afternoon school hours (12 pm–3 pm). When collecting saliva, 9th graders were asked to refrain from eating or drinking anything except water for approximately 1 h before sample collection. Upon arrival to the testing room, the participants were instructed to rinse their mouth thoroughly with water 5–10 min before the sample was collected to minimize potential pH variability and bacterial contamination.

Specimens were collected using a passive drool approach to collect saliva in a cryo vial using a saliva collection aid for a period of 3 min while under the principal investigator's supervision" (Williams et al., 2017, p. 25).

STUDY QUESTIONS

1. What types of reliability testing are commonly presented in nursing research reports to demonstrate the consistency of instruments in measuring study variables? Why is reliability testing important? Document your answer.

2. What statistical techniques are most commonly used to determine internal consistency or homogeneity reliability for scales with interval- or ratio-level data and for scales with nominal-level data? Provide a rationale for your answer.

3. If Cronbach's alpha coefficient was 0.55 for a multi-item pain perception scale to measure pain in adolescents, is this value acceptable? Provide a rationale for your answer that includes a calculation of the percentage of measurement error for this scale.

4. What level of measurement is achieved by the CESD-10 scale? What type of reliability testing is appropriate to conduct on this scale? Provide a rationale for your answer.

5. What reliability value was reported for the CESD-10 scale in this study and was this reliability value satisfactory? Provide a rationale for your answer.

6. Calculate the percentage of random error for the CESD-10 scale in the Williams et al. (2017) study. Show your calculations and round to the nearest whole percent.

7. What type of scale is the PECK? Was this scale appropriate to gather data on bullying from adolescents? Provide a rationale for your answer.

8. What is stability reliability and what was the stability reliability value reported for the verbal/relational bullying subscale of the PECK reported in the Williams et al. (2017) study? Was this reliability value acceptable? Provide a rationale for your answer.

9. "When collecting saliva, 9th graders were asked to refrain from eating or drinking anything except water for approximately 1 h before sample collection" (Williams et al., 2017, p. 25). Discuss the importance of this statement in this study.

10. Why is the readability level or value of a measurement method important to include in a research report? Discuss the relevance of Williams et al. (2017), including a readability level for the PECK scale used in their study.

Answers to Study Questions

1. The three most common types of reliability testing reported in nursing studies are (1) stability reliability, (2) equivalence reliability, and (3) internal consistency or homogeneity (see Table 4-1; Gray et al., 2017). Reliability testing determines the consistency of an instrument in measuring a variable and the potential for measurement or random error. An instrument with strong reliability and limited potential for error provides consistent data about a concept or variable. If an instrument has limited reliability in a study, reviewers need to question the results and findings related to the instrument (DeVon et al., 2007; Waltz et al., 2017).

2. Cronbach's alpha coefficient (α) is calculated to determine the homogeneity or internal consistency of multi-item scales with interval- or ratio-level of data in a study. The α value should be determined for every multi-item scale and its subscales used in a study, since a scale should be reliable for a particular study sample. The Kuder-Richardson formula (*KR 20*) is calculated to determine the internal consistency of instruments with data measured at the nominal level. Researchers also need to discuss the reliability of the scales used in their study based on previous research (Gray et al., 2017; Grove & Gray, 2019).

3. If Cronbach's alpha coefficient is $\alpha = 0.55$, then the scale has a 0.55 internal consistency reliability and a 0.698 (69.8%) measurement error. The error calculations is: $1.00 - (0.55)^2 = 1.00 - 0.3025 = 0.6975 = 0.698$, and multiple $100\% \times 0.698 = 69.8\%$ error. This high potential for error means that researchers should question the results obtained from the adolescents in this study using this pain perception scale. In addition, the reliability of this scale should be reported as a limitation in the study (Gray et al., 2017). Further research is needed to identify a reliable scale to measure pain perception in adolescents (Waltz et al., 2017).

4. The CESD-10 is a 10-item Likert scale developed to measure depression in adolescents. Multi-item scales are tested for internal consistency reliability (see Table 4-1) using Cronbach's alpha coefficient (Bialocerkowski et al., 2010; Waltz et al., 2017). Multi-item scales are considered interval-level measurement, so Cronbach's alpha is the appropriate statistic to conduct for internal consistency (see Exercise 1; Grove & Gray, 2019).

5. The CESD-10 had a reliability $\alpha = 0.86$ for the Williams et al. (2017) study. A reliability value greater than 0.80 is strong and indicates the scale had evidence of adequate reliability in this study (Armenta et al., 2014; Bialocerkowski et al., 2010; Waltz et al., 2017).

6. The percentage of random error for the CESD-10 scale in the Williams et al. (2017) study was 26%. The calculations are: $1.00 - (0.86)^2 = 1.00 - 0.7396 = 0.2604$, and multiple by $100\% \times 0.2604 = 26.04\% = 26\%$ error.

7. Yes, the PECK is a Likert scale that is appropriate to gather data on bullying from adolescents. Williams et al. (2017, p. 25) reported, "Bullying was measured using the PECK, a 32-item Likert scale instrument that was previously used with adolescents' age 8 to 15 years (Hunt, Peters, & Rapee, 2012)." The reliability for the PECK in this study was $\alpha = 0.94$. Thus, the PECK has a history of being used with adolescents, and the internal consistency reliability was very strong in this study.

8. Stability reliability is concerned with the consistency of repeated measures of the same variable or concept with the same scale or measurement method over time. Stability is commonly referred to as test-retest reliability due to the repeated measurement of a variable over time (see Table 4-1). The test-retest coefficient for verbal/relational bullying was $r = 0.75$. This is an acceptable reliability value for test-retest, which is usually lower than internal consistency values, since the scale is administered over time (DeVon et al., 2007; Waltz et al., 2017).

9. This statement indicates how precision was achieved in the collection of the saliva specimens. Precision is the degree of consistency or reproducibility of measurements obtained with physiological instruments or devices. Williams et al. (2017) documented the protocol that was followed to ensure consistent collection of specimens in this study (Ryan-Wenger, 2017).

10. Researchers reporting appropriate reading levels or readability scores for their measurement methods in a study enhance the reliability and validity of the instruments. Study participants must be able to read and understand the items on an instrument in order to complete it consistently and accurately. The measurement section for the PECK scale would have been strengthened by Williams et al. (2017) reporting the readability level of the PECK scale to ensure the reading level was below the ninth grade level. Study participants have varying levels of reading capability, so a sixth to seventh grade level of reading might have strengthened the reliability and validity of the PECK in this study (Gray et al., 2017; Waltz et al., 2017).

Questions to Be Graded

Name: _____ Class: _____

Date: _____

Follow your instructor's directions to submit your answers to the following questions for grading. Your instructor may ask you to write your answers below and submit them as a hard copy for grading. Alternatively, your instructor may ask you to submit your answers online.

1. Based on the information provided from the Williams et al. (2017) study, which of the two scales have the higher Cronbach's alpha coefficient for this study? Which scale has the greater random error? Provide rationales for your answers.

2. Would you consider the CESD-10 a reliable measure of depression in this population of ninth grade adolescents? Provide a rationale for your answer.

3. What types of reliability testing were provided for the cyberbullying subscale of the PECK? Were the reliability values acceptable? Provide a rationale for your answer.

4. Calculate the percentage of random error for the cyberbullying subscale of the PECK? Show your calculations and round to the nearest whole percent.

5. What are the Cronbach's alphas for the four subscales for the PECK used to measure bullying in the Williams et al. (2017) study? Did these subscales have adequate reliability in this study? Provide a rationale for your answer.

6. Which subscale of the PECK had the lowest Cronbach's alpha? What is the random error for this subscale? Show your calculations and round to the nearest whole percent.

7. Williams et al. (2017, p. 25) reported the PECK "was previously used in adolescents' ages 8 to 15." Based on readability, do you think the PECK is acceptable for the population in this study? Provide a rationale for your answer.

8. Could you assume that the PECK would be a reliable scale to measure bullying in college students? Provide a rationale for your answer.

9. Did Williams et al. (2017) provide a clear discussion of the reliability of the CESD-10 and PECK scales in their study? Provide a rationale for your answer.

10. Was the collection of saliva for cortisol values precise? Provide a rationale for your answer.

Understanding Validity of Measurement Methods

STATISTICAL TECHNIQUE IN REVIEW

Validity of Measurement Methods

A measurement method has **validity** if it accurately reflects the concept it was developed to measure. In examining validity, we focus on the appropriateness, meaningfulness, and usefulness of the measurement method in capturing the aspects of a selected concept. Validity, like reliability, is not an all-or-nothing phenomenon; it is measured on a continuum. No instrument is completely valid, so researchers determine the degree of validity of an instrument rather than whether validity exists or not (DeVon et al., 2007; Waltz, Strickland, & Lenz, 2017).

Many types of validity exist, but this text will focus on the types most commonly reported in nursing studies, which include content validity, construct validity, and criterion-related validity (Bannigan & Watson, 2009; Goodwin, 2002; Polit & Yang, 2016; Waltz et al., 2017). Table 5-1 provides a brief overview of content, construct, and criterion-related validity that are discussed in more depth in the following paragraphs.

Content validity examines the extent to which the measurement method includes all the major elements relevant to the concept being measured. The evidence for content validity of an instrument or scale includes the following: (1) how well the items of the scale reflect the description of the concept in the literature (or face validity); (2) the content experts' evaluation of the relevance of items on the scale that might be reported as an index; and (3) the study participants' responses to scale items (Gray, Grove, & Sutherland, 2017; Waltz et al., 2017).

Construct validity focuses on determining whether the instrument actually measures the theoretical construct that it purports to measure, which involves examining the fit between the conceptual and operational definitions of a variable (see Chapter 8, Grove & Gray, 2019). Construct validity is developed using several methods such as convergent validity, divergent validity, validity from factor analysis, validity from contrasting groups, and successive verification validity (see Table 5-1; Waltz et al., 2017). **Convergent validity** is examined by comparing a newer instrument with an existing instrument that measures the same concept or construct. The two instruments are administered to a sample at the same time, and the results are evaluated with correlational analyses. If the measures are strongly positively correlated, the validity of each instrument is strengthened. For example, the Center for Epidemiological Studies Depression Scale (CES-D) has shown positive correlations ranging from 0.40 to 0.80 with the Hamilton Rating Scale for Depression, which supports the convergent validity of both scales (Locke & Putnam, 2002; Sharp & Lipsky, 2002). **Divergent validity** is examined when the scores from an existing instrument are correlated with the scores from an instrument measuring an opposite concept. For example, two different scales, one measuring hope and the other measuring

TABLE 5-1	EXAMINING THE VALIDITY OF MEASUREMENT METHODS
Quality Indicator	**Description**
Validity	**Content validity:** Examines the extent to which a measurement method includes all the major elements relevant to the construct being measured.
	Construct validity: Focuses on determining whether the instrument actually measures the theoretical construct that it purports to measure, which involves examining the fit between the conceptual and operational definitions of a variable.
	Convergent validity: Two scales measuring the same concept are administered to a group at the same time and the subjects' scores on the scales should be positively correlated. For example, subjects completing two scales to measure depression should have positively correlated scores.
	Divergent validity: Two scales that measure opposite concepts, such as hope and hopelessness, administered to subjects at the same time should result in negatively correlated scores on the scales.
	Validity from factor analysis examines if an instrument includes the elements of the concept being measured by conducting exploratory and/or confirmatory factor analysis to determine if the items in an instrument are related and cluster together to form factors that reflect the elements or sub-concepts of the concept being measured.
	Validity from contrasting (known) groups: An instrument or scale is given to two groups that are expected to have opposite or contrasting scores, where one group scores high on the scale and the other scores low.
	Successive verification validity is achieved when an instrument is used in several studies with a variety of study participants.
	Criterion-related validity: Validity that is strengthened when a study participant's score on an instrument can be used to infer his or her performance on another variable or criterion.
	Predictive validity: The extent to which an individual's score on a scale or instrument can be used to predict future performance or behavior on a criterion.
	Concurrent validity: Focuses on the extent to which an individual's score on an instrument or scale can be used to estimate his or her present or concurrent performance on another variable or criterion.
Accuracy	**Accuracy of physiological measure**: Addresses the extent to which the physiological instrument or equipment measures what it is supposed to measure in a study; comparable to validity for multi-item scales.

hopelessness, could be examined for divergent validity. If the two measurement strategies have a moderate to strong negative correlation (such as –0.40 to –0.80), the divergent validity of both scales is strengthened (Waltz et al., 2017).

Validity tested by factor analysis examines if an instrument includes the elements of the concept being measured. A researcher uses exploratory and/or confirmatory factor analysis to determine if the items in an instrument are related and cluster together to form factors that reflect the elements or sub-concepts of the concept being measured (Gray et al., 2017; Plichta & Kelvin, 2013). The factors identified with factor analysis can then be compared with the sub-concepts of the concept identified through the review of literature for content validity. If the factor analysis results identify the essential elements of the concept to be measured by an instrument, then the validity of the instrument is strengthened (Gray et al., 2017; Plichta & Kelvin, 2013; Waltz et al., 2017).

Validity from contrasting groups is tested by identifying groups that are expected or known to have contrasting scores on an instrument and then asking the groups to complete the instrument (see Table 5-1). If the two groups have contrasting scores on the instrument, then the validity of the instrument is strengthened. For example, researchers could compare the scores on the CES-D scale (Radloff, 1977) for a group of patients diagnosed with depression and a group of individuals who do not have a depression diagnosis. If the groups have contrasting scores, then the depression scale is thought to measure the concept of depression, and the validity of the scale is strengthened (DeVon et al., 2007; Gray et al., 2017). **Successive verification validity** is achieved when an instrument is used in several studies with a variety of study participants in various settings (Grove & Gray, 2019). The validity of instruments are determined over time, with some of the strongest instruments developed over 20 to 30 years ago, resulting in older sources for scales often used in studies.

Criterion-related validity is examined by using a study participant's score on an instrument or scale to infer his or her performance on a criterion. Criterion validity is strengthened when the participants' scores on a scale are successful in determining their behaviors on a variable or criterion. Criterion-related validity includes validity from the prediction of future events and prediction of concurrent events. **Validity from the prediction of future events** is achieved when the scores on an instrument can be used to predict future behaviors, attitudes, and events. For example, fall risk assessment scales have been developed to predict the fall potential of elderly patients. The positive relationship of the scale score with the incidence of falls in the elderly strengthens the validity of this scale to determine the risk for falling. Thus, elderly with high fall risk assessment scores require additional interventions to prevent their falling. **Validity from prediction of concurrent events** can be tested by examining the ability to predict the concurrent value of one instrument on the basis of the value obtained on an instrument to measure another concept. For example, researchers might use the results from a self-esteem scale to predict the results on a coping scale. Thus, if study participants with high self-esteem scores had high coping scores, this would add to the validity of the self-esteem scale (Goodwin, 2002; Gray et al., 2017; Waltz et al., 2017).

In summary, there are a variety of ways to add to the validity of an instrument, and an instrument's validity needs to be presented in the measurement section of a study. The validity of an instrument is often provided from previous research, but sometimes a study might focus on examining an instrument's validity. An instrument must be both valid and reliable to provide a quality measurement of a concept in a study (Bannigan & Watson, 2009; Goodwin, 2002; Waltz et al., 2017).

Accuracy of Physiological Measures

The accuracy of physiological and biochemical measures is similar to the validity of scales used in research. **Accuracy** involves determining the closeness of the agreement between the measured value and the true value of the physiological variable being measured. New measurement devices are compared with existing standardized methods of measuring a biophysical property or concept (Gray et al., 2017; Ryan-Wenger, 2017). For example, measures of oxygen saturation with a pulse oximeter were correlated with arterial blood gas measures of oxygen saturation to determine the accuracy of the pulse oximeter. There should be a very strong, positive correlation (≥ 0.95) between pulse oximeter and blood gas measures of oxygen saturation to support the accuracy of the pulse oximeter. Accuracy of physiological measures depends on the quality of the measurement equipment or device, detail of the data collection plan, and expertise of the data collector (Ryan-Wenger, 2017). Researchers need to report the accuracy of the physiological and biochemical measures used in their studies.

RESEARCH ARTICLE

Source

Williams, S. G., Turner-Henson, A., Langhinrichsen-Rohling, J., & Azuero, A. (2017). Depressive symptoms in 9th graders: Stress and physiological contributors. *Applied Nursing Research, 34*(1), 24–28.

Introduction

Williams, Turner-Henson, Langhinrichsen-Rohling, and Azuero (2017) conducted a predictive correlational study to determine if stressful life events, perceived stress, and bullying were predictive of depressive symptoms in ninth graders. In addition, cortisol values and cortisol diurnal rhythm were examined in these adolescents. "A non-probability, convenience sampling method was used; the resulting sample consisted of 143 9th graders recruited from two public suburban southeastern U.S. high schools" (Williams et al., 2017, p. 25). Nurses may encounter adolescents with depressive symptoms in many settings, but school is an optimal site to screen for these symptoms.

The Williams et al.'s (2017) article was the focus of Exercise 4 and included content relevant to the reliability of some of the measurement methods in the study. This exercise includes relevant content focused on the validity of the measurement methods for depressive symptoms, stressful life events, and cortisol values that are presented in the following study excerpt.

Relevant Study Results

"Depressive symptoms were measured with The Center for Epidemiologic Studies Depression Survey (CESD-10) that has been used to measure four factors related to depressive symptoms including: positive/negative affect, somatic symptoms, retarded activity, and interpersonal issues. CESD-10 scores range from 0 to 30 with scoring from 0 to 3: 0 (rarely), 1 (some of the time), 2 (occasionally or moderate amount), 3 (all the time) for each item. A score of 10 or greater indicates need for referral (clinically meaningful). The CESD-10 was chosen due to the applicability for adolescent populations and the length of the measure (10 questions) . . . Reliability for the current study was $\alpha = 0.86$.

Stressful life events (SLE) and the impact of these events or Life Change Units (LCU) were measured with The Coddington (1972) Life Events Scale for Adolescents (CLES-A). The CLES-A, designed for adolescents aged 13–19 years, had validity and reliability determined with test-retest reliability ($\alpha = 0.84$) (Thompson & Morris, 1994) and interclass correlation ($r = 0.63$) (Villalonga-Olives et al., 2011). Reliability for the current study was $\alpha = 0.76$.

Cortisol diurnal rhythm (cortisol change from morning to afternoon) was assessed by collecting salivary specimens during an elective course in the morning school hours (8 am–11 am) and again in the afternoon school hours (12 pm–3 pm). When collecting saliva, 9th graders were asked to refrain from eating or drinking anything except water for approximately 1 h before sample collection. Upon arrival to the testing room, the participants were instructed to rinse their mouth thoroughly with water 5–10 min before the sample was collected to minimize potential pH variability and bacterial contamination. Specimens were collected using a passive drool approach to collect saliva in a cryo vial using a saliva collection aid for a period of 3 min while under the principal investigator's supervision. Specimens were kept on ice during data collection and then frozen at −20 °C until shipped to Salimetrics, LLC on dry ice. Duplicate analysis of saliva was completed with an ELISA/EIA assay, calibration range of 0.012–3.00 µg/dL and a sensitivity of <0.003 µg/dL to determine the cortisol levels. The expected range of salivary cortisol for adolescents aged 12–18 years is 0.021–0.883 µg/dL for morning and 0.0–0.259 µg/dL for afternoon, and the correlation between saliva and serum cortisol is $r (47) = 0.91, p < 0.0001$ (Salimetrics LLC, 2013)" (Williams et al., 2017, p. 25).

STUDY QUESTIONS

1. Define validity for measurement methods. What are the three different categories of measurement validity discussed in this exercise?

2. Identify the types of validity that contribute to the construct validity of an instrument or scale? Which of these types of validity involves comparing the values from two scales? Provide a rationale for your answer.

3. What type of validity is examined when a scale is initially developed? Provide a rationale for your answer.

4. A measurement method that predicts the potential for pressure ulcer development in hospitalized patients has which type of validity? Provide a rationale for your answer.

5. Which scale would have stronger validity for the measurement of the concept of depression in the Williams et al. (2017) study: (1) The CESD scale developed by Radloff in 1977, refined for use with different age groups, and used frequently in studies; or (2) a depression scale developed 15 years ago for young adults? Provide a rationale for your answer.

6. What scale was used to measure stressful life events in the Williams et al. (2017) study? What type of validity information was provided for this scale?

7. Was the validity information provided for the CLES-A adequate in this research report? Provide a rationale for your answer.

8. Give an example of how validity from contrasting groups might have been developed for the CLES-A?

9. The CLES-A had a reliability of $\alpha = 0.76$ for this study. Is there link between reliability and validity for a scale used in a study? Provide a rationale for your answer.

10. Williams et al. (2017, p. 27) reported, "This study results identify that 9th graders' perception of stress, bullying, and sexual orientation explained 59% of the variance of depressive symptoms" (for results from regression analysis see Exercise 15). Review Williams et al.'s (2017) article in the Resource Library for this text and discuss how the findings from this study might be used in clinical practice.

Answers to Study Questions

1. The validity of a measurement method is determined by how accurately it measures the abstract concept it was developed to measure. The three categories of measurement validity presented in this text are content validity, construct validity, and criterion-related validity (see Table 5-1; Gray et al., 2017; Grove & Gray, 2019; Waltz et al., 2017).

2. Construct validity includes convergent validity, divergent validity, validity from factor analysis, validity from contrasting groups, and successive verification validity (Gray et al., 2017). Convergent validity involves determining the relationship between two instruments that measure the same concept, such as two scales to measure depression. Divergent validity is examined by comparing the scores from an existing instrument with the scores from an instrument that measures an opposite concept, such as scales measuring hope and hopelessness.

3. Content validly is examined during the initial development of a scale. Researchers identify a concept like hope that they want to measure. They review the literature to define and identify possible sub-concepts of hope. Using this content, they develop possible items for a scale to measure hope. The scale items are reviewed by experts for completeness, conciseness, clarity, and readability and refined as needed (Gray et al., 2017).

4. Criterion-related validity is examined when an instrument, such as the Braden Scale, is used to predict the future event of pressure ulcers in hospitalized patients. The predictive criterion validity of the Braden Scale is strengthened if it can be used to successfully predict the potential for pressure ulcer development (Waltz et al., 2017). Identifying patients at risk enables nurses to implement interventions to prevent pressure ulcer development in at risk patients.

5. The CESD scale probably has stronger validity than the 15-year-old depression scale because it was developed and refined over 40 years to measure depression (Radloff, 1977). In addition, the CESD scale has been refined for use with different age groups, and the CESD-10 is considered "applicable for adolescent populations" (Williams et al., 2017, p. 25). A depression scale for young adults would probably not be as valid as the CESD-10 in measuring depression in adolescents (Waltz et al., 2017). The CESD-10 also has stronger successive verification validity with its use in a variety of studies with different populations in various settings than a depression scale developed 15 years ago (Gray et al., 2017).

6. The Life Events Scale for Adolescents (CLES-A) was used to measure stressful life events in this study. Content validity was addressed by indicating the CLES-A measured "Stressful life events (SLE) and the impact of these events or Life Change Units (LCU)" (Williams et al., 2017, p. 25). The CLES-A was designed for adolescents 13 to 19 years of age, which adds to the scale's validity. In addition, the CLES-A has successive verification validity, since it was used in previous studies.

7. The validity information provided for the CLES-A was not adequate in this study. Only limited, vague information on content and successive verification validity was provided. The researchers indicated the scale had validity but no specific information was provided, so the validity of the scale cannot be evaluated (Grove & Gray, 2019; Waltz et al., 2017).

8. Answers will vary. You need to identify two groups that you think would have different or contrasting values on the CLES-A (Waltz et al., 2017). For example, you might contrast the scores of the CLES-A for ninth graders in private school versus those in public schools. Students who are home schooled might be contrasted with those in formal school settings using the CLES-A. These groups might be expected to have different stressful life events.

9. Yes, there is a link between reliability and validity for a scale in a study. A scale must be reliable or consistently measuring something in order to be valid. The CLES-A had an acceptable (0.76) but not strong ($\geq$ 0.80) reliability in this study (see Exercise 4; Grove & Gray, 2019). The acceptable reliability in this study was essential for the CLES-A to be valid.

10. Williams et al. (2017, p. 27) made the following recommendations for clinical practice: "It is important for nurses to recognize that 9th graders may be vulnerable and to seek them out for inquiry. Nurses should also advocate for screening of depressive symptoms in settings where 9th graders are readily accessible to try and identify and to refer for post screening follow-up and treatment if necessary."

Questions to Be Graded

Name: _____ Class: _____

Date: _____

Follow your instructor's directions to submit your answers to the following questions for grading. Your instructor may ask you to write your answers below and submit them as a hard copy for grading. Alternatively, your instructor may ask you to submit your answers online.

1. Discuss the importance of a measurement method's validity in a study.

2. Does the CESD-10 scale have evidence of successive verification validity in the Williams et al. (2017) study? Provide a rationale for your answer.

3. Did the CESD-10 have evidence of criterion-related validity in the Williams et al. (2017) study? Provide a rationale for your answer.

4. Discuss the evidence of validity obtained by factor analysis that is provided for the CESD-10 in the Williams et al. (2017) study.

5. Provide an example of how convergent validity might have been examined for the CESD-10.

6. What types of validity were discussed related to the CESD-10 scale in the Williams et al. (2017) study?

7. Was the information on validity provided for the CESD-10 scale adequate in this study? Provide a rationale for your answer.

8. Williams et al. (2017, p. 25) reported, "Specimens were collected . . . under the principal investigator's supervision. Specimens were kept on ice during data collection and then frozen at −20 °C until shipped to Salimetrics, LLC on dry ice." What does this statement indicate about the precision and accuracy of the saliva specimens collected?

9. How was accuracy determined in the measurement of cortisol levels in the Williams et al. (2017) study?

10. Was the description of the measurement of cortisol diurnal rhythm adequate in this study? Provide a rationale for your answer.

Understanding Frequencies and Percentages

EXERCISE 6

STATISTICAL TECHNIQUE IN REVIEW

Frequency is the number of times a score or value for a variable occurs in a set of data. **Frequency distribution** is a statistical procedure that involves listing all the possible values or scores for a variable in a study. Frequency distributions are used to organize study data for a detailed examination to help determine the presence of errors in coding or computer programming (Gray, Grove, & Sutherland, 2017). In addition, frequencies and percentages are used to describe demographic and study variables measured at the nominal or ordinal levels. (see Exercise 1; Waltz, Strickland, & Lenz, 2017)

Percentage can be defined as a portion or part of the whole or a named amount in every hundred measures. For example, a sample of 100 subjects might include 40 females and 60 males. In this example, the whole is the sample of 100 subjects, and gender is described as including two parts, 40 females and 60 males. A percentage is calculated by dividing the smaller number, which would be a part of the whole, by the larger number, which represents the whole. The result of this calculation is then multiplied by 100%. For example, if 14 nurses out of a total of 62 are working on a given day, you can divide 14 by 62 and multiply by 100% to calculate the percentage of nurses working that day. Calculations: $(14 \div 62) \times 100\% = 0.2258 \times 100\% = 22.58\% = 22.6\%$. The answer also might be expressed as a whole percentage, which would be 23% in this example.

A **cumulative percentage distribution** involves the summing of percentages from the top of a table to the bottom. Therefore, the bottom category has a cumulative percentage of 100% (Grove & Gray, 2019). Cumulative percentages can also be used to determine percentile ranks, especially when discussing standardized scores. For example, if 75% of a group scored equal to or lower than a particular examinee's score, then that examinee's rank is at the 75th percentile. When reported as a percentile rank, the percentage is often rounded to the nearest whole number. **Percentile ranks** can be used to analyze ordinal data that can be assigned to categories that can be ranked. Percentile ranks and cumulative percentages might also be used in any frequency distribution where subjects have only one value for a variable. For example, demographic characteristics are usually reported with the frequency (f) or number (n) of subjects and percentage (%) of subjects for each level of a demographic variable. Income level is presented as an example for 200 subjects:

Income Level	Frequency (f)	Percentage (%)	Cumulative %
1. <$40,000	20	10%	10%
2. $40,000–$59,999	50	25%	35%
3. $60,000–$79,999	80	40%	75%
4. $80,000–$100,000	40	20%	95%
5. >$100,000	10	5%	100%

In data analysis, percentage distributions can be used to compare findings from different studies that have different sample sizes, and these distributions are usually arranged in tables in order either from greatest to least or least to greatest percentages (Kim & Mallory, 2017; Plichta & Kelvin, 2013).

RESEARCH ARTICLE

Source

Eckerblad, J., Tödt, K., Jakobsson, P., Unosson, M., Skargren, E., Kentsson, M., & Theander, K. (2014). Symptom burden in stable COPD patients with moderate to severe airflow limitation. *Heart & Lung, 43*(4), 351–357.

Introduction

Eckerblad and colleagues (2014, p. 351) conducted a descriptive comparative study to examine the symptoms of "patients with stable chronic obstructive pulmonary disease (COPD) and determine whether symptom experience differed between patients with moderate or severe airflow limitations." The Memorial Symptom Assessment Scale (MSAS) was used to measure the symptoms of 42 outpatients with moderate airflow limitations and 49 patients with severe airflow limitations. The results indicated that the mean number of symptoms was 7.9 (±4.3) for both groups combined, with no significant differences found in symptoms between the patients with moderate and severe airflow limitations. For patients with the highest MSAS symptom burden scores in both the moderate and the severe limitations groups, the symptoms most frequently experienced included shortness of breath, dry mouth, cough, sleep problems, and lack of energy. The researchers concluded that patients with moderate or severe airflow limitations experienced multiple severe symptoms that caused high levels of distress. Quality assessment of COPD patients' physical and psychological symptoms is needed to improve the management of their symptoms. (Note: This article does not use American Psychological Association [APA, 2010] format to report means and standard deviations). Using APA format, the results would be reported as follows: ($M = 7.9$, $SD = 4.3$).)

Relevant Study Results

Eckerblad et al. (2014, p. 353) noted in their research report that "In total, 91 patients assessed with MSAS met the criteria for moderate ($n = 42$) or severe airflow limitations ($n = 49$). Of those 91 patients, 47% were men, and 53% were women, with a mean age of 68 (±7) years for men and 67 (±8) years for women. The majority (70%) of patients were married or cohabitating. In addition, 61% were retired, and 15% were on sick leave. Twenty-eight percent of the patients still smoked, and 69% had stopped smoking. The mean BMI (kg/m^2) was 26.8 (±5.7).

There were no significant differences in demographic characteristics, smoking history, or BMI between patients with moderate and severe airflow limitations (Table 1). A lower proportion of patients with moderate airflow limitation used inhalation treatment with glucocorticosteroids, long-acting β$_2$-agonists and short-acting β$_2$-agonists, but a higher proportion used analgesics compared with patients with severe airflow limitation.

Symptom prevalence and symptom experience

The patients reported multiple symptoms with a mean number of 7.9 (±4.3) symptoms (median = 7, range 0–32) for the total sample, 8.1 (±4.4) for moderate airflow limitation and 7.7 (±4.3) for severe airflow limitation ($p = 0.36$).... Highly prevalent physical

TABLE 1 BACKGROUND CHARACTERISTICS AND USE OF MEDICATION FOR PATIENTS WITH STABLE CHRONIC OBSTRUCTIVE LUNG DISEASE CLASSIFIED IN PATIENTS WITH MODERATE AND SEVERE AIRFLOW LIMITATION

	Moderate $n = 42$	Severe $n = 49$	p Value
Sex, *n* (%)			0.607
Women	19 (45)	29 (59)	
Men	23 (55)	20 (41)	
Age (yrs), mean (*SD*)	66.5 (8.6)	67.9 (6.8)	0.396
Married/cohabitant *n* (%)	29 (69)	34 (71)	0.854
Employed, *n* (%)	7 (17)	7 (14)	0.754
Smoking, *n* %			0.789
Smoking	13 (31)	12 (24)	
Former smokers	28 (67)	35 (71)	
Never smokers	1 (2)	2 (4)	
Pack years smoking, mean (*SD*)	29.1 (13.5)	34.0 (19.5)	0.177
BMI (kg/m^2), mean (*SD*)	27.2 (5.2)	26.5 (6.1)	0.555
FEV_1 % of predicted, mean (*SD*)	61.6 (8.4)	42.2 (5.8)	<0.001
SpO^2 % mean (*SD*)	95.8 (2.4)	94.5 (3.0)	0.009
Physical health, mean (*SD*)	3.2 (0.8)	3.0 (0.8)	0.120
Mental health, mean (*SD*)	3.7 (0.9)	3.6 (1.0)	0.628
Exacerbation previous 6 months, *n* (%)	14 (33)	15 (31)	0.781
Admitted to hospital previous year, *n* (%)	10 (24)	14 (29)	0.607
Medication use, *n* (%)			
Inhaled glucocorticosteroids	30 (71)	44 (90)	0.025
Systemic glucocorticosteroids	3 (6.3)	0 (0)	0.094
Anticholinergic	32 (76)	42 (86)	0.245
Long-acting β_2-agonists	30 (71)	45 (92)	0.011
Short-acting β_2-agonists	13 (31)	32 (65)	0.001
Analgesics	11 (26)	5 (10)	0.046
Statins	8 (19)	11 (23)	0.691

Eckerblad, J., Tödt, K., Jakobsson, P., Unosson, M., Skargren, E., Kentsson, M., & Theander, K. (2014). Symptom burden in stable COPD patients with moderate to severe airflow limitation. *Heart & Lung, 43*(4), p. 353.

symptoms (≥50% of the total sample) were shortness of breath (90%), cough (65%), dry mouth (65%), and lack of energy (55%). Five additional physical symptoms, feeling drowsy, pain, numbness/tingling in hands/feet, feeling irritable, and dizziness, were reported by between 25% and 50% of the patients. The most commonly reported psychological symptom was difficulty sleeping (52%), followed by worrying (33%), feeling irritable (28%) and feeling sad (22%). There were no significant differences in the occurrence of physical and psychological symptoms between patients with moderate and severe airflow limitations" (Eckerblad et al., 2014, p. 353).

STUDY QUESTIONS

1. What are the frequency and percentage of women in the moderate airflow limitation group?

2. What were the frequencies and percentages of the moderate and the severe airflow limitation groups who experienced an exacerbation in the previous 6 months?

3. What is the total sample size of COPD patients included in this study? What number or frequency of the subjects is married/cohabitating? What percentage of the total sample is married or cohabitating? Show your calculations.

4. Were the moderate and severe airflow limitation groups significantly different regarding married/cohabitating status? Provide a rationale for your answer.

5. List at least three other relevant demographic variables the researchers might have gathered data on to describe this study sample.

6. For the total sample, what physical symptoms were experienced by ≥50% of the subjects? Identify the physical symptoms and the percentages of the total sample experiencing each symptom.

7. Were the physical symptoms identified in the study what you might expect for patients with moderate to severe COPD? Provide a rationale for your answer with documentation.

8. What frequency and percentage of the total sample used inhaled glucocorticosteroids? Show your calculations and round to the nearest tenth of a percent.

9. Is there a significant difference between the moderate and severe airflow limitation groups regarding the use of inhaled glucocorticosteriods? Provide a rationale for your answer.

10. Was the percentage of COPD patients with moderate and severe airflow limitations using inhaled glucocorticosteriods what you expected? Provide a rationale for your answer with documentation.

Answers to Study Questions

1. The moderate airflow limitation group included 19 women, which means 45% of this group was female (see Table 1).

2. A frequency of 14 (33%) of the moderate airflow limitation group and a frequency of 15 (31%) of the severe airflow limitation group experienced an exacerbation in the previous 6 months (see Table 1).

3. The total sample was $N = 91$ patients with COPD in the Eckerblad et al. (2014) study (see the narrative of study results). The number or frequency of subjects' who were married/cohabitating is calculated by adding the frequencies from the two groups in Table 1.

   Calculation: Frequency married/cohabitating = 29 moderate group + 34 severe group = 63. The percentage of the sample married/cohabitating is 70% (see narrative of study results) or can be calculated by (frequency married/cohabitating ÷ sample size) × 100% = (63 ÷ 91) × 100% = 69.23% = 69%. The researchers might have rounded to next higher whole percent of 70% (see the study narrative), but 69% is a more accurate percentage of the married/cohabitating for the sample.

4. No, the moderate and severe airflow limitation groups were not significantly different regarding married/cohabitating status as indicated by $p = 0.854$ (see Table 1). The level of significance or alpha (α) in most nursing studies is set at $\alpha = 0.05$ (Grove & Gray, 2019). Since the p value is >0.05, the two groups were not significantly different in this study.

5. Additional demographic variables that might have been described in this study include race/ethnicity, socioeconomic status or income level, years diagnosed with COPD, and other co-morbid medical diagnoses of these study participants. You might have identified other relevant demographic variables to be included in this study.

6. "Highly prevalent physical symptoms (≥50% of the total sample) were shortness of breath (90%), cough (65%), dry mouth (65%), and lack of energy (55%)" (Eckerblad et al., 2014, p. 353; see study narrative of results).

7. Yes, the physical symptoms of shortness of breath, cough, dry mouth, and lack of energy or fatigue are extremely common in patients with COPD who have moderate to severe airflow limitations. The Global Initiative for Chronic Obstructive Lung Disease website is an excellent resource at https://goldcopd.org/wp-content/uploads/2018/11/GOLD-2019-POCKET-GUIDE-FINAL_WMS.pdf. This website include the the GOLD 2019 Pocket Guide for the diagnosis, management, and prevention of COPD. The Centers for Disease Control and Prevention (CDC) also provide current empirical information about COPD at https://www.cdc.gov/copd/index.html. You might document with other websites, research articles, or textbooks.

8. Frequency = 74 and percent = 81.3%. In this study, 30 of the moderate airflow limitation group and 44 of the severe group used inhaled glucocorticosteroids. Calculations: Frequency = 30 + 44 = 74. Percentage total sample = (74 ÷ 91) × 100% = 0.8132 × 100% = 81.32% = 81.3%, rounded to the nearest tenth of a percent.

9. Yes, the moderate and severe airflow limitation groups were significantly different regarding the use of inhaled glucocorticosteroids as indicated by $p = 0.025$ (see Table 1). The level of significance or alpha (α) in most nursing studies is set at 0.05. Since the p value is <0.05, the two groups were significantly different for the use of inhaled glucocorticosteroids in this study (Gray et al., 2017; Kim & Mallory, 2017).

10. In this study, 30 (71%) of the patients with moderate airflow limitation and 44 (90%) of the patients with severe airflow limitation were treated with glucocorticosteroids. The mean percentage for the total sample who used glucocorticosteroids is (71% + 90%) ÷ 2 = 161 ÷ 2 = 80.5%, or 81%. The use of inhaled glucocorticosteroids is very common for patients with moderate to severe COPD, in fact, recommended by national evidence-based guidelines, particularly for those with severe airflow limitation. Thus, you might expect that a large number of COPD patients in this study were using inhaled glucocorticosteroids. The Gold Standard for the management of COPD can be found at the Global Initiative for Chronic Obstructive Lung Disease website at: https://goldcopd.org/wp-content/uploads/2018/11/GOLD-2019-POCKET-GUIDE-FINAL_WMS.pdf.

Questions to Be Graded

> Name: _____ Class: _____
>
> Date: _____

Follow your instructor's directions to submit your answers to the following questions for grading. Your instructor may ask you to write your answers below and submit them as a hard copy for grading. Alternatively, your instructor may ask you to submit your answers online.

1. What are the frequency and percentage of the COPD patients in the severe airflow limitation group who are employed in the Eckerblad et al. (2014) study?

2. What percentage of the total sample is retired? What percentage of the total sample is on sick leave?

3. What is the total sample size of this study? What frequency and percentage of the total sample were still employed? Show your calculations and round your answer to the nearest whole percent.

4. What is the total percentage of the sample with a smoking history—either still smoking or former smokers? Is the smoking history for study participants clinically important? Provide a rationale for your answer.

5. What are pack years of smoking? Is there a significant difference between the moderate and severe airflow limitation groups regarding pack years of smoking? Provide a rationale for your answer.

6. What were the four most common psychological symptoms reported by this sample of patients with COPD? What percentage of these subjects experienced these symptoms? Was there a significant difference between the moderate and severe airflow limitation groups for psychological symptoms?

7. What frequency and percentage of the total sample used short-acting β_2-agonists? Show your calculations and round to the nearest whole percent.

8. Is there a significant difference between the moderate and severe airflow limitation groups regarding the use of short-acting β_2-agonists? Provide a rationale for your answer.

9. Was the percentage of COPD patients with moderate and severe airflow limitation using short-acting β_2-agonists what you expected? Provide a rationale for your answer with documentation.

10. Are these findings ready for use in practice? Provide a rationale for your answer.

Interpreting Line Graphs

STATISTICAL TECHNIQUE IN REVIEW

Tables and figures are commonly used to present findings from studies or to provide a way for researchers to become familiar with research data. Using figures, researchers are able to illustrate the results from descriptive data analyses, assist in identifying patterns in data, identify changes over time, and interpret exploratory findings (American Psychological Association, 2010). A **line graph** is a figure that is developed by joining a series of plotted points with a line to illustrate how a variable changes over time or how one variable changes in relation to another (Kim & Mallory, 2017). A line graph figure includes a horizontal scale, or x-axis, and a vertical scale, or y-axis. The x-axis is often used to document time, and the y-axis is used to document the mean scores or values for a variable (Gray, Grove, & Sutherland, 2017; Plichta & Kelvin, 2013). For example, researchers might include a line graph to compare the values for anxiety and pain variables in a sample of post-surgical patients or to identify the changes in group(s) for a selected variable over time. Figure 7-1 presents a line graph that documents time in weeks on the x-axis and mean weight loss in pounds on the y-axis for an experimental group consuming a low carbohydrate diet and a control group consuming a standard diet. This line graph illustrates the trend of a strong, steady increase in the mean weight lost by the experimental or intervention group and minimal mean weight loss by the control group.

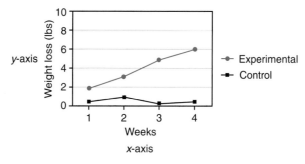

FIGURE 7-1 ■ **LINE GRAPH COMPARING EXPERIMENTAL AND CONTROL GROUPS FOR WEIGHT LOSS OVER FOUR WEEKS.**

It is important to note that sometimes, the slope of a line (or the amount by which a line deviates from the horizontal axis) in a line graph does not represent significant effects. Alternatively, sometimes lines do not indicate large changes, but may represent significant effects in large samples (Gray et al., 2017; Kim & Mallory, 2017).

RESEARCH ARTICLE

Source

Azzolin, K., Mussi, C. M., Ruschel, K. B., de Souza, E. N., Lucena, A. D., & Rabelo-Silva, E. R. (2013). Effectiveness of nursing interventions in heart failure patients in home care using NANDA-I, NIC, and NOC. *Applied Nursing Research, 26*(4), 239–244.

Introduction

Azzolin and colleagues (2013) analyzed data from a larger randomized clinical trial to determine the effectiveness of 11 nursing interventions from the Nursing Interventions Classification (NIC) on selected nursing outcomes from the Nursing Outcomes Classification (NOC; Moorhead, Swanson, Johnson, & Maas, 2018) in a sample of patients with heart failure (HF) receiving home care. A total of 23 patients with HF were followed for 6 months after hospital discharge and provided four home visits and four telephone calls. The home visits and phone calls were organized using the nursing diagnoses from the North American Nursing Diagnosis Association International (NANDA-I) classification list. The researchers found that eight nursing interventions significantly improved the nursing outcomes for these HF patients. Those interventions included "health education, self-modification assistance, behavior modification, telephone consultation, nutritional counselling, teaching: prescribed medications, teaching: disease process, and energy management" (Azzolin et al., 2013, p. 243). The researchers concluded that the NANDA-I, NIC, and NOC linkages were useful in managing patients with HF in their home. They recommended additional studies using the nursing taxonomies be conducted in clinical settings.

Relevant Study Results

Azzolin and colleagues (2013, p. 240) presented their results in a line graph format to display the nursing outcome changes over the 6 months of the home visits and phone calls. "The activities and interventions implemented at each home care visit varied according to patient needs. The indicators of each outcome were evaluated by the principle investigator at each visit using a five-point Likert scale (1 = worst and 5 = best)."

"Of the eight outcomes selected and measured during the visits, four belonged to the health & knowledge behavior domain (50%), as follows: knowledge: treatment regimen; compliance behavior; knowledge: medication; and symptom control. Significant increases were observed in this domain for all outcomes when comparing mean scores obtained at visits no. 1 and 4 (Figure 1; $p < 0.001$ for all comparisons).

The other four outcomes assessed belong to three different NOC domains, namely, functional health (activity tolerance and energy conservation), physiologic health (fluid balance), and family health (family participation in professional care). The scores obtained for activity tolerance and energy conservation increased significantly from visit no. 1 to visit no. 4 ($p = 0.004$ and $p < 0.001$, respectively). Fluid balance and family participation in professional care did not show statistically significant differences ($p = 0.848$ and $p = 0.101$, respectively) (Figure 2)" (Azzolin et al., 2013, p. 241). The significance level or alpha (α) was set at 0.05 for this study.

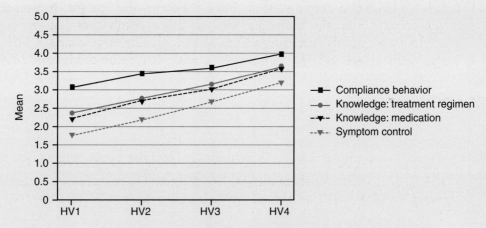

FIGURE 1 ■ **NURSING OUTCOMES MEASURED OVER 6 MONTHS (HEALTH & KNOWLEDGE BEHAVIOR DOMAIN):** Knowledge: medication (95% CI −1.66 to −0.87, $p < 0.001$); knowledge: treatment regimen (95% CI −1.53 to −0.98, $p < 0.001$); symptom control (95% CI −1.93 to −0.95, $p < 0.001$); and compliance behavior (95% CI −1.24 to −0.56, $p < 0.001$).

HV = home visit.

CI = confidence interval for the mean change over time.

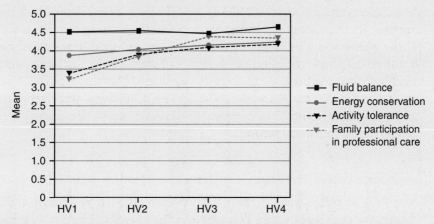

FIGURE 2 ■ **NURSING OUTCOMES MEASURED OVER 6 MONTHS (OTHER DOMAINS):** Activity tolerance (95% CI −1.38 to −0.18, $p = 0.004$); energy conservation (95% CI −0.62 to −0.19, $p < 0.001$); fluid balance (95% CI −0.25 to 0.07, $p = .848$); family participation in professional care (95% CI −2.31 to −0.11, $p = 0.101$).

HV = home visit.

CI = confidence interval for the mean change over time.

Azzolin, K., Mussi, C. M., Ruschel, K. B., de Souza, E. N., Lucena, A. D., & Rabelo-Silva, E. R. (2013). Effectiveness of nursing interventions in heart failure patients in home care using NANDA-I, NIC, and NOC. *Applied Nursing Research, 26*(4), p. 242.

STUDY QUESTIONS

1. What is the purpose of a line graph? What elements are included in a line graph?

2. Review Figure 1 and identify the focus of the x-axis and the y-axis. What is the time frame for the x-axis? What variables are presented on this line graph?

3. In Figure 1, did the nursing outcome compliance behavior change over the 6 months of home visits? Provide a rationale for your answer.

4. State the null hypothesis for the nursing outcome compliance behavior.

5. Was there a significant difference in compliance behavior from the first home visit (HV1) to the fourth home visit (HV4)? Was the null hypothesis accepted or rejected? Provide a rationale for your answer.

6. In Figure 1, what outcome had the lowest mean at HV1? Did this outcome improve over the four home visits? Provide a rationale for your answer.

7. Was there a significant change in the outcome knowledge: medication over the four home visits? Provide a rationale for your answer. What does this result mean?

8. Was there a significant change in the outcome knowledge: treatment regimen over the four home visits? Provide a rationale for your answer. What does this result mean?

9. Was the sample size adequate in this study? Provide a rationale for your answer.

10. Are the findings from this study ready for generalization to the population of patients with heart failure? Provide a rationale for your answer.

Answers to Study Questions

1. A line graph is a figure developed to illustrate the results from descriptive data analyses, to identify patterns in data over time, or to demonstrate how one variable changes in relation to another (Kim & Mallory, 2017; King & Eckersley, 2019). A line graph might include an *x*-axis to document time in a study and a *y*-axis to identify the mean scores or values for a variable. The mean scores for variables are plotted and connected with a line to show change over time. More than one variable can be included in a line graph as shown in Figures 1 and 2.

2. In Figure 1, the *x*-axis represents the four home visits (HVs) provided study participants over 6 months. The *y*-axis represents the means for the 23 HF patients on the nursing outcomes measured in this study. The variables included in Figure 1 were compliance behavior, knowledge: medication, knowledge: treatment regimen, and symptom control (Moorhead et al., 2018).

3. Yes, the outcome compliance behavior did change over the 6 months of the study from a mean of 3 to a mean of approximately 4 (see Figure 1).

4. Null hypothesis: *There is no change in the nursing outcome compliance behavior for patients with HF receiving four HVs and telephone calls over 6 months.*

5. Yes, there was a statistically significant change in the outcome compliance behavior from HV1 to HV4 as indicated by $p < 0.001$ (see the footnote under Figure 1 and the study results section). The null hypothesis is rejected since $\alpha = 0.05$ in this study and the p value was less than α. The results of studies are statistically significant when the p values are less than α set by the researcher for the study (Grove & Gray, 2019).

6. The outcome symptom control had the lowest mean at HV1. The means increased for symptom control over the four HVs from approximately 1.6 at HV1 to 3.1 at HV4 as illustrated on the line graph. This change was statistically significant at $p < 0.001$.

7. Yes, there was a statistically significant change in the outcome knowledge: medication from HV1 to HV4 as indicated by $p < 0.001$, which is less than $\alpha = 0.05$ set for the study. This result means that following the 4 HVs and telephone calls the 23 HF patients demonstrated a significant increase in their knowledge of medications.

8. Yes, there was a statistically significant change in the outcome knowledge: treatment regimen from HV1 to HV4 as indicated by $p < 0.001$, which is less than $\alpha = 0.05$ set for the study. This result means that following the 4 HVs and telephone calls the 23 HF patients demonstrated a significant increase in their knowledge of treatment regimen.

9. Answers may vary. The sample size was small with 23 participants, and some of the results were nonsignificant, indicating that a Type II error might have occurred due to the limited sample size. The researchers did conduct a power analysis and determined a sample of 17 was needed for their study if they had a moderate effect size of 0.50. However, they did not determine the power for their nonsignificant findings, and post hoc power analyses are warranted (Aberson, 2019; Cohen, 1988; Gray et al., 2017).

10. We would not recommend generalizing these study findings. This is a single study focused on the changes in nursing outcomes with HVs and phone calls, and the sample size was small with only 23 patients with HF. The study results were mixed with nonsignificant findings for the energy conservation, fluid balance, and family participation in professional care variables. In addition, the principle investigator evaluated the outcomes at each visit, which promotes consistent data collection but might have created a bias. Replication of this study with a larger sample size is needed before generalizing the findings. Azzolin et al. (2013) also recommended additional research in this area.

Questions to Be Graded

Name: _____ Class: _____

Date: _____

Follow your instructor's directions to submit your answers to the following questions for grading. Your instructor may ask you to write your answers below and submit them as a hard copy for grading. Alternatively, your instructor may ask you to submit your answers online.

1. What is the focus of the example Figure 7-1 in the section introducing the statistical technique of this exercise?

2. In Figure 2 of the Azzolin et al. (2013, p. 242) study, did the nursing outcome activity tolerance change over the 6 months of home visits (HVs) and telephone calls? Provide a rationale for your answer.

3. State the null hypothesis for the nursing outcome activity tolerance.

4. Was there a significant difference in activity tolerance from the first home visit (HV1) to the fourth home visit (HV4)? Was the null hypothesis accepted or rejected? Provide a rationale for your answer.

5. In Figure 2, what nursing outcome had the lowest mean at HV1? Did this outcome significantly improve over the four HVs? Provide a rationale for your answer.

6. What nursing outcome had the highest mean at HV1 and at HV4? Was this outcome significantly different from HV1 to HV4? Provide a rationale for your answer.

7. State the null hypothesis for the nursing outcome family participation in professional care.

8. Was there a statistically significant difference in family participation in professional care from HV1 to HV4? Was the null hypothesis accepted or rejected? Provide a rationale for your answer.

9. Was Figure 2 helpful in understanding the nursing outcomes for patients with heart failure (HF) who received four HVs and telephone calls? Provide a rationale for your answer.

10. What nursing interventions significantly improved the nursing outcomes for these patients with HF? What implications for practice do you note from these study results?

Measures of Central Tendency: Mean, Median, and Mode

STATISTICAL TECHNIQUE IN REVIEW

Mean, median, and mode are the three **measures of central tendency** used to describe study variables. These statistical techniques are calculated to determine the center of a distribution of data, and the central tendency that is calculated is determined by the level of measurement of the data (nominal, ordinal, interval, or ratio; see Exercise 1). The **mode** is a category or value that occurs with the greatest frequency in a distribution of data. The mode is the only acceptable measure of central tendency for analyzing nominal-level data, which are not continuous and cannot be ranked (Grove & Gray, 2019). Most distributions of values in a study are **unimodal**, or have one mode, and frequencies progressively decline as they move away from the mode. A **symmetrical curve**, like the one in Figure 8-1, is unimodal, and the left side of the curve is a mirror image of the right side of the curve. The mode, median, and mean are essentially equal. If a distribution has two scores that occur more frequently than others (two modes), the distribution is called **bimodal**. A distribution with more than two modes is **multimodal** (Gray, Grove, & Sutherland, 2017).

The **median** (*MD*) is a score that lies in the middle of a rank-ordered list of values of a distribution. If a distribution consists of an odd number of scores, the *MD* is the middle score that divides the rest of the distribution into two equal parts, with half of the values falling above the middle score and half of the values falling below this score. In a distribution with an even number of scores, the *MD* is half of the sum of the two middle scores

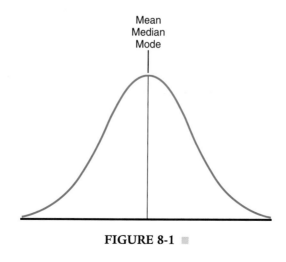

FIGURE 8-1 ■

of that distribution. If several scores in a distribution are of the same value, then the *MD* will be the value of the middle score.

The *MD* is the most precise measure of central tendency for ordinal-level data and for non-normally distributed or skewed interval- or ratio-level data. Curves that are not symmetrical are referred to **asymmetrical or skewed**. A curve may be positively skewed, which means that the largest portion of data is below the mean (Figure 8-2). For example, data on length of enrollment in hospice are **positively skewed**. Most people die within the first few days or weeks of enrollment, whereas increasingly smaller numbers survive as time increases. A curve can also be negatively skewed, which means that the largest portion of data is above the mean (see Figure 8-2). For example, data on the occurrence of chronic illness by age in a population are **negatively skewed**, with most chronic illnesses occurring in older age groups. In a **skewed distribution**, the mean, median, and mode are not equal. In a positively skewed distribution the mean is greater than the median, which is greater than the mode. In a negatively skewed distribution the mean is less than the median, which is less than the mode (see Figure 8-2).

The following calculation can be conducted to locate the median in a distribution of values.

$$\text{Median}\,(MD) = (N+1) \div 2$$

N is the number of scores

Example: $N = 31$ Median $= \dfrac{31+1}{2} = 32 \div 2 = 16^{\text{th}}$ score

Example: $N = 40$ Median $= \dfrac{40+1}{2} = 41 \div 2 = 20.5^{\text{th}}$ score

In the first example, the sample includes an odd number of subjects ($N = 31$) so the median is an actual score in the distribution (16th score). In the second example, the sample includes an equal number of subjects ($N = 40$) so, the median is halfway between the 20th and the 21st scores in the sampling distribution (Grove & Gray, 2019; Kim & Mallory, 2017)

The **mean** ($\overline{X}$) is the arithmetic average of all scores of a sample, that is, the sum of its individual scores divided by the total number of scores. The mean is the most accurate measure of central tendency for normally distributed data measured at the interval and ratio levels and is only appropriate for these levels of data (Gray et al., 2017). In a normal distribution as presented in Figure 8-1, the mean, median, and mode are essentially equal (see Exercise 26 for determining the normality of a distribution). The mean is sensitive to

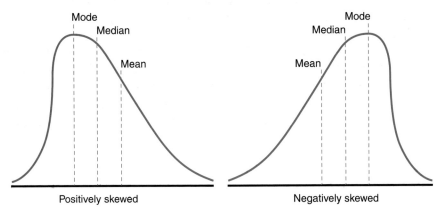

FIGURE 8-2 ▥

extreme values such as outliers. An **outlier** is a value in a sample data set that is unusually low or unusually high in the context of the rest of the sample data. Outliers can result in skewed distributions of data and skewness interferes with the validity of many statistical analyses; therefore statistical procedures have been developed to measure the skewness of the distribution of the sample being studied (see Exercise 26 focused on determining the normality of a distribution). If a study has outliers, the mean is most affected by these, so the median might be the measure of central tendency included in the research report (Kim & Mallory, 2017; Plichta & Kelvin, 2013).

The formula for the mean is:

$$\text{Mean} = \bar{X} = \frac{\sum X}{n}$$

$\sum X$ is the sum of the raw scores in a study
N is the sample size or number of scores in the study

Example: Raw scores = 8, 9, 9, 10, 11, 11 $n = 6$ Mean = 58 ÷ 6 = 9.666 = 9.67

RESEARCH ARTICLE

Source

Winkler, C., Funk, M., Schindler, D. M., Hemsey, J. Z., Lampert, R., & Drew, B. J. (2013). Arrhythmias in patients with acute coronary syndrome in the first 24 hours of hospitalization. *Heart & Lung, 42*(6), 422–427.

Introduction

Winkler and colleagues (2013) conducted their study to describe the arrhythmias of a population of patients with acute coronary syndrome (ACS) during their first 24 hours of hospitalization and to explore the link between arrhythmias and patients' outcomes. The patients with ACS were admitted through the emergency department (ED), where a Holter recorder was attached for continuous 12-lead electrocardiographic (ECG) monitoring. The ECG data from the Holter recordings of 278 patients with ACS were analyzed. The researchers found that "approximately 22% of patients had more than 50 premature ventricular contractions (PVCs) per hour. Non-sustained ventricular tachycardia (VT) occurred in 15% of the patients.... Only more than 50 PVCs/hour independently predicted an increased length of stay ($p < 0.0001$). No arrhythmias predicted mortality. Age greater than 65 years and a final diagnosis of acute myocardial infarction (AMI) independently predicted more than 50 PVCs per hour ($p = 0.0004$)" (Winkler et al., 2013, p. 422).

Winkler and colleagues (2013, p. 426) concluded: "Life-threatening arrhythmias are rare in patients with ACS, but almost one quarter of the sample experienced isolated PVCs. There was a significant independent association between PVCs and a longer length of stay (LOS), but PVCs were not related to other adverse outcomes. Rapid treatment of the underlying ACS should remain the focus, rather than extended monitoring for arrhythmias we no longer treat."

Relevant Study Results

The demographic and clinical characteristics of the sample and the patient outcomes for this study are presented in this exercise. "The majority of the patients ($n = 229$; 83%) had a near complete Holter recording of at least 20 h [hours] and 171 (62%) had a full 24 h recorded. We included recordings of all patients in the analysis. The mean duration of continuous 12-lead Holter recording was 21 ± 6 (median 24) h.

The mean patient age was 66 years and half of the patients identified White as their race (Table 1). There were more males than females and most patients (92%) experienced chest pain as one of the presenting symptoms to the ED. Over half of the patients experienced shortness of breath (68%) and jaw, neck, arm, or back pain (55%). Hypertension was the most frequently occurring cardiovascular risk factor (76%), followed by hypercholesterolemia (63%) and family history of coronary artery disease (53%). A majority had a personal history of coronary artery disease (63%) and 19% had a history of arrhythmias" (Winkler et al., 2013, pp. 423–424).

TABLE 1 DEMOGRAPHIC AND CLINICAL CHARACTERISTICS OF THE SAMPLE (N = 278)		
Characteristic	**N**	**%**
Gender		
Male	158	57
Female	120	43
Race		
White	143	51
Asian	60	22
Black	50	18
American Indian	23	8
Pacific Islander	2	<1
Presenting Symptoms to the ED (May Have >1)		
Chest pain	255	92
Shortness of breath	189	68
Jaw, neck, arm, or back pain	152	55
Diaphoresis	116	42
Nausea and vomiting	96	35
Syncope	11	4
Cardiovascular Risk Factors (May Have >1)		
Hypertension	211	76
Hypercholesterolemia	175	63
Family history of CAD	148	53
Diabetes	81	29
Smoking (current)	56	20
Cardiovascular Medical History (May Have >1)		
Personal history of CAD	176	63
History of unstable angina	124	45
Previous acute myocardial infarction	114	41
Previous percutaneous coronary intervention	85	31
Previous CABG surgery	54	19
History of arrhythmias	53	19
Final Diagnosis		
Unstable angina	180	65
Non-ST elevation myocardial infarction	74	27
ST elevation myocardial infarction	24	9
Interventions during 24-h Holter Recording		
PCI ≤ 90 min of ED admission	14	5
PCI > 90 min of ED admission	3	1
Thrombolytic medication	3	1
Interventions Any Time during Hospitalization		
PCI	76	27
Treated with anti-arrhythmic medication	16	6
CABG surgery	22	8

	Mean (SD)	**Median**	**Range**
Age (years)	66 (14)	66	30–102
ECG recording time (hours)	21 (6)	24	2–25

ED, emergency department; CAD, coronary artery disease; CABG, coronary artery bypass graft; PCI, percutaneous coronary intervention; SD, standard deviation; ECG, electrocardiogram.

Winkler, C., Funk, M., Schindler, D. M., Hemsey, J. Z., Lampert, R., & Drew, B. J. (2013). Arrhythmias in patients with acute coronary syndrome in the first 24 hours of hospitalization. *Heart & Lung, 42*(6), p. 424.

Winkler et al. (2013, p. 424) also reported: "We categorized patient outcomes into four groups: 1) inpatient complications (of which some patients may have experienced more than one); 2) inpatient length of stay; 3) readmission to either the ED or the hospital within 30-days and 1-year of initial hospitalization; and 4) death during hospitalization, within 30-days, and 1-year after discharge (Table 2). These are outcomes that are reported in many contemporary studies of patients with ACS. Thirty-two patients (11.5%) were lost to 1-year follow-up, resulting in a sample size for the analysis of 1-year outcomes of 246 patients" (Winkler et al., 2013, p. 424).

TABLE 2   OUTCOMES DURING INPATIENT STAY, AND WITHIN 30 DAYS AND 1 YEAR OF HOSPITALIZATION ($N = 278$)

Outcomes	N	%
Inpatient complications (may have >1)		
AMI post admission for patients admitted with UA	21	8
Transfer to intensive care unit	17	6
Cardiac arrest	7	3
AMI extension (detected by 2nd rise in CK-MB)	6	2
Cardiogenic shock	5	2
New severe heart failure/pulmonary edema	2	1
Readmission*		
30-day		
To ED for a cardiovascular reason	42	15
To hospital for ACS	13	5
1-year ($N = 246$)		
To ED for a cardiovascular reason	108	44
To hospital for ACS	24	10
All-cause mortality[†]		
Inpatient	10	4
30-day	13	5
1-year ($N = 246$)	27	11

	Mean (*SD*)	Median	Range
Length of stay (days)	5.37 (7.02)	4	1–93

AMI, acute myocardial infarction; UA, unstable angina; CK-MB, creatinine kinase-myocardial band; ED, emergency department; ACS, acute coronary syndrome; *SD*, standard deviation.
*Readmission: 1-year data include 30-day data.
[†]All-cause mortality: 30-day data include inpatient data; 1-year data include both 30-day and inpatient data.

Winkler, C., Funk, M., Schindler, D. M., Hemsey, J. Z., Lampert, R., & Drew, B. J. (2013). Arrhythmias in patients with acute coronary syndrome in the first 24 hours of hospitalization. *Heart & Lung, 42*(6), p. 424.

STUDY QUESTIONS

1. In Table 1, what is the mode for cardiovascular risk factors? Provide a rationale for your answer. What percentage of the patients experienced this risk factor?

2. Which measure of central tendency always represents an actual score of the distribution? Provide a rationale for your answer.

   a. Mean

   b. Median

   c. Mode

   d. Range

3. What is the mode for the variable presenting symptoms to the ED? What percentage of the patients had this symptom? Do the presenting symptoms have a single mode or is this distribution bimodal or multimodal? Provide a rationale for your answer.

4. What are the three most common presenting symptoms to the ED, and why is this clinically important? What symptom was the least common in this study?

5. For this study, what are the mean and median ages in years for the study participants?

6. Are the mean and median ages similar or different? What does this indicate about the distribution of the sample? Draw the curve for the distribution of age data in the Winkler et al. (2013) study.

7. What are the mean and median ECG recording times in hours? What is the range for ECG recordings? Does this distribution of data include an outlier? Provide a rationale for your answer.

8. What is the effect of outliers on the mean? If the study data have extreme outliers (either high or low scores) in the data, what measure(s) of central tendency might be reported in a study? Provide a rationale for your answer.

9. In the following example, 10 ACS patients were asked to rate their pain in their jaw and neck on a 0–10 scale: 3, 4, 7, 7, 8, 5, 6, 8, 7, 9. What are the range and median for the pain scores?

10. Calculate the mean ($\bar{X}$) for the pain scores in Question 9. Does this distribution of scores appear to be normal? Provide a rationale for your answer.

Answers to Study Questions

1. Hypertension (HTN) is the mode for the cardiovascular risk factors since it is the most frequent risk factor experienced by 211 of the study participants. A total of 76% of the study participants had HTN.

2. Answer: c. Mode. The mode is the most frequently occurring score in a distribution; thus, it will always be an actual score of the distribution. The mean is the average of all scores, so it may not be an actual score of the distribution. Median is the middle score of the distribution, which, with an even number of items, may not be an actual score in the distribution. The range is a measure of dispersion, not a measure of central tendency (Gray et al., 2017; Kim & Mallory, 2017).

3. Chest pain was the mode for the variable presenting symptoms to the ED, with 255 or 92% of the participants experiencing it (see Table 1). The variable presenting symptoms to the ED has one mode, chest pain, which was the most reported symptom.

4. Chest pain (92%); shortness of breath (68%); and jaw, neck, arm, or back pain (55%) are the three most commonly reported presenting symptoms to the ED by study participants. This is clinically important because nurses and other healthcare providers need to rapidly assess for these symptoms, diagnose the problem, and appropriately manage patients presenting with ACS at the ED. Since 92% of the participants had chest pain, it is clinically important to note this symptom is common for both males and females in this study. Syncope was the least reported symptom, with only 11 (4%) of the patients reporting it.

5. Both the mean ($\bar{X}$) and median (MD) values were equal to 66 years, as identified at the bottom of Table 1.

6. In this study, the $\bar{X}$ age = MD age = 66 years, so they are the same value. In a normal distribution of scores, the mode = MD = $\bar{X}$ (Gray et al., 2017). Since the MD = $\bar{X}$ = 66 years, age seems to be normally distributed in this sample. The shape of the curve would be similar to Figure 8-1, and the line down the middle of the curve would have a value of 66.

7. ECG recording time has $\bar{X}$ = 21 hours and MD = 24 hours, with a range of 2–25 hours (see Table 1). The 2 hours of ECG Holter monitoring seems to be an outlier, which resulted in the difference between the mean and median ($\bar{X}$ = 21 hours and MD = 24 hours) numbers of monitoring hours. Winkler et al. (2013) reported that 83% of the study participants had a near complete Holter recording of at least 20 hours, and 62% of the participants had a full 24 hours recorded, which supports the 2 hours of monitoring as an outlier. You would need to examine the study data to determine more about possible outliers. All ECG data were analyzed regardless of the monitoring time, and more explanation is needed about outliers and the reasons for including all recordings in the study analyses.

91

8. An unusually low score or outlier decreases the value of the mean as in this study (see the answer to Question 7), and an unusually high score increases the mean value (see Figure 8-2). The mean in a study is most affected by outliers (Gray et al., 2017; Kim & Mallory, 2017). If the outliers cause the data to be skewed or not normally distributed, it is best to report the median. If the data are normally distributed, then the mean is the best measure of central tendency to report.

9. Place the pain scores in order from the least to the greatest score = 3, 4, 5, 6, 7, 7, 7, 8, 8, 9. In this example, the range of pain scores = 3–9. The mode = 7 and the *MD* or middle score = 7.

10. $\bar{X} = (3 + 4 + 5 + 6 + 7 + 7 + 7 + 8 + 8 + 9) \div 10 = 64 \div 10 = 6.4$. The mode = median = approximately the mean, so this is a normal distribution of scores that forms a symmetrical curve as shown in Figure 8-1. Exercise 26 provides the steps for determining the normality of a distribution of scores or values.

Questions to Be Graded

Name: _____ Class: _____

Date: _____

Follow your instructor's directions to submit your answers to the following questions for grading. Your instructor may ask you to write your answers below and submit them as a hard copy for grading. Alternatively, your instructor may ask you to submit your answers online.

1. The number of nursing students enrolled in a particular nursing program between the years of 2013 and 2020, respectively, were 563, 593, 606, 540, 563, 610, and 577. Determine the mean ($\bar{X}$), median (*MD*), and mode of the number of the nursing students enrolled in this program. Show your calculations.

2. What is the mode for the variable inpatient complications in Table 2 of the Winkler et al. (2013) study? What percentage of the study participants had this complication?

3. Identify the mean, median, and range for the electrocardiographic (ECG) recording time (hours) for the patients in the Winkler et al. (2013) study. Is the distribution of the data normal, positively skewed, or negatively skewed? Provide a rationale for your answer.

4. As reported in Table 1, what are the three most common cardiovascular medical history events in this study, and why is it clinically important to know the frequency of these events?

5. What are the mean and median lengths of stay (LOS) for the study participants?

6. Are the mean and median for LOS similar or different? What might this indicate about the distribution of the sample? Is the distribution normal, positively skewed, or negatively skewed? Provide a rationale for your answer.

7. Examine the study results and determine the mode for arrhythmias experienced by the participants. What was the second most common arrhythmia in this sample?

8. Was the most common arrhythmia in Question 7 related to LOS? Was this result statistically significant? Provide a rationale for your answer.

9. What study variables were independently predictive of the 50 premature ventricular contractions (PVCs) per hour in this study?

10. In Table 1, what race is the mode for this sample? Should these study findings be generalized to American Indians with ACS? Provide a rationale for your answer.

Measures of Dispersion: Range and Standard Deviation

STATISTICAL TECHNIQUE IN REVIEW

Measures of dispersion, or measures of variability, are descriptive statistical techniques conducted to identify individual differences of the scores or values in a sample. These techniques give some indication of how values in a sample are dispersed, or spread, around the mean. The measures of dispersion indicate how different the scores on a particular scale are or the extent that individual scores deviate from one another. If the individual scores are similar, dispersion or variability values are small and the sample is relatively **homogeneous**, or similar, in terms of these scores or values. A **heterogeneous** sample has a wide variation in the scores, resulting in increased values for the measures of dispersion. Range and standard deviation are the most common measures of dispersion included in research reports (Gray, Grove, & Sutherland, 2017).

The simplest measure of dispersion is the **range**. In published studies, range is presented in two ways: (1) the range includes the lowest and highest values obtained for a variable, or (2) the range is calculated by subtracting the lowest score from the highest score. For example, the range for the following scores, 8, 9, 9, 10, 11, 11, might be reported as 8 to 11 (8–11), which identifies outliers or extreme values for a variable. The range can also be calculated as follows: $11 - 8 = 3$. In this form, the range is a difference score that uses only the two extreme values in a sample for the comparison. The range is generally reported in published studies but is not used in further analyses (Grove & Gray, 2019; Kim & Mallory, 2017).

The **standard deviation** (*SD*) is a measure of dispersion that is the average number of points by which the scores or values of a distribution vary from the mean. It indicates the degree of error that would result if the mean alone were used to interpret the data for a variable in a study. The *SD* indicates the variability of values in the normals curve. Figure 9-1 presents the normal curve, where the mean is zero (0) and each $SD = 1$. Values that are greater than +1.96 or −1.96 *SD* from the mean are significantly different from the mean at $p = 0.05$ when alpha = 0.05. Values that are greater than +2.58 or −2.58 are significant at $p = 0.01$.

The *SD* is an important statistic, both for understanding dispersion within a distribution and for interpreting the relationship of a particular value to the distribution. When the scores of a distribution deviate from the mean considerably, the *SD* or spread of scores is large. When the degree of deviation of scores from the mean is small, the *SD* or spread of the scores is small. *SD* is a measure of dispersion that is the square root of the variance (Grove & Gray, 2019; King & Eckersley, 2019). The equation and steps for calculating the standard deviation are presented in Exercise 27, which is focused on calculating descriptive statistics.

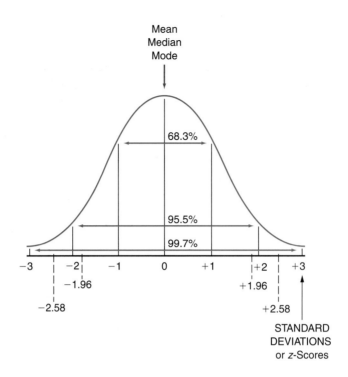

RESEARCH ARTICLE

Source

Roch, G., Dubois, C. A., & Clarke, S. P. (2014). Organizational climate and hospital nurses' caring practices: A mixed-methods study. *Research in Nursing & Health, 37*(3), 229–240.

Introduction

Roch and colleagues (2014) conducted a two-phase mixed methods study (Creswell & Clark, 2018) to describe the elements of the organizational climate of hospitals that directly affect nursing practice. The first phase of the study was quantitative and involved surveying nurses (*N* = 292), who described their hospital organizational climate and their caring practices. The second phase was qualitative and involved a study of 15 direct-care registered nurses (RNs), nursing personnel, and managers. The researchers found the following: "Workload intensity and role ambiguity led RNs to leave many caring practices to practical nurses and assistive personnel. Systemic interventions are needed to improve organizational climate and to support RNs' involvement in a full range of caring practices" (Roch et al., 2014, p. 229).

Relevant Study Results

The survey data were collected using the Psychological Climate Questionnaire (PCQ) and the Caring Nurse-Patient Interaction Short Scale (CNPISS). The PCQ included a five-point Likert-type scale that ranged from *strongly disagree* to *strongly agree*, with the high scores corresponding to positive perceptions of the organizational climate. The CNPISS included a five-point Likert scale ranging from *almost never* to *almost always*, with the higher scores indicating higher frequency of performing caring practices. The return rate for the surveys was 45%. The survey results indicated that "[n]urses generally assessed overall organizational climate as moderately positive (Table 2). The job dimension relating to autonomy, respondents' perceptions of the importance of their work, and the feeling of being challenged at work was rated positively. Role perceptions (personal workload, role clarity, and role-related conflict), ratings of manager leadership, and work groups were significantly more negative, hovering around the midpoint of the scale, with organization ratings slightly below this midpoint of 2.5.

Caring practices were regularly performed; mean scores were either slightly above or well above the 2.5 midpoint of a 5-point scale. The subscale scores clearly indicated, however, that although relational care elements were often carried out, they were less frequent than clinical or comfort care" (Roch et al., 2014, p. 233).

TABLE 2 NURSES' RESPONSES TO ORGANIZATIONAL CLIMATE SCALE AND SELF-RATED FREQUENCY OF PERFORMANCE OF CARING PRACTICES ($N = 292$)

Scale and Subscales (Possible Range)	M	SD	Observed Range
Organizational Climate			
Overall rating (1–5)	3.13	0.56	1.75–4.67
Job (1–5)	4.01	0.49	1.94–5.00
Role (1–5)	2.99	0.66	1.17–4.67
Leadership (1–5)	2.93	0.89	1.00–5.00
Work group (1–5)	3.36	0.88	1.08–5.00
Organization (1–5)	2.36	0.74	1.00–4.67
Caring Practices			
Overall rating (1–5)	3.62	0.66	1.95–5.00
Clinical care (1–5)	4.02	0.57	2.44–5.00
Relational care (1–5)	2.90	1.01	1.00–5.00
Comforting care (1–5)	4.08	0.72	1.67–5.00

Roch, G., Dubois, C., & Clarke, S. P. (2014). *Research in Nursing & Health, 37*(3), p. 234.

STUDY QUESTIONS

1. Organizational climate was measured with which type of scale? What level of measurement was achieved with this scale? Provide a rationale for your answer.

2. The mean ($\bar{X}$) is a measure of _____ _____ of a distribution, while the standard deviation (SD) is a measure of _____ of its scores. Both $\bar{X}$ and SD are _____ statistics.

3. What is the purpose of the range, and how is it determined in a distribution of scores?

4. What subscales were included in the description of organizational climate? Do these seem relevant? Provide a rationale for your answer with documentation.

5. Which organizational climate subscale had the lowest mean? What is your interpretation of this result?

6. What were the dispersion results for the organization subscale in Table 2? What do these results indicate?

7. Which aspect or subscale of organizational climate has the lowest dispersion or variation of scores? Provide a rationale for your answer.

8. Is the dispersion or variation of the ratings on jobs more homogeneous or heterogeneous than the other subscales? Provide a rationale for your answer.

9. Which subscale of organization climate had the greatest dispersion of scores? Provide a rationale for your answer.

10. Ledoux, Forchuk, Higgins, and Rudnick (2018, p. 17) conducted a predictive correlational study to "examine how structural empowerment, psychological empowerment, and inter-professional collaboration affect nurse compassion." These variables were measured with 5-point Likert scales, and Table 1 includes the mean, SD, range, and reliability alphas for these variables. Which scale's scores or values had the smallest dispersion? Provide a rationale for your answer.

TABLE 1 MEAN, STANDARD DEVIATION (SD), RANGE, RELIABILITY (α) OF VARIABLES				
Variable	Mean	SD	Range	α
Structural empowerment	3.09	0.58	1.75-4.68	0.89
Psychological empowerment	3.80	0.51	2.25-5	0.84
Interprofessional collaboration	3.51	0.53	1.97-4.94	0.96
Compassion	4.20	0.43	3-5	0.84

From Ledoux, K., Forchuk, C., Higgins, C., & Rudnick, A. (2018). The effect of organizational and personal variables on the ability to practice compassionately. *Applied Nursing Research, 41*(1), 15–20.

Answers to Study Questions

1. Organizational climate was measured with the Psychological Climate Questionnaire (PCQ), which is a 5-point Likert scale. This scale has multiple items, and the participants mark their responses to each item using a scale of 1 = *strongly disagree* to 5 = *strongly agree*. The data obtained from multiple-item Likert scales are combined and usually analyzed as though they are interval-level data as in this study (Gray et al., 2017). Some sources might describe Likert scale data as ordinal because the 5-point rating scale used in a Likert scale lacks continuous values. However, most nursing and healthcare researchers analyze data from multiple-item Likert scales as interval-level data (see Exercise 1; Waltz, Strickland, & Lenz, 2017).

2. The $\bar{X}$ is a measure of central tendency, and the SD is a measure of dispersion. Both $\bar{X}$ and SD are descriptive or summary statistics.

3. Range is the simplest measure of dispersion or variability, obtained by identifying the lowest and highest scores in a distribution or by subtracting the lowest score from the highest score in the distribution of scores (Grove & Gray, 2019).

4. The subscales included in organizational climate were job, role, leadership, work group, and organization (see Table 2). Yes, these subscales seem relevant because the items used to measure job were related to perceived autonomy, importance of work, and being challenged. The role subscale included personal workload, role clarity, and role-related conflict (see narrative of results). Thus, the items of these five subscales are important in understanding the organizational climate in a hospital. The American Hospital Association (AHA) promotes research to improve the climates in hospitals. For more information on AHA, review their website at http://www.aha.org/research/index.shtml. A subsidiary of AHA is the American Organization of Nurses Executives, which is focused on improving nursing leadership in the current healthcare system (AONE; http://www.aone.org/). You might document with other research articles, texts, and websites.

5. Organization had the lowest mean at 2.36, indicating this is the most negatively perceived of the subscales included in the PCQ scale. The lower the mean the more negative the nurses' perception of their organization. The results identified a problem area that requires additional investigation and management to improve the relationships between the nurses and their organization.

6. The dispersion results for the organization subscale included range = 1.00−4.67 and SD = 0.74. The score for each item on the organization subscale could range from 1.00−5.00 based on the Likert scale used in the PCQ. Both the range and SD seemed similar to the other subscales, indicating the dispersion of scores was similar for the organization subscale (King & Eckersley, 2019).

7. The job subscale had the lowest dispersion with range = 1.94–5.00 or, when calculating the range by subtracting the lowest score from the highest score, 5.00 − 1.94 = 3.06. The *SD* = 0.49 was also the lowest for organizational climate, indicating the scores for job had the lowest variation of the subscales. Focusing on the subscales' results rather than just on the overall organizational climate rating provides readers with a richer understanding of the nurses' perceptions of their organization.

8. Job scores were the most homogeneous or had the least variation of the organization climate subscales as indicated by the lowest range and *SD* results discussed in Question 7 (Grove & Gray, 2019).

9. When compared with the other subscales, leadership scores had the greatest dispersion or variation among the subscales as indicated by the largest *SD* (*SD* = 0.89) and range (1.00–5.00 or 5.00 − 1.00 = 4).

10. The compassion variable has the lowest dispersion or variation of values in this study. The *SD* (0.43) and the range (3–5) were the lowest values of the four scales indicating the lowest dispersion (Grove & Gray, 2019; Kim & Mallory, 2017)

Questions to Be Graded

Name: _____	Class: _____
Date: _____	

Follow your instructor's directions to submit your answers to the following questions for grading. Your instructor may ask you to write your answers below and submit them as a hard copy for grading. Alternatively, your instructor may ask you to submit your answers online.

1. What were the name and type of measurement method used to measure caring practices in the Roch, Dubois, and Clarke (2014) study?

2. The data collected with the scale identified in Questions 1 were at what level of measurement? Provide a rationale for your answer.

3. What were the subscales included in the CNPISS used to measure RNs' perceptions of their caring practices? Do these subscales seem relevant? Document your answer.

4. What were the dispersion results for the relational care subscale of the caring practices in Table 2? What do these results indicate?

5. Which subscale of caring practices has the lowest dispersion or variation of scores? Provide a rationale for your answer.

6. Which subscale of caring practices had the highest mean? What do these results indicate?

7. Compare the overall rating for organizational climate with the overall rating of caring practices. What do these results indicate?

8. The response rate for the survey in this study was 45%. Is this a study strength or limitation? Provide a rationale for your answer.

9. What conclusions did the researchers make regarding the caring practices of the nurses in this study? How might these results affect your practice?

10. What additional research is needed in the areas of organizational climate and caring practices?

Description of a Study Sample

STATISTICAL TECHNIQUE IN REVIEW

Most research reports describe the subjects or participants who comprise the study sample. This description of the sample is called the **sample characteristics.** These characteristics are often presented in the narrative and a table within the research report. Data are collected for demographic and clinical variables to describe the sample. **Demographic variables** are attribute variables such as age, gender, and ethnicity collected to describe a sample and as a basis for comparison with the demographic characteristics in other studies. **Clinical variables** are selective physical, emotional, and cognitive variables collected and analyzed to describe the specific clinical characteristics of the study sample. The sample characteristics might be presented for the entire sample or for the different groups in a study (i.e., intervention and control groups) (Gray, Grove, & Sutherland, 2017).

Descriptive statistics are calculated to generate sample characteristics, and the type of statistic conducted depends on the level of measurement of the demographic and clinical variables included in a study (see Exercise 1; Grove & Gray, 2019; Kim & Mallory, 2017). For example, data collected on gender is nominal level and can be described using frequencies, percentages, and mode (see Exercises 6 and 8). Measuring an educational level usually produces ordinal data that can be described using frequencies, percentages, mode, median, and range (see Exercise 27). Obtaining each participant's specific age is an example of ratio data that can be described using mean, median, range, and standard deviation (see Exercises 9 and 27). Interval and ratio data are analyzed with the same statistical techniques and are sometimes referred to as interval/ratio-level data in this text.

RESEARCH ARTICLE

Source

Riegel, B., Dickson, V. V., Lee, C. S., Daus, M., Hill, J., Irani, E., ... Bove, A. (2018). A mixed methods study of symptom perception in patients with chronic heart failure. *Heart & Lung, 47*(2), 107–114.

Introduction

Riegel and colleagues (2018) conducted a longitudinal sequential explanatory mixed methods study to examine the symptom perceptions of patients with chronic heart failure (HF). A mixed methods study includes both quantitative and qualitative research methods. An exploratory sequential design begins with the collection and analysis of qualitative data, followed by the collection of quantitative data. Often, findings of the qualitative data analyses are used to design the quantitative phase (Gray et al., 2017). Riegel et al. (2018) enrolled a small sample of 36 HF patients to allow depth rather than

105

breadth of data collection (Creswell & Clark, 2018). "Maximum variability was sought in participant age, gender, HF duration and severity, and comorbidity" to promote understanding of HF patients' perceptions and management of their symptoms (Riegel et al., 2018, p. 108). The researchers collected demographic data such as age, gender, education, socioeconomic status, race, employment, marital status, and self-reported income. Likert scales were used to collect data on depression, decision-making, and self-care maintenance and management. "Clinical characteristics (e.g. such as HF duration, type, ejection fraction) were abstracted from the medical record" (Riegel et al., 2018, p. 109). Other clinical data such as cognitive function, comorbidity, and New York Heart Association (NYHA) class were also collected to describe the patients with HF.

Riegel et al. (2018, p. 113) determined "that although some HF patients had systems in place for monitoring their symptoms, problems with symptom detection were evident, interpretation was poor, and problems in management delayed response ... Notably, even the most savvy patients in this sample were not able to avoid a HF hospitalization." The researchers encouraged further research to promote rapid response to signs and symptoms with early intervention to decrease HF hospitalization.

Relevant Study Results

"The enrolled sample of 36 was predominately male (67%), older (64 ± 15.2 years), White (61%), and functionally compromised (56% NYHA class III), with a moderate level of comorbidity (42%). See Table 1. Seven participants withdrew or were lost to follow-up before the final home visit, but only one withdrew early, so a rich dataset was available on each of these participants.

At enrollment, self-care was poor overall. Self-care maintenance scores were barely adequate (mean 69.8 ± 13.5, range 33–93). Self-care management scores (64.4 ± 18.9, range 35–90) and self-care confidence were low (mean 68.4 ± 19.1, range 17–100) as well. The HFSPS [Heart Failure Somatic Perception Scale] total score was low (mean 8.1 ± 10.6, range 0–51), the HFSPS Dyspnea subscale score was also low (mean 1.8 ± 3.7, range 0–15), as was the daily diary fatigue score (mean 4.1 ± 6.6, range 0–24), indicating that few were symptomatic on enrollment. Within the 3-month follow-up period, four participants were admitted to the hospital for HF; two of these four were admitted twice" (Riegel et al., 2018, p. 109).

TABLE 1 DEMOGRAPHIC AND CLINICAL CHARACTERISTICS OF THE FULL SAMPLE (N = 36)

	Mean ± SD	N. Percentage
Patient Characteristics		
Age (years)	63.8 ± 15.2	
Socioeconomic status (Barratt Simplified Measure of Social Status)	43.8 ± 11.1	
Depression (PHQ-9)	4.5 ± 4.1	
MoCA Score	25.28 ± 3.1	
Charlson Comorbidity Index (CCI) Score	3.36 ± 2.0	
Ejection Fraction (%)	37.4 ± 16.8	
HF duration in months	135.4 ± 102.2	
Total number of medication	10.9 ± 4.8	
Male		24 (66.7)
Race		
African American		9 (25.0)
Caucasian		22 (61.1)
Mixed or other		5 (13.9)

TABLE 1	DEMOGRAPHIC AND CLINICAL CHARACTERISTICS OF THE FULL SAMPLE (N = 36)—cont'd		
		Mean ± SD	N. Percentage
Education			
High school or less			6 (16.7)
Some trade or college education (e.g., vocational, associate degree)			16 (44.4)
College (bachelor degree or higher)			14 (38.9)
Employment			
Employed full or part-time			12 (33.3)
Unemployed (sick leave, disability, retired)			23 (63.9)
Other (e.g., student)			1 (2.8)
Marital Status			
Single			4 (11.1)
Married			24 (66.7)
Divorced or Separated			6 (16.7)
Widowed			2 (5.6)
Self-reported Income			
More than enough to make ends meet			20 (55.6)
Enough to make ends meet			13 (36.1)
Not enough to make ends meet			3 (8.3)
Quality of Support			
Satisfactory			2 (5.6)
Good			6 (16.7)
Very Good			28 (77.8)
Perceived Health			
Poor			5 (14.3)
Fair			16 (45.7)
Good			8 (22.9)
Very Good			6 (17.1)
Abnormal MoCA score (<26)			19 (52.8)
Categorized Charlson Comorbidity (CCI) Score			
Low level (CCI 1-2)			13 (36.1)
Moderate level (CCI 3-4)			15 (41.7)
High level (CCI ≥5)			8 (22.2)
Common Comorbid Conditions			
Atrial Fibrillation			15 (41.7)[a]
Myocardial infarction			14 (38.9)
Sleep disordered breathing			14 (38.9)
Diabetes			13 (36.1)
Chronic pain			8 (22.2)
Chronic Obstructive Pulmonary Disease			8 (22.2)
Cerebrovascular Accident			7 (19.4)
Renal Disease			6 (16.7)
NYHA Class			
I			3 (8.6)
II			11 (31.4)
III			20 (57.1)
IV			1 (2.9)

HF=heart failure; PHQ-9=Patient Health Questionaire; MoCA=Montreal Cognitive Assessment; NYHA=New York Heart Association.

[a]Percentages were calculated by the formula: n/36 x 100 (each disease was treated individually, so the sum of percentages under "common comorbidity conditions" are not 100).

From Riegel, B., Dickson, V. V., Lee, C. S., Daus, M., Jill, J., Irani, E., ... Bove, A. (2018). A mixed methods study of symptom perception in patients with chronic heart failure. *Heart & Lung, 47*(2), p. 110.

STUDY QUESTIONS

1. What type of variables are age, gender, education, and socioeconomic status in the Riegel et al. (2018) study. Are these variables commonly described in nursing studies? Provide a rationale for your answer.

2. What levels of measurement are the age and gender variables identified in Table 1? Provide a rationale for your answer.

3. What analysis techniques were conducted to describe age and gender? Were these analysis techniques appropriate? Provide a rationale for your answer.

4. What was the mode for race in this study? Provide a rationale for your answer.

5. Could a mean be calculated on the education demographic variable? Provide a rationale for your answer.

6. What level of measurement is the quality of support variable? Provide a rationale for your answer.

7. What statistics were conducted to describe quality of support? Were these appropriate? Provide a rationale for your answer.

8. Describe the dyspnea score for this sample of patients with heart failure. Were there outliers in these data? Provide a rationale for your answer.

9. Were the HF patients' self-care confidence scores strong in the study? Provide a rationale for your answer. What do these scores indicate clinically about this sample?

10. Are the findings from the Riegel et al. (2018) study ready for use in practice? Provide a rationale for your answer and document your response.

Answers to Study Questions

1. Age, gender, education, and socioeconomic status are demographic variables that were described in the study. Riegel et al. (2018) identified these as demographic variables in the study narrative and in Table 1. Yes, these are common demographic variables collected by nurses and other health professionals to describe the samples in their studies. Researchers can compare their sample characteristics with those of other studies using these demographic results (Gray et al., 2017). Federal grant guidelines often encourage researchers to describe their sample with these common demographic variables (see National Institute of Nursing Research website at https://www.ninr.nih.gov/researchandfunding/desp/oep/fundingopportunities).

2. Age is measured at the ratio level because the specific age of each patient in years was obtained. Age in years is a continuous variable where each year equals 12 months or 365 days. Age has an absolute zero where zero years old indicates the absence of age (see Exercise 1; Gray et al., 2017; Waltz, Strickland, & Lenz, 2017). The data collected for gender in this study include two categories, male and female. These categories are basically exhaustive and mutually exclusive, because all study participants fit into only one category. Male and female gender cannot be ranked, so the data are nominal versus ordinal level (Grove & Gray, 2019).

3. Mean and standard deviation (*SD*) were computed to describe the variable age because it was measured at the ratio level. Ratio-level data are best analyzed with parametric statistics, such as mean and *SD* (Grove & Gray, 2019; Kim & Mallory, 2017). Frequencies and percentages were used to describe the variable gender. Because the data are nominal, frequencies and percentages were appropriate (see Exercise 6). The researchers might have also identified the mode, which was male (66.7% or 67%) for this sample.

4. The mode for race was Caucasian ($n = 22$; 61.1%). The mode is the most frequently occurring value for a variable, which was Caucasian in this study (see Exercise 8; Grove & Gray, 2019).

5. No, a mean cannot be calculated on the education demographic variable, which is at the ordinal level (Grove & Gray, 2019; Waltz et al., 2017). The education variable was organized into three categories (high school or less, some trade or college education, and college [bachelor degree or higher]) that are exhaustive and exclusive. The levels of education can be ranked from a low of high school or less to a high of bachelor degree or higher. However, education is not a continuous variable in this study, so a mean cannot be calculated.

6. The quality of support variable is measured at the ordinal level. Quality support was described with four categories of poor, fair, good, and very good that can be ranked from a low of poor to a high of very good (see Exercise 1; Grove & Gray, 2019).

7. The quality of support variable was described with frequencies and percentages. Frequencies and percentages are acceptable analyses, but the quality support data are at the ordinal level and stronger analyses of median and range could have been conducted to expand the description of this variable.

8. "The dyspnea subscale score was also low (mean 1.8 ± 3.7, range 0-15)" (Riegel et al., 2018, p. 109). Yes, the distribution of dyspnea data appears to have an outlier because the mean is 1.8 and the top score in the range is 15. The score of 15 is very different than the mean of this distribution and is likely an outlier. However, the distribution of scores needs to be examined for outliers and the distribution tested for skewness (see Exercise 26).

9. No, the self-care confidence scores in this study were not strong. Riegel et al. (2018, p. 109) stated the "self-care confidence scores were low (mean 68.4 ± 19.1, range 17-100)." Low self-confidence scores are clinically important because they indicated the uncertainty and probable problems these patients and family members are having in assessing and managing their HF symptoms. These patients need additional support and education to improve their self-confidence and possibly decrease their HF symptoms.

10. Answers might be varied. These findings are not ready for use in practice because the focus of this mixed methods study was to describe HF patients' perception and management of their symptoms (Creswell & Clark, 2018). The knowledge gained from this study provides a basis for future research with a larger sample to improve responses to signs and symptoms of HF and to implement early treatment to reduce hospitalization (Riegel et al., 2018). However, nurses might use the findings about the HF patients' self-care problems with symptom detection and delayed management to focus and expand their education of these patients (see heartfailure.org).

Questions to Be Graded

Name: _____ Class: _____

Date: _____

Follow your instructor's directions to submit your answers to the following questions for grading. Your instructor may ask you to write your answers below and submit them as a hard copy for grading. Alternatively, your instructor may ask you to submit your answers online.

1. In the Riegel et al. (2018) study, what level of measurement is the marital status variable? Provide a rationale for and document your answer.

2. What statistics were calculated to describe marital status in this study? Were these appropriate? Provide a rationale for your answer.

3. In the Riegel et al. (2018) study, depression was measured with the Patient Health Questionnaire (PHQ-9). What level of measurement is the depression variable? Provide a rationale for your answer.

4. What statistics were calculated to describe depression in this study? Were these appropriate? Provide a rationale for your answer.

5. What is the mode for the New York Heart Association (NYHA) class in the Riegel et al. (2018) study? Why is this clinically important?

6. What statistics were calculated to describe the NYHA class in this study? Were these appropriate? Provide a rationale for your answer.

7. Describe the fatigue score for this sample of patients with HF. Were there outliers in these data? Provide a rationale for your answer.

8. Was the sample size adequate for this study? Provide a rationale for your answer.

9. Describe the HF patients' self-care maintenance and self-care management scores. Discuss the clinical importance of these scores.

10. Was the sample for the Riegel et al. (2018) study adequately described? Provide a rationale for your answer.

Interpreting Scatterplots

STATISTICAL TECHNIQUE IN REVIEW

Scatterplots or scatter grams are used to describe relationships between two variables and to provide a graphic representation of data from a study. Variables are illustrated on two axes, x and y. The x-axis is the horizontal axis, and the y-axis is the vertical axis (see Figure 11-1). To provide a visual image of the data, each point on the graph is a subject's values for variables x and y, thus representing the relationship between the x and y variables on the graph. Each subject's values on the two variables are plotted on the graph, and the number of points on the graph depends on the study sample size (Gray, Grove, & Sutherland, 2017). In the example scatterplot in Figure 11-1, there are 20 points, so this example includes a sample of 20 participants.

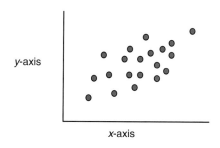

FIGURE 11-1 ■ **EXAMPLE SCATTERPLOT.**

The display of points on the graph indicates the direction (positive or negative) and strength (weak, moderate, or strong) of the relationship between the two variables studied. Scatterplot points moving from the lower left corner to the upper right corner illustrate a positive or direct relationship. Figure 11-2 identifies a positive relationship between the variables of total cholesterol and grams of dietary fat consumed a day: As the grams of fat consumed increase, so does the total cholesterol value. Scatterplot points moving from the upper left corner to the lower right corner indicate a negative or inverse relationship. Figure 11-3 demonstrates a negative relationship between the variables of low-density lipoprotein (LDL) cholesterol and weight loss in pounds per month. A decrease in LDL cholesterol values is associated with increased weight loss in pounds per month.

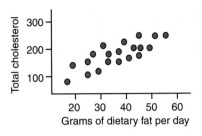

FIGURE 11-2 ■ **POSITIVE OR DIRECT RELATIONSHIP.**

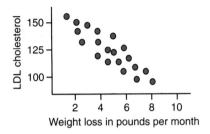

FIGURE 11-3 ■ **NEGATIVE OR INVERSE RELATIONSHIP.**

The strength of the relationships shown in a scatterplot ranges from −1 to +1, with −1 indicating a perfect negative relationship between two variables and +1 indicating a perfect positive relationship between two variables. Pearson *r* is calculated or computed to determine the strength of the relationship between two continuous variables or variables measured at the interval or ratio level (see Exercise 1). A weak relationship is approximately <0.30 or <−0.30, a moderate relationship is 0.30 to 0.50 or −0.30 to −0.50, and a strong relationship is >0.50 or >−0.50 (Cohen, 1988; Gray et al., 2017; Plichta & Kelvin, 2013). The closer the plotted points are to each other and the more they form a straight line, the stronger the linear relationship between the two variables (see Figures 11-2 and 11-3). Conversely, if the plotted points are further away from each other and widespread across the graph, this indicates a weak relationship that is closer to 0. The widespread data points in Figure 11-4 demonstrate a weak positive relationship between minutes of exercise per day and pain perception scores (Kim & Mallory, 2017). A scatterplot visually represents a relationship between two variables, but Pearson *r* correlational analysis must be calculated to determine the specific value for the strength of the relationship (see Exercises 13 and 28).

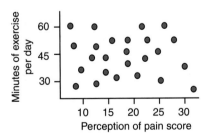

FIGURE 11-4 ■ **WEAK RELATIONSHIP WITH OUTLIERS.**

When looking at scatterplots, it is important to identify outliers. **Outliers** are extreme values in the data set that occur with inherent variability, measurement error, sampling error, and errors in study implementation. Outliers skew the data set or affect the normality of the frequency distribution and are exceptions to the overall findings of a study.

Figure 11-4 has examples of two outliers, one in the upper left corner and the other in the lower right corner. Researchers use scatterplots to identify linear and nonlinear relationships, but the focus of this exercise is understanding linear relationships (Kim & Mallory, 2017).

RESEARCH ARTICLE

Source

Kriikku, P., Wilhelm, L., Jenckel, S., Rintatalo, J., Hurme, J., et al. (2014). Comparison of breath-alcohol screening test results with venous blood-alcohol concentration in suspected drunken drivers. *Forensic Science International, 239*(0379-0738), 57–61.

Introduction

Kriikku and colleagues (2014) conducted a correlational study to determine the relationship between breath-alcohol screening test levels and the venous blood-alcohol concentrations (BAC) of suspected drunk drivers. "Hand-held electronic breath-alcohol analyzers are widely used by police authorities in their efforts to detect drunken drivers and to improve road-traffic safety" (Kriikku et al., 2014, p. 57). However, it is important that the breath-alcohol screening instrument provide results that are comparable to the venous BAC results to ensure accurate identification of drunk drivers. The study results indicated that the breath-alcohol test on average reads 15% lower than the venous BAC. Thus, the researchers concluded that the breath-alcohol screening test was affective in identifying drivers' alcohol levels that were above the statutory limit.

Relevant Study Results

Kriikku and colleagues (2014) described their sample and presented the relationship between breath-alcohol screening results and venous BAC in a scatterplot (Figure 2). "The apprehended [drunk] drivers were predominantly male (87%) with mean age (range) of 40 y (14–81 y)....The mean, median, and highest BAC ($N = 1,875$) was 1.82 g/kg, 1.85 g/kg, and 4.36 g/kg, respectively. The mean BAC was higher in men (1.94 ± 0.83 g/kg) than women (1.76 ± 0.85 g/kg) although the correlation between age and BAC was low (Pearson $r = 0.16$)" (Kriikku et al., 2014, p. 58).

"Blood—Breath Alcohol Relationship

Figure 2 shows a scatterplot of a high [strong] correlation (Pearson $r = 0.86$) between venous BAC (*x*-variate) and BAC estimated by analysis of breath (*y*-variate)" (Kriikku et al., 2014, p. 58). The correlation coefficient of $r = 0.86$ is shown in the scatterplot without correction for the metabolism of alcohol between sampling blood and breath.

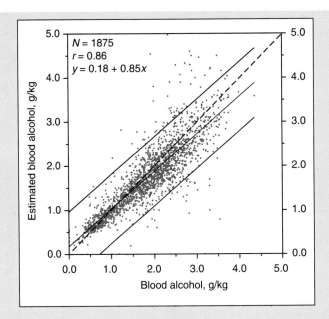

FIGURE 2 ■ **SCATTERPLOT AND CORRELATION-REGRESSION ANALYSIS OF THE RELATIONSHIP BETWEEN VENOUS BLOOD-ALCOHOL CONCENTRATIONS (BAC) AND THE CORRESPONDING ESTIMATE OF BAC WITH HAND-HELD BREATH-ALCOHOL INSTRUMENTS. THE DIAGONAL LINES IN THE GRAPH REPRESENT THE LEAST SQUARES REGRESSION LINE AND 95% PREDICTION INTERVAL AND THE DASHED LINE IS THE LINE OF IDENTITY.**
(Kriikku, P., Wilhelm, L., Jenckel, S., Rintatalo, J., Hurme, J., et al. (2014). Comparison of breath-alcohol screening test results with venous blood-alcohol concentration in suspected drunken drivers. *Forensic Science International, 239*(0379-0738), p. 59.)

STUDY QUESTIONS

1. What is a scatterplot? What elements are included in a figure of a scatterplot?

2. What type of relationship (positive or negative) does Figure 11-3 illustrate? Provide a rationale for your answer. What is the meaning of this relationship?

3. By looking at the scatterplot shown in Figure 11-3, can you tell if the relationship is strong, moderate, or weak? Provide a rationale for your answer.

4. What is the strength of the relationship presented in Figure 11-4? Does this scatterplot have outliers? Provide a rationale for your answer.

5. In Figure 11-2, what variable is on the *x*-axis and what variable is on the *y*-axis? What type of relationship is shown in Figure 11-2?

6. Examine the scatterplots from this exercise, and then provide your own example of a positive relationship between two variables in a scatterplot that includes 30 participants.

7. In the Kriikku et al. (2014) study, were the drunk drivers apprehended predominantly female or male? Is this an expected or unexpected result? Provide a rationale for your answer.

8. Was the mean venous BAC higher in men or women? Provide a rationale for your answer.

9. What was the relationship between age and BAC in the Kriikku et al. (2014) study? How would you describe the strength of this relationship?

10. Figure 2 provides results from regression analysis. What do the diagonal lines represent in Figure 2?

Answers to Study Questions

1. A scatterplot or scatter gram is used to describe a relationship between two variables and provides a graphic representation of the data collected on these two variables from the study participants. The elements included in a scatterplot are presented in Figure 11-1. These elements include an x-axis with the name of one variable and a y-axis with the name of the other variable and the points that represent the study participants' values for the two variables plotted on the scatterplot (Kim & Mallory, 2017).

2. Figure 11-3 shows a negative or inverse relationship between the LDL cholesterol and weight loss in pounds per month. The plotted points move from the left upper corner to the right lower corner, indicating a negative relationship. A decrease in LDL cholesterol is associated with an increase in weight loss in pounds.

3. Yes, by looking at a scatterplot you can usually identify the strength of the relationship as strong, moderate, or weak based on the closeness of the plotted points and if the points form close to a straight line. Thus, Figure 11-3 demonstrates a strong relationship based on the closeness of the points and the fairly straight line formed by the points that extends from the left upper corner of the graph to the right lower corner. However, the specific strength of the relationship between two variables is determined with correlational analysis (Gray et al., 2017).

4. Figure 11-4 approximates a weak relationship since the plotted points are widespread and do not clearly form a straight line. One would expect these two variables, minutes of exercise per day and perception of pain score, to have a limited relationship or association. The scatterplot also has two outliers with values very different from the other values that decrease the strength of the relationship (Kim & Mallory, 2017).

5. In Figure 11-2 the variable on the x-axis is grams of dietary fat per day, and the variable on the y-axis is total cholesterol. These might also be referred to as the x-variable and y-variable. Figure 11-2 is a positive relationship because the data points extend from the left lower corner of the graph to the right upper corner of the graph.

6. The scatterplot you develop will look similar to Figure 11-2 but needs to include 30 plotted points (see the example that follows).

Example Positive Relationship for 30 Study Participants

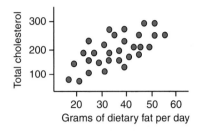

7. The drunk drivers apprehended were predominantly male (87%). Yes, this is an expected finding because most of the statistics in the research and clinical literature indicate that males are apprehended more often than females for drunk driving.

8. The mean venous BAC was higher in men than women. The mean BAC for men was 1.94 and for women was 1.76.

9. The relationship between age and BAC was Pearson $r = 0.16$. This is a weak or small relationship indicating limited association between age and BAC in this study because the r is less than 0.30 (Gray et al., 2017).

10. The diagonal lines in the graph represent the least squares regression line and 95% prediction interval, and the dashed line is the line of identity (see the narrative under Figure 2 from the Kriikku et al. [2014] study). The line of identity is also referred to as the line of best fit in regression analysis (Gray et al., 2017). Exercises 14 and 15 provide more details on linear regression analysis results.

Questions to Be Graded

Name: _____ Class: _____

Date: _____

Follow your instructor's directions to submit your answers to the following questions for grading. Your instructor may ask you to write your answers below and submit them as a hard copy for grading. Alternatively, your instructor may ask you to submit your answers online.

1. Why might researchers choose to include a scatterplot in the publication of their study?

2. Identify the x-variable and the y-variable presented in the Figure 2 of the Kriikku et al. (2014) study.

3. What type of relationship (positive or negative) does Figure 2 illustrate? Provide a rationale for your answer.

4. Describe the pattern of plotted points in Figure 2 (Kriikku et al., 2014). What is the strength of the relationship shown in this figure? Provide a rationale for your answer.

5. What is an outlier? What are the ways in which an outlier might occur in a study?

6. Are there any outliers in Figure 2 from the Kriikku et al. (2014) study? Provide a rationale for your answer.

7. Do outliers increase or decrease the strength of the relationship between the variables breath-alcohol screening results (estimated blood-alcohol levels) and the venous blood-alcohol levels? Provide a rationale for your answer.

8. Review Figure 2 from the Kriikku et al. (2014) study and identify how many points are on this scatterplot. What does each point represent?

9. Did this study have an adequate sample size? Provide a rationale for your answer.

10. Based on the results of Kriikku and colleagues (2014) study, what do you think is the most appropriate method for determining if an individual is driving while intoxicated or drunk? Provide a rationale for your answer.

Algorithm for Determining the Appropriateness of Inferential Statistical Techniques

STATISTICAL TECHNIQUE IN REVIEW

Multiple factors are involved in determining the appropriateness or suitability of the inferential statistical techniques conducted in nursing studies. **Inferential statistics** are conducted to examine relationships, make predictions, and determine differences among groups or variables in studies. When conducting data analyses for their studies, researchers consider many aspects of the study, including the study purpose, hypotheses or questions, level of measurement of the variables, design, and number of groups studied. Determining the appropriateness of the various inferential statistics reported for a particular study is not straightforward. Often, there is not necessarily *one right statistical technique* for a study.

One approach for judging the appropriateness of a statistical technique in a study is to use an **algorithm** or decision tree. The algorithm directs you by gradually narrowing the number of statistical techniques as you make judgments about the nature of the study and the data. An algorithm for judging the suitability of statistical procedures in studies is presented in Figure 12-1 that was developed by Cipher (Grove & Gray, 2019). This algorithm identifies four key factors related to the appropriateness of a statistical technique: (1) nature of the research question or hypothesis (differences or associations) for a study; (2) level of measurement (nominal, ordinal, or interval/ratio) of the dependent or research variables; (3) number of groups studied, and (4) a research design element (independent or paired samples).

Evaluating the statistical techniques reported in a study requires you to make a number of judgments about the nature of the data and what the researcher wanted to know. The study purpose and research questions or hypotheses need to be examined to determine if the focus of the study was examining associations or relationships, making predictions, or determining group differences. Research questions are often used to direct descriptive and correlational studies. However, quasi-experimental and experimental studies, focused on determining the effectiveness of an intervention or treatment, are best directed by hypotheses (Grove & Gray, 2019; Shadish, Cook, & Campbell, 2002).

You also need to determine whether the study variables were measured at the nominal, ordinal, interval, or ratio level (see Figure 12-1; review Exercise 1). You might see statistical techniques identified as parametric or nonparametric, depending on the level of measurement of the study variables. If study variables are measured at the nominal or ordinal levels, then **nonparametic statistics** are conducted (Pett, 2016). If the study variables are measured at either the interval or ratio levels and the values of the subjects for the variable studied are normally distributed, then **parametric statistics** are conducted (see Exercise 1; Kim & Mallory, 2017). Interval/ratio levels of data are often included together

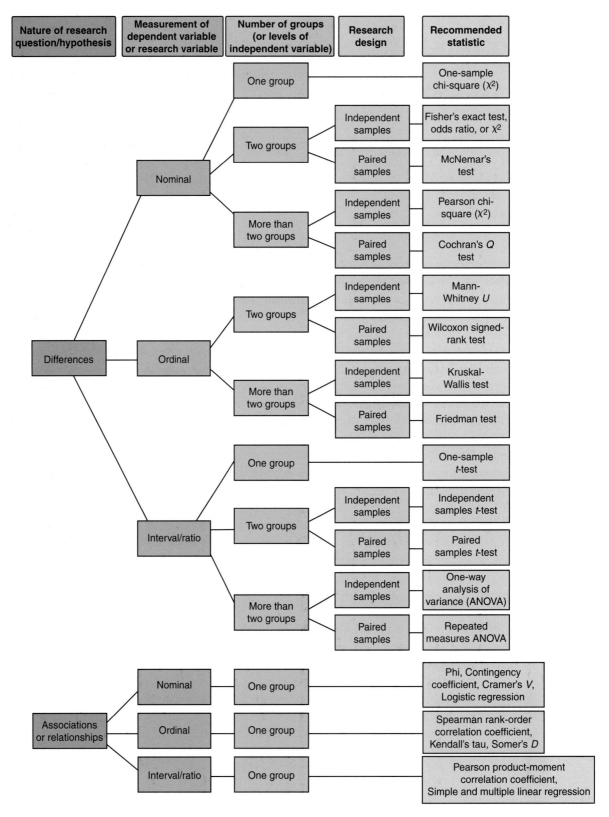

FIGURE 12-1 ■ ALGORITHM OR DECISION TREE FOR DETERMINING APPROPRIATE STATISTICAL TECHNIQUES FOR NURSING STUDIES.
(Adapted from Grove, S. K., & Gray, J. R. (2019). *Understanding nursing research: Building an evidence-based practice* (7th ed.). St. Louis, MO: Saunders, p. 311.)

because the analysis techniques are the same whether the data are interval or ratio level of measurement. Researchers run a computer program to determine if the dependent variables' frequency distributions are normally distributed (see Exercise 26). If the distribution of values or scores collected for a dependent variable are not normally distributed or are skewed, then nonparametric statistics are conducted even though the variables were measured at the interval/ratio level.

In Figure 12-1, examination of the research design element involves determining if the samples or groups in a study are independent or paired. With **independent samples or groups**, the assignment of one subject to a group is unrelated to the assignment of other subjects to groups. For example, if subjects are randomly assigned to the intervention and control groups, the samples are independent. In **paired samples or groups** (also called dependent samples or groups), subjects or observations selected for data collection are related in some way to the selection of other subjects or observations. For example, if subjects serve as their own control by using their pretest data as a control group, the observations (and therefore the groups) are considered to be paired. Some studies require repeated measures of the dependent variable on the same group of subjects, resulting in paired samples or groups (Gray, Grove, & Sutherland, 2017; Shadish et al., 2002).

To apply the algorithm in Figure 12-1, you would perform the following steps: (1) determine whether the research question or hypothesis focuses on differences or associations (relationships); (2) determine the level of measurement (nominal, ordinal, or interval/ratio) of the study variables; (3) select the number of groups that were included in the study; and (4) determine the design, with either independent or paired samples, that most closely fits the study you are critically appraising. The lines on the algorithm are followed through each selection to identify an appropriate statistical technique for the data being analyzed. The recommended statistic is identified in the far right column in Figure 12-1.

Regression analysis is focused on the prediction of a dependent variable using one or more independent variables. A study with one dependent variable and one independent variable (predictor) is analyzed using simple linear regression (see Exercises 14 and 29). If the study has one dependent variable and more than one independent variable, then the data are analyzed with multiple linear regression (see Exercises 15 and 30; Gray et al., 2017; Kim & Mallory, 2017; Plichta & Kelvin, 2013).

STUDY QUESTIONS

Directions: Answer the following questions using the algorithm or decision tree in Figure 12-1 and its description.

1. What are the reasons for conducting inferential statistics in nursing research?

2. Discuss the independent and paired samples or groups reported in studies. Why is knowing the type of samples or groups important in critically appraising the statistical technique in a research report?

3. Which statistic was probably conducted for a study focused on examining differences that had variables measured at the ordinal level and included two independent samples or groups? Provide a rationale for your answer.

4. Which statistic was probably conducted for a study focused on examining relationships that had variables measured at the ratio level? Provide a rationale for your answer.

5. Which statistic was probably conducted for a study focused on examining differences that had variables measured at the nominal level and included one group? Provide a rationale for your answer.

6. A study was focused on examining differences among the randomly assigned intervention, placebo, and standard care groups and the dependent variable perception of pain was measured at the interval level with a Likert pain scale. However, the data on pain perception were skewed or not normally distributed. What statistic was probably conducted to analyze the study pain perception data? Provide a rationale for your answer.

7. Study hypothesis: Women taking calcium 1,200 mg plus vitamin D_3 2,000 International Units (INU) have higher bone density scores than women taking only calcium 1,200 mg. The women were randomly selected and assigned to the intervention and standard care groups. Which statistical technique would researchers probably conduct to test this hypothesis? Provide a rationale for your answer.

8. Robinson et al. (2018) examined the effectiveness of a coloring intervention on the anxiety levels of parents at two points in time, before and after surgery for their child. Anxiety was measured with the Spielberger State Trait Anxiety Inventory (STAI), which is a Likert scale that produces a total anxiety score for each subject. What statistical technique did these researchers conduct in analyzing the parents' anxiety scores? Provide a rationale for your answer.
Source: Robinson, E. M., Baker, R., & Hossain, M. (2018). Randomized trial evaluating the effectiveness of coloring on decreasing anxiety among parents in a pediatric surgical waiting area. *Journal of Pediatric Nursing, 41*(1), 80–83.

9. Guvenc et al. (2013) randomly selected and assigned women to receive an educational program to promote Pap smear testing or to receive standard care. The two groups were examined for differences and the data collected were "yes—I got a Pap smear" or "no—I did not get a Pap smear" over the past 12 months. What statistical technique did these researchers conduct to analyze the Pap smear data? Provide a rationale for your answer.
   Source: Guvenc, G., Akyuz, A., & Yenen, M. C. (2013). Effectiveness of nursing interventions to increase Pap smear test screening. *Research in Nursing & Health*, 36(2), 146–157.

10. Eckhardt and colleagues (2014) conducted a study to determine if age, income, history of smoking, and depressive symptoms were predictive of fatigue intensity in individuals with coronary heart disease. What statistical technique did these researchers conduct to analyze these data and predict fatigue? Provide a rationale for your answer.
   Source: Eckhardt, A. L., DeVon, H. A., Piano, M. R., Ryan, C. J., & Zerwic, J. J. (2014). Fatigue in the presence of coronary heart disease. *Nursing Research*, 63(2), 83–93.

Answers to Study Questions

1. Inferential statistics are conducted to analyze data in nursing studies for the following purposes: (1) to examine relationships (associations), (2) to make predictions, and (3) to determine differences among groups. Inferential statistics are usually conducted to analyze data in quantitative, mixed-methods, and outcomes studies (Gray et al., 2017; Leedy & Ormrod, 2019; Shadish et al., 2002).

2. Independent samples or groups exist when the assignment of a subject to a group is unrelated to the assignment of other subjects to groups. For example, samples are independent when participants are randomly assigned to the intervention or control groups. With paired samples or groups, the subjects or observations selected for data collection are related in some way, such as participants serving as their own control in a one-group pretest–posttest design or repeated measures design. The analysis techniques conducted vary based on whether the groups are independent or paired in a study (see Figure 12-1; Grove & Gray, 2019).

3. The statistical technique conducted in this study was probably the Mann-Whitney U (see Exercise 21 for more details; Kim & Mallory, 2017; Pett, 2016). Applying the algorithm in Figure 12-1, you note the research question or hypothesis is focused on differences, the variables are measured at the ordinal level, the study has two groups, and the samples or groups are independent. This information assists you in identifying the Mann-Whitney U as an appropriate analysis technique.

4. The statistical technique conducted in this study was probably the Pearson product-moment correlation coefficient (see Exercises 13 and 28 for more details). Applying the algorithm in Figure 12-1, you note the research question is focused on relationships or associations and the variables are measured at the ratio level. This information assists you in identifying the Pearson correlation as an appropriate analysis technique.

5. The statistical technique conducted in this study was probably the one-sample chi-square test. Using the algorithm in Figure 12-1, you note the research question is focused on differences, the variables are measured at the nominal level, and the study included one group. This information assists you in identifying the one-sample chi-square test as the appropriate analysis technique (Kim & Mallory, 2017; Pett, 2016).

6. The statistical technique conducted in this study was probably the Kruskal-Wallis test. Applying the algorithm in Figure 12-1, you note the study hypothesis is focused on differences, the variable pain perception is measured at the interval level, and the study included three independent groups (intervention, placebo, and standard care). This information assists you in identifying the one-way analysis of variance (ANOVA) statistical technique; however, the data were not normally distributed so the nonparametric Kruskal-Wallis test is the most appropriate analysis technique (Kim & Mallory, 2017; Pett, 2016).

7. The statistical technique conducted in this study was probably the independent samples t-test (see Exercises 16 and 31 for more details). Applying the algorithm in Figure 12-1, you note

the hypothesis is focused on differences, the dependent variable bone density value is measured at the ratio level, and the study included two independent groups (subjects randomly assigned to either the intervention or standard care group). This information assists you in identifying the independent samples *t*-test as an appropriate analysis technique to test this hypothesis (Gray et al., 2017).

8. The paired sample *t*-test was conducted to analyze the anxiety data in this study (see Exercises 17 and 32 for more details). Applying the algorithm in Figure 12-1, you note the study hypothesis is focused on differences, the dependent variable (anxiety scores before and after surgery) is measured at the interval level, and the study included one sample or group. This information supports the researchers analyzing their data with a paired sample *t*-test.

9. A chi-square test or a Fisher's exact test could be conducted to analyze the Pap smear data. Applying the algorithm in Figure 12-1, you note the study hypothesis is focused on differences, Pap smear was measured at the nominal level (yes I got a Pap smear or no I did not get a Pap smear), and the study had two groups (one receiving the educational intervention and the other receiving standard care). This information supports the researchers analyzing their data with the chi-square test (Kim & Mallory, 2017; Pett, 2016).

10. Multiple linear regression was conducted to analyze the study data and predict fatigue in patients with coronary heart disease (CHD). Eckhardt et al. (2014) used four independent variables (age, income, history of smoking, and depressive symptoms) to predict the dependent variable fatigue intensity in a single sample of CHD patients. This information supports Eckhardt et al.'s (2014) analysis of their data with multiple linear regression. You can review Exercises 15 and 30 in this text for more information on multiple linear regression.

Questions to Be Graded

Name: _____ Class: _____

Date: _____

Follow your instructor's directions to submit your answers to the following questions for grading. Your instructor may ask you to write your answers below and submit them as a hard copy for grading. Alternatively, your instructor may ask you to submit your answers online.

Directions: Answer the following questions by reviewing the statistical content and applying the algorithm in Figure 12-1 of this exercise.

1. Discuss the differences between parametric and nonparametric statistical techniques. Provide an example of a parametric statistical technique and a nonparametric statistical technique applying the algorithm in Figure 12-1.

2. What statistical technique was probably conducted for a study focused on examining associations or relationships that had variables measured at the ordinal level? Provide a rationale for your answer.

3. What statistical technique was probably conducted for a study focused on examining differences that had variables measured at the ratio level and included three independent groups (intervention, placebo, and control)? Provide a rationale for your answer.

4. What statistical technique was probably conducted for a study focused on predicting a dependent variable using one independent variable that was measured at the interval/ratio level in a sample of patients with heart failure? Provide a rationale for your answer.

5. What statistical technique was probably conducted for a study focused on examining differences that had variables measured at the ordinal level and included three paired samples or groups? Provide a rationale for your answer.

6. Study hypothesis: *Nurses working in healthcare organizations with magnet status have higher job satisfaction than nurses working in organizations without magnet status.* Job satisfaction was measured with a multi-item Likert scale. What statistical technique would researchers probably conduct to test this hypothesis? Provide a rationale for your answer.

7. Lee et al. (2018) examined selective symptoms (dyspnea, anxiety, depression, and fatigue) to predict their contribution to impaired physical performance in patients with chronic obstructive pulmonary disease (COPD). Dyspnea was measured with FEV1 (forced expiratory volume in 1 second) and anxiety, depression, and fatigue were measured with multi-item Likert scales. Physical performance was measured with the 6-minute walk test (6MWT), which was the distance patients could walk in six minutes. What is the level of measurement for each of the study variables? Provide a rationale for your answer.
Source: Lee, H., Nguyen, H. Q., Jarrett, M. E., Mitchell, P. H., Pike, K. C., & Fan, V. S. (2018). Effect of symptoms on physical performance in COPD. *Heart & Lung, 47*(2), 149–156.

8. The focus of the Lee et al. (2018) study was presented in Question 7. What type of inferential statistical technique did Lee and colleagues conduct in their study? Provide a rationale for your answer.

9. Smith and colleagues (2014, p. 68) developed the following question to guide their study: "What are the relationships among the variables of perceived stress, sleep quality, loneliness, and self-esteem among obese young adult women?" The variables were measured with multi-item Likert scales, and the data were considered at the interval level. What inferential statistical technique did these researchers conduct to analyze their study data? Provide a rationale for your answer. Source: Smith, M. J., Theeke, L., Culp, S., Clark, K., & Pinto, S. (2014). Psychosocial variables and self-rated health in young adult obese women. *Applied Nursing Research, 27*(1), 67–71.

10. Hersch et al. (2018) conducted a randomized controlled trial (RCT) that examined the effect of a web-based stress management intervention on nurses' stress. The study included 104 subjects that were randomized into an intervention or control group. Nurses' stress was measured with the Nursing Stress Scale, a multi-item Likert scale, that provided a total stress score. What inferential statistical technique was conducted to examine the effect of the web-based intervention? Provide a rationale for your answer. Source: Hersch, R. K., Cook, R. F., Deitz, D. K., Kaplan, S., Hughes, D., Friesen, M. A., & Vezina, M. (2016). Reducing nurses' stress: A randomized controlled trial of a web-based stress management program for nurses. *Applied Nursing Research, 32*(1), 18–25.

Understanding Pearson Product-Moment Correlation Coefficient

STATISTICAL TECHNIQUE IN REVIEW

Many studies are conducted to identify relationships between two or more variables. The correlational coefficient is the mathematical expression of the relationship or association studied. Two common analysis techniques are used to examine relationships in healthcare studies: Pearson product-moment correlation coefficient, or r; and Spearman rank-order correlation coefficient, or *rho* (see the algorithm in Exercise 12). The **Pearson correlation coefficient** is a parametric analysis technique conducted to examine bivariate correlations between continuous variables measured at the interval or ratio level (Gray, Grove, & Sutherland, 2017; Kim & Mallory, 2017). **Bivariate correlation** measures the extent of the relationship between two variables at a time in a study. The purpose of Pearson r is to examine associations or relationships and *not to determine cause and effect* between independent and dependent variables (Grove & Gray, 2019; Shadish, Cook, & Campbell, 2002). The Spearman correlation coefficient (see Exercise 20) is a nonparametric analysis technique conducted to examine relationships when variables are measured at the ordinal level or do not meet the normality assumption of the Pearson r (Pett, 2016).

Relationships are interpreted in terms of direction and strength. The direction of the relationship is expressed as either positive or negative. A **positive or direct relationship** exists when one variable increases as the other variable increases or when one variable decreases as the other decreases. For example, a moderate increase in calorie intake per day is related to an increase in weight gain. Conversely, a **negative or inverse relationship** exists when one variable increases as the other variable decreases. For example, an increase in minutes of exercise per day is related to a decrease in weight.

The strength or magnitude of a relationship is described as weak, moderate, or strong. Pearson r is never less than -1.00 or greater than $+1.00$, so an r value of -1.00 or $+1.00$ indicates the strongest possible relationship, either negative or positive, respectively. An r value of 0.00 indicates no relationship or association between two variables. To describe a relationship, the labels *weak* $(r < 0.3)$, *moderate* $(r = 0.3$ to $0.5)$, and *strong* $(r > 0.5)$ are used in conjunction with both positive and negative values of r. Thus, the magnitude of the negative relationships would be weak with $r < -0.3$, moderate with $r = -0.3$ to -0.5, and strong with $r > -0.5$ (Cohen, 1988; Kim & Mallory, 2017; Plichta & Kelvin, 2013).

The significance of r values can be determined by examining the Table of Critical Values for r for the Pearson product-moment correlation coefficient in Appendix B at the back of this text. To use this table, you need to know the level of significance or alpha for the study, which is usually set at 0.05. The degrees of freedom (*df*) for Pearson r is the sample size minus 2 $(N - 2)$. For example, if a study had $r = 0.36$, a sample size of 50,

TABLE 13-1 MIRROR-IMAGE PEARSON R CORRELATION TABLE			
Variables	**1**	**2**	**3**
1. Hours of class attended per week	–	0.34	0.52
2. Hours studying per week	0.34	–	0.58
3. Final grade as a percentage	0.52	0.58	–

and $\alpha = 0.05$, is the r value statistically significant? The answer is yes because the $r = 0.36$ with a $df = 48$ is larger than the critical table value 0.2787 at $\alpha = 0.05$ for a two-tailed test. The significance of r values can also be determined with an independent samples t-test (see Exercise 28 for the process of calculating Pearson r and determining the significance).

Mirror-Image Table of Pearson r Results

A **mirror-image table**, as the name implies, has the same labels for variables in the same order for both the x- and y-axes (see Exercise 7 for a discussion of x- and y-axes). Frequently, numbers or letters are assigned to each variable, and only the letter or number designator is used to label one of the axes. To find the r value for a pair of variables, look both along the labeled or y-axis in Table 13-1 and then along the x-axis, using the number designator assigned to the variable you want to know the relationship for, and find the cell in the table with the r value. Table 13-1 is an example of a mirror-image table that displays the relationships among the variables hours of class attended per week, hours studying per week, and final grade as a percentage. The results in the table are intended as an example of a mirror-image table and are not based on research. If you were asked to identify the r value for the relationship between hours of class attended per week and the final grade as a percentage, the answer would be $r = 0.52$; for between hours studying per week and final grade as a percentage, the answer would be $r = 0.58$. The dash (–) marks located on the diagonal line of the table represent the variable's correlation with itself, which is always a perfect positive correlation $r = +1.00$. Because the results are the same in both sides of the mirror-image table, most researchers only include half of the table in their final report (Gray et al. 2017).

Effect Size of an r Value

The Pearson r value is equal to the effect size (ES) or the strength of a relationship between two continuous variables. In the previous table, the association between hours of class attended per week and hours of studying per week is $r = 0.34$; thus the $r = ES = 0.34$ for this relationship. The ES is used in power analysis to determine sample size and examine the power of study results (Aberson, 2019). (Exercise 24 describes the elements of power analysis, and Exercise 25 includes the steps for conducting a power analysis for different statistical techniques.) The strength of the ES is the same as that for the r values, with a weak effect size as one <0.30 or <-0.30, a moderate effect size 0.3 to 0.5 or -0.3 to -0.5, and a strong effect size >0.5 or >-0.5. The smaller the ES, the greater the sample size needed to detect significant relationships in studies. A large ES or association between two variables usually requires a smaller sample size to identify a significant relationship. Correlational studies usually involve examining relationships among multiple variables, so a large sample size is important (Cohen, 1988; Gray et al., 2017).

Percentage of Variance Explained in a Relationship

There is some variation in the relationship between the values for the two variables for individual participants. Some of the variation in values is explained by the relationship

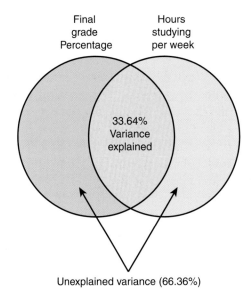

FIGURE 13-1 ■ **PERCENTAGES OF EXPLAINED AND UNEXPLAINED VARIANCES IN A RELATIONSHIP.**

between the two variables and is called **explained variance**, which is indicated by r^2 and is expressed as a percentage. To calculate the percentage of variance explained, square the r value and multiply by 100% to determine a percentage (Cohen, 1988; Grove & Gray, 2019).

$$\text{Formula: } \% \text{ variance explained} = r^2 \times 100\%$$

Example: $r = 0.58$ (correlation between hours studying and final grade as a percentage)
$(0.58)^2 \times 100\% = 0.3364 \times 100\% = 33.64\%$ variance explained

In this example, the hours studying per week explains 33.64% of the variance in the final course grade. However, part of the variation is the result of factors other than the relationship and is called **unexplained variance**. In the example provided, 100% − 33.64% (explained variance) = 66.36% (unexplained variance). Figure 13-1 demonstrates the concepts of explained and unexplained variance in this example.

Calculating the percentage of variance explained helps researchers and consumers of research understand the practical implications of reported results. The stronger the r value, the greater the percentage of variance explained. For example, if $r = 0.50$, then 25% of the variance in one variable is explained by another variable; if $r = 0.6$, then 36% of the variance is explained. All Pearson r values need to be examined for clinical importance, but the potential for clinical importance increases with moderate and strong relationships, where $r \geq 0.3$ and yields a 9% or higher percentage of variance explained. Keep in mind that a result may be statistically significant ($p \leq 0.05$), but it may not represent a clinically important finding. The r values in a study need to be examined for statistical significance and clinical importance (Gray et al., 2017; Grove & Gray, 2019; Kim & Mallory, 2017).

RESEARCH ARTICLE

Source

Hartson, K. R., Gance-Cleveland, B., Amura, C. R., & Schmiege, S. (2018). Correlates of physical activity and sedentary behaviors among overweight Hispanic school-aged children. *Journal of Pediatric Nursing, 40*(1), 1–6.

Introduction

Hartson and colleagues (2018) examined the correlates of physical activity (PA) and sedentary screen time behaviors among overweight Hispanic children ages 7 to 14 years. The PA (days/week moderate PA $\geq$ 60 minutes), sedentary screen time behavior (hours/week), body mass index (BMI) percentile, body esteem, and self-esteem were examined for the child, and the fruit intake (servings/day) and vegetable intake (servings/day) were examined for both the child and parent. The sample consisted of 40 child–parent dyads. The parental education was largely high school or lower, and 75% of the sample was from lower-income households. Hartson et al. (2018, p. 1) concluded: "Understanding the correlates of physical activity and sedentary screen time behaviors in this underrepresented population allows nurses to better understand the connections between physical activity and other aspect of well-being in children. Further investigation is needed to determine how these relationships can be incorporated into physical activity interventions that improve the health of over-weight Hispanic school-aged children."

Relevant Study Results

"On average, the children participated in at least 60 min of moderate PA on 3.19 (SD = 2.40) days per week and reported 7.09 (SD = 6.30) hours per week of sedentary screen time behaviors. Mean fruit intakes for children (mean = 2.24, SD = 1.47) and parents (mean = 2.26, SD = 1.31) were slightly above the recommended 2 cup-equivalents per day, while the mean vegetable intakes for children (mean = 1.56, SD = 1.00) and parents (mean = 1.91, SD = 1.60) were below the recommended 2.5 cup-equivalents per day, based on recommended amounts of fruits and vegetables required for a healthy nutrient–rich pattern of eating (Health and Human Services & U.S. Department of Agriculture, 2015). The mean child BMI percentile of the sample was 95.23% (SD = 5.78), which placed the sample mean BMI in the obese category, based on the Centers for Disease Control (CDC, 2015) growth reference curves. See Table 2 for additional baseline characteristics of the sample.

TABLE 2 BASELINE CHARACTERISTICS			
	n (%)	**Mean**	**SD**
Child variable			
PA (days/week moderate PA $\geq$ 60 min)	37 (92.5)	3.19	2.40
Sedentary screen time behavior (hours/week)	38 (95.0)	7.09	6.30
BMI%	40 (100.0)	95.23	5.78
Fruit intake (servings/day)	39 (97.5)	2.24	1.47
Vegetable intake (servings/day)	37 (92.5)	1.54	1.00
Body esteem	38 (95.0)	13.00	4.92
Self-esteem	39 (97.5)	21.64	5.93
Parental variable			
Fruit intake (servings/day)	39 (97.5)	2.26	1.31
Vegetable intake (servings/day)	37 (92.5)	1.91	1.60

From Hartson, KR et al. (2018). Correlates of physical activity and sedentary behaviors among overweight Hispanic school-aged children. *Journal of Pediatric Nursing, 40*(2018), 3.

Correlations With Physical Activity and Sedentary Behavior

"Child self-esteem (r = 0.34, p < .05) and parental vegetable intake (r = 0.36, p < .05) had a positive association of moderate size with PA in this coed sample of overweight Hispanic school-aged children . . . Interestingly, BMI percentile, sedentary screen time behaviors, and body esteem were not associated with child PA. None of the potential correlates were associated with sedentary screen time behavior, except for body esteem which was negatively associated with sedentary screen time behavior in males . . . See Table 3 for Pearson's correlations" (Hartson et al., 2018, p. 3).

TABLE 3   PARENT- AND CHILD-CORRELATES OF CHILD PA AND SEDENTARY BEHAVIOR (PEARSON'S CORRELATIONS, r)

	PA	Sedentary Behavior	BMI%	Fruit intake	Veg intake	Body esteem	Self-esteem	Parent Fruit	Parent veg
PA	-								
Sedentary behavior	0.05	-							
BMI%	0.08	0.13	-						
Fruit intake	0.31	-0.08	-0.12	-					
Veg intake	0.05	-0.26	0.16	**0.55****					
Body esteem	0.06	-0.04	**-0.40***	0.22	-0.04	-			
Self esteem	**0.34***	0.06	-0.14	**0.34***	0.12	**0.44****	-		
Parent fruit	0.19	0.09	0.14	**0.53****	0.25	0.06	0.10	-	
Parent veg	**0.36***	0.05	0.15	**0.60****	0.15	-0.08	0.09	**0.78****	-

Note: *$p < .05$, **$p < .01$, two-tailed.

From Hartson, KR et al. (2018). Correlates of physical activity and sedentary behaviors among overweight Hispanic school-aged children. *Journal of Pediatric Nursing, 40*(2018), 4.

STUDY QUESTIONS

1. Identify the descriptive results for the BMI percentile in this sample. What do these results indicate clinically for these children?

2. What is the value of the Pearson r for the relationship between child PA and sedentary behavior? Is the relationship between PA and sedentary behavior positive or negative? What is the strength of this relationship? Provide rationales for your answers.

3. Identify the type of Table 3 in the Hartson et al. (2018) study. What values are presented in this table? What do the dashes (–) along the diagonal of this table indicate?

4. Is the relationship between child PA and child self-esteem statistically significant? Provide a rationale for your answer.

5. State the null hypothesis for the relationship between child PA and self-esteem. Was the null hypothesis accepted or rejected? Provide a rationale for your answer.

6. What is the Pearson r and effect size (ES) for the association between parent fruit intake and child fruit intake? Describe this relationship using words rather than numbers.

7. What percentage of variance is explained by the relationship between the variables parent fruit intake and child fruit intake? Show your calculations and round your answer to two decimal places.

8. Is the relationship in Question 7 clinically important? Provide a rationale for your answer.

9. Discuss the quality of the sample size in this study. Document your answer.

10. Do the results in Table 3 support the statement that the child BMI percentile causes reduced body esteem? Provide a rationale for your answer.

Answers to Study Questions

1. The BMI percentile, based on all 40 children in the sample, had a mean of 95.23% and a *SD* of 5.78. As indicated in the study narrative, the 95.23% BMI placed these children in the obese category based on the CDC (2015) growth reference curve. This type of study to promote understanding of the correlates of PA is important to the development of future interventions to increase PA in Hispanic school-aged children to promote weight loss and improve their health.

2. $r = 0.05$. The r value is listed in Table 3 and can be identified by locating where variable 1 PA intersects with variable 2, sedentary behavior. This r value is positive (no minus sign) but is so close to zero that there is essentially no relationship between PA and sedentary behavior (Grove & Gray, 2019; Knapp, 2017).

3. Table 3 is a mirror-image correlational table used to present the Pearson r results in research reports (Kim & Mallory, 2017). The dashes along the diagonal of Table 3 indicate that each variable is correlated with itself, such as the dash for the relationship of PA with PA. When a variable is correlated with itself the $r = +1.00$, a perfect positive relationship and researchers put either the dashes or 1.00 along the table diagonal.

4. $r = 0.34*$ is a statistically significant, moderate, positive relationship between child PA and self-esteem. The * indicates that the r value is statistically significant because its probability is $p < 0.05$ as identified in the footnote for Table 3. Most nurse researchers set their level of significance or alpha (α) = 0.05. Since $p < 0.05$ is smaller than α, the relationship is statistically significant (Grove & Gray, 2019; Kim & Mallory, 2017).

5. Null hypothesis: *There is no relationship between PA and self-esteem in overweight school-aged Hispanic children.* This null hypothesis was rejected because there is a significant relationship (0.34*) between PA and self-esteem in this study. When a result is statistically significant, the null hypothesis is rejected (Gray et al., 2017).

6. Pearson $r = 0.53 = ES$. The r value is the ES in correlational studies (Cohen, 1988; Gray et al., 2017). There is a statistically significant, large, positive relationship between parent fruit intake and child fruit intake, where an increase in parent fruit intake is associated with or related to an increase in child fruit intake.

7. The percentage of variance = 28.09%. The percent of variance = $r^2 \times 100\% = 0.53^2 \times 100\% = 0.2809 \times 100\% = 28.09\%$.

8. Yes, the strong, positive relationship between parent and child fruit intake is clinically important because this relationship explains 28.09% of the variance between these two variables (Gray et al., 2017; Kim & Mallory, 2017). In addition, it is clinically important for nurses to encourage parents to increase their fruit intake because it is positively associated with their child's fruit intake (Hartson et al., 2018).

9. The sample size is $N = 40$ child–parent dyads. This is a small sample size because several variables were correlated in the Hartson et al. (2018) study. Several of the relationships in Table 3 were not significant, which might be due to a Type II error with the limited sample size in this study. Correlational studies need large sample sizes to detect small associations between variables, which was not accomplished in this study (Aberson, 2019; Cohen, 1988; Gray et al., 2017).

10. No. Pearson r is calculated to examine a relationship or association between two variables and does not determine causality between the variables (Grove & Gray, 2019; Knapp, 2017). A relationship indicates that two variables are linked to each other but not that one variable causes the other. Causality indicates a strong relationship between two variables, but one of the variables must precede the other in time and be present when the effect occurs (Shadish et al., 2002).

Questions to Be Graded

Name: _____ Class: _____

Date: _____

Follow your instructor's directions to submit your answers to the following questions for grading. Your instructor may ask you to write your answers below and submit them as a hard copy for grading. Alternatively, your instructor may ask you to submit your answers online.

1. Were the vegetable intakes for both the parents and children in this study adequate? Provide a rationale for your answer.

2. What is the value of the Pearson r for the relationship between child self-esteem and body esteem? Describe this relationship and discuss its statistical significance.

3. What is the largest relationship in Table 3? What percentage of variance was explained by this relationship? Show your calculations and round your answer to two decimal places.

4. Is the relationship in Question 3 clinically important? Is the relationship statistically significant? Provide rationales for your answers.

5. Describe the correlation $r = -0.40*$ using words. Is this a statistically significant correlation? Provide a rationale for your answer.

6. State the null hypothesis for Question 5. Was the hypothesis accepted or rejected? Provide a rationale for your answer.

7. What Pearson r value was calculated for the relationship between sedentary behavior and BMI%? What were the effect size (ES) and strength of this relationship? Provide a rationale for your answer.

8. Is the relationship between sedentary behavior and BMI% statistically significant? Is the relationship clinically important? Provide a rationale for your answers.

9. In a hypothetical study, BMI and perceived quality of life were correlated at Pearson $r = 0.41$. The sample size was $N = 87$, $\alpha = 0.05$, and the data were examined with a two-tailed test. Using the Table of Critical Values for Pearson r in Appendix B, determine if $r = 0.41$ is statistically significant. Provide a rationale for your answer.

10. Are the findings from the Hartson et al. (2018) study ready for use in practice? Provide a rationale for your answer.

Understanding Simple Linear Regression

STATISTICAL TECHNIQUE IN REVIEW

In nursing practice, the ability to predict future events or outcomes is crucial, and researchers calculate and report linear regression results as a basis for making these predictions. **Linear regression** provides a means to estimate or predict the value of a dependent variable based on the value of one or more independent variables or predictors (Gray, Grove, & Sutherland, 2017). The regression equation is a mathematical expression of a theorized influential association between a variable (predictor) and an outcome. The linkage between the theoretical statement and the equation is made prior to data collection and analysis. Linear regression is a statistical method of estimating the expected value of one variable, y, given the value of another variable, x. The focus of this exercise is **simple linear regression**, which involves the use of one independent variable, x, to predict one dependent variable, y.

The regression line developed from simple linear regression is usually plotted on a graph, with the horizontal axis representing x (the independent or predictor variable) and the vertical axis representing the y (the dependent or predicted variable; see Figure 14-1). The value represented by the letter a is referred to as the y intercept, or the point where the regression line crosses or intercepts the y-axis. At this point on the regression line, $x = 0$. The value represented by the letter b is referred to as the slope, or the coefficient of x. The slope determines the direction and angle of the regression line within the graph. The slope expresses the extent to which y changes for every one-unit change in x. The score on variable y (dependent variable) is predicted from the subject's known score on variable x (independent variable). The predicted score or estimate is referred to as $\hat{Y}$ (expressed as y-hat) (Kim & Mallory, 2017; King & Eckersley, 2019; Zar, 2010).

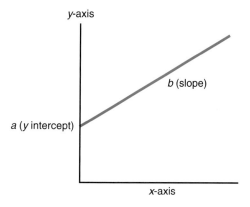

FIGURE 14-1 ■ GRAPH OF A SIMPLE LINEAR REGRESSION LINE.

Simple linear regression is an effort to explain the dynamics within a scatterplot (see Exercise 11) by drawing a straight line through the plotted scores or values. No single regression line can be used to predict, with complete accuracy, every *y* value from every *x* value. However, the purpose of the regression equation is to develop the line to allow the highest degree of prediction possible, the **line of best fit**. The procedure for developing the line of best fit is the **method of least squares**. If the data were perfectly correlated, all data points would fall along the straight line or line of best fit. However, not all data points fall on the line of best fit in studies, but the line of best fit provides the best equation for the values of *y* to be predicted by locating the intersection of points on the line for any given value of *x*.

The algebraic equation for the regression line of best fit is $y = bx + a$, where:

y = dependent variable (outcome)

x = independent variable (predictor)

b = **slope of the line** (beta, or what the increase in value is along the *x*-axis for every unit of increase in the *y* value), also called the regression coefficient.

a = *y* – **intercept** (the point where the regression line intersects the *y*-axis), also called the regression constant (Zar, 2010).

Research reports often present linear regression results in a table and/or narrative format (American Psychological Association, 2010). The formula developed from the regression results and a figure of the line of best fit for the study data might also be included. In Figure 14-2, the *x*-axis represents Gestational Age in weeks and the *y*-axis represents Birth Weight in grams. As gestational age increases from 20 weeks to 34 weeks, birth weight also increases. In other words, the slope of the line is positive. This line of best fit can be used to predict the birth weight (dependent variable) for an infant based on his or her gestational age in weeks (independent variable). Figure 14-2 is an example of a line of best fit that was developed from hypothetical data. In addition, the *x*-axis was started at 22 weeks rather than 0, which is the usual start in a regression figure focused on gestational age. Using the formula $y = bx + a$, the birth weight of a baby born at 28 weeks of gestation is calculated as follows.

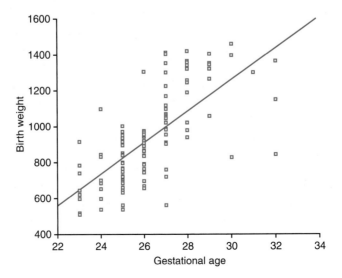

FIGURE 14-2 ■ **EXAMPLE LINE OF BEST FIT FOR GESTATIONAL AGE AND BIRTH WEIGHT.**

Formula: $y = bx + a$

In this example, $a = 500$, $b = 20$, and $x = 28$ weeks

$$y = 20(28) + 500 = 560 + 500 = 1,060 \text{ grams}$$

The regression line represents y for any given value of x. As you can see, some data points fall above the line, and some fall below the line. If we substitute any x value in the regression equation and solve for y, we will obtain a $\hat{y}$ that will be somewhat different from the actual values. The distance between the $\hat{y}$ and the actual value of y is called **residual**, and this represents the degree of error in the regression line as well as error of prediction. The regression line or the line of best fit for the data points is the unique line that will minimize error and yield the smallest residual (Zar, 2010). The step-by-step process for calculating simple linear regression in a study is presented in Exercise 29.

RESEARCH ARTICLE

Source

Flannigan, C., Bourke, T. W., Sproule, A., Stevenson, M., & Terris, M. (2014). Are APLS formulae for estimating weight appropriate for use in children admitted to PICU? *Resuscitation, 85*(7), 927–931.

Introduction

Medications and other therapies often necessitate knowing a patient's weight. However, a child may be admitted to a pediatric intensive care unit (PICU) without a known weight, and instability and on-going resuscitation may prevent obtaining this needed weight. Clinicians would benefit from a tool that could accurately estimate a patient's weight when such information is unavailable. Thus Flannigan et al. (2014) conducted a retrospective observational study for the purpose of determining "if the revised APLS UK [Advanced Paediatric Life Support United Kingdom] formulae for estimating weight are appropriate for use in the paediatric care population in the United Kingdom" (Flannigan et al., 2014, p. 927). The sample included 10,081 children (5,622 males and 4,459 females), who ranged from term-corrected age to 15 years of age, admitted to the PICU during a 5-year period. Because this was a retrospective study, no geographic location, race, and ethnicity data were collected for the sample. A paired samples *t*-test was used to compare mean sample weights with the APLS UK formula weight. "The formula 'Weight = (0.05 × age in months) + 4' significantly overestimates the mean weight of children under 1 year admitted to PICU by between 10% [and] 25.4%. While the formula 'Weight = (2 × age in years) + 8' provides an accurate estimate for 1-year-olds, it significantly underestimates the mean weight of 2–5-year-olds by between 2.8% and 4.9%. The formula 'Weight = (3 × age in years) + 7' significantly overestimates the mean weight of 6–11-year-olds by between 8.6% and 20.7%" (Flannigan et al., 2014, p. 927). Therefore, the researchers concluded that the APLS UK formulas were not appropriate for estimating the weight of children admitted to the PICU. Our novel formula provides a more accurate "method of weight estimation specifically developed for the PICU population" (Flannigan et al., 2014, p. 930.

Relevant Study Results

"Simple linear regression was used to produce novel formulae for the prediction of the mean weight specifically for the PICU population" (Flannigan et al., 2014, p. 927). The three novel formulas are presented in Figures 1, 2, and 3, respectively. The new formulas' calculations are more complex than the APLS UK formulas. "Although a good estimate of mean weight can be obtained by our newly derived formula, reliance on mean weight alone will still result in significant error as the weights of children admitted to PICU in each age and sex [gender] group have a large standard deviation…Therefore as soon as possible after admission a weight should be obtained, e.g., using a weight bed" (Flannigan et al., 2014, p. 929).

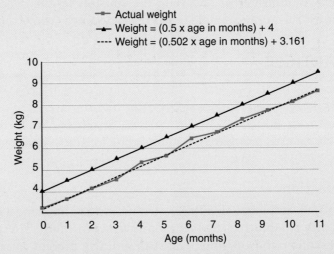

FIGURE 1 ▪ **COMPARISON OF ACTUAL WEIGHT WITH WEIGHT CALCULATED USING APLS FORMULA "WEIGHT IN KG = (0.5 × AGE IN MONTHS) + 4" AND NOVEL FORMULA "WEIGHT IN KG = (0.502 × AGE IN MONTHS) + 3.161".**
Flannigan, C., Bourke, T. W., Sproule, A., Stevenson, M., & Terris, M. (2014). Are APLS formulae for estimating weight appropriate for use in children admitted to PICU? *Resuscitation*, *85*(7), p. 928.

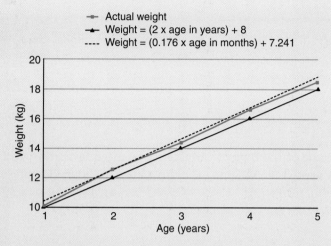

FIGURE 2 ■ COMPARISON OF ACTUAL WEIGHT WITH WEIGHT CALCULATED USING APLS FORMULA "WEIGHT IN KG = (2 × AGE IN YEARS) + 8" AND NOVEL FORMULA "WEIGHT IN KG = (0.176 × AGE IN MONTHS) + 7.241".

Flannigan, C., Bourke, T. W., Sproule, A., Stevenson, M., & Terris, M. (2014). Are APLS formulae for estimating weight appropriate for use in children admitted to PICU? *Resuscitation, 85*(7), p. 928.

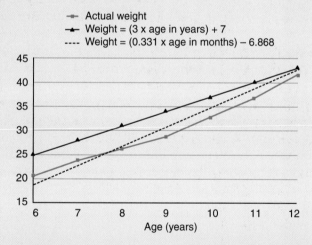

FIGURE 3 ■ COMPARISON OF ACTUAL WEIGHT WITH WEIGHT CALCULATED USING APLS FORMULA "WEIGHT IN KG = (3 × AGE IN YEARS) + 7" AND NOVEL FORMULA "WEIGHT IN KG = (0.331 × AGE IN MONTHS) − 6.868".

Flannigan, C., Bourke, T. W., Sproule, A., Stevenson, M., & Terris, M. (2014). Are APLS formulae for estimating weight appropriate for use in children admitted to PICU? *Resuscitation, 85*(7), p. 929.

STUDY QUESTIONS

1. What are the variables on the *x*- and *y*-axes in Figure 1 from the Flannigan et al. (2014) study?

2. What is the name of the type of variable represented by *x* and *y* in Figure 1? Is *x* or *y* the score or value to be predicted? What do the three lines in Figure 1 represent?

3. What is the purpose of simple linear regression analysis and the regression equation? What is the novel formula in Figure 1?

4. What is the point where the regression line meets the *y*-axis called? Is there more than one term for this point and what is the value of *x* at that point?

5. In the formula $y = bx + a$, is *a* or *b* the slope? What does the slope represent in regression analysis?

6. Using the values $a = 3.161$ and $b = 0.502$ with the novel formula in Figure 1, what is the predicted weight in kilograms for a child at 4 months of age? Show your calculations.

7. What are the variables on the x-axis and the y-axis in Figures 2 and 3? Describe these variables and how they might be entered into the regression novel formulas identified in Figures 2 and 3.

8. Using the values $a = 7.241$ and $b = 0.176$ with the novel formula in Figure 2, what is the predicted weight in kilograms for a child at 4 years of age? Show your calculations.

9. Does Figure 1 have a positive or negative slope? Provide a rationale for your answer. Discuss the meaning of the slope of Figure 1.

10. According to the study narrative, why are estimated child weights important in a pediatric intensive care (PICU) setting? Are the findings from the Flannigan et al. (2014) study ready for use in practice. Provide a rationale for your answer. Which formula in Figure 1 is the most representative of actual weight?

Answers to Study Questions

1. The x variable is age in months, and the y variable is weight in kilograms in Figure 1.

2. x is the independent or predictor variable. y is the dependent or outcome variable that is to be predicted by the independent variable, x (Gray et al., 2017). The colored line represents actual weight, the solid line with small triangles represents the weight calculated with the APLS formula, and the dotted line represents the novel formula weight (see the key to Figure 1 and its title).

3. Simple linear regression is conducted to estimate or predict the values of one dependent variable based on the values of one independent variable. Regression analysis is used to calculate a line of best fit based on the relationship between the independent variable x and the dependent variable y (King & Eckersley, 2019). The formula developed with regression analysis can be used to predict the dependent variable (y) values based on values of the independent variable x (Kim & Mallory, 2017; Plichta & Kelvin, 2013). The novel formula in Figure 1 is: Weight in Kg = (0.502 × age in months) + 3.161.

4. The point where the regression line meets the y-axis is called the y intercept and is also represented by a (see Figure 14-1). a is also called the regression constant. At the y intercept, $x = 0$.

5. b is the slope of the line of best fit (see Figure 14-1). The slope of the line indicates the amount of change in y for each one unit of change in x. b is also called the regression coefficient (Gray et al., 2017; Plitchta & Kelvin, 2013).

6. Use the following formula to calculate your answer: $y = bx + a$

   $y = 0.502 (4) + 3.161 = 2.008 + 3.161 = 5.169$ kilograms

   Note: Flannigan et al. (2014) expressed the novel formula of weight in kilograms = (0.502 × age in months) + 3.161 in the title of Figure 1 and is also presented in the narrative of the study.

7. Age in years is displayed on the x-axis and is used for the APLS UK formulas in Figures 2 and 3. Figure 2 includes children 1 to 5 years of age, and Figure 3 includes children 6 to 12 years of age. However, the novel formulas developed by simple linear regression are calculated with age in months. Therefore, the age in years must be converted to age in months before calculating the y values with the novel formulas provided for Figures 2 and 3. For example, a child who is 2 years old would be converted to 24 months (2 × 12 mos./year = 24 mos.). Then the formulas in Figures 2 and 3 could be used to predict y (weight in kilograms) for the different aged children. The y-axis on both Figures 2 and 3 is weight in kilograms (kg).

155

8. First calculate the child's age in months, which is 4 × 12 months/year = 48 months.

$$y = bx + a = 0.176 (48) + 7.241 = 8.448 + 7.241 = 15.689 \text{ kilograms}$$

Note the x value needs to be age in months and Flannigan et al. (2014) expressed the novel formula of weight in kilograms = (0.176 × age in months) + 7.241.

9. Figure 1 has a positive slope since the line extends from the lower left corner to the upper right corner and shows a positive relationship. This line shows that the increase in x (independent variable) is associated with an increase in y (dependent variable). In the Flannigan et al. (2014) study, the independent variable age in months is used to predict the dependent variable of weight in kilograms. As the age in months increases, the weight in kilograms also increases, which is the positive relationship illustrated in Figure 1.

10. According to Flannigan et al. (2014, p. 927), "The gold standard for prescribing therapies to children admitted to Paediatric Intensive Care Units (PICU) requires accurate measurement of the patient's weight.... An accurate weight may not be obtainable immediately because of instability and on-going resuscitation. An accurate tool to aid the critical care team estimate the weight of these children would be a valuable clinical tool." Accurate patient weights are an important factor in preventing medication errors particularly in pediatric populations. The American Academy of Pediatrics (AAP)'s policy on Prevention of Medication Errors in the Pediatric Inpatient Setting can be obtained from the following website: https://www.aap.org/en-us/advocacy-and-policy/federal-advocacy/Pages/Federal-Advocacy.aspx#SafeandEffectiveDrugsandDevicesforChildren. The Centers for Medicare & Medicaid Services, Partnership for Patients provides multiple links to Adverse Drug Event (ADE) information including some resources specific to pediatrics at https://partnershipforpatients.cms.gov/p4p_resources/tsp-adversedrugevents/tooladversedrugeventsade.html. The novel formula 'Weight in kg = (0.502 × age in months) + 3.161" is more similar to actual weight than the APLS. Flannigan et al. (2014, p. 927) reported "the APLS formulae are not appropriate for estimating the weight of children admitted to PICU."

Name: _____ Class: _____

Date: _____

Follow your instructor's directions to submit your answers to the following questions for grading. Your instructor may ask you to write your answers below and submit them as a hard copy for grading. Alternatively, your instructor may ask you to submit your answers online.

1. According to the study narrative and Figure 1 in the Flannigan et al. (2014) study, does the APLS UK formula under- or overestimate the weight of children younger than 1 year of age? Provide a rationale for your answer.

2. Using the values $a = 3.161$ and $b = 0.502$ with the novel formula in Figure 1, what is the predicted weight in kilograms (kg) for a child at 7 months of age? Show your calculations.

3. Using the values $a = 3.161$ and $b = 0.502$ with the novel formula in Figure 1, what is the predicted weight in kilograms for a child at 10 months of age? Show your calculations.

4. In Figure 2, the formula for calculating y (weight in kg) is Weight in kg = (0.176 × Age in months) + 7.241. Identify the y intercept and the slope in this formula.

5. Using the values $a = 7.241$ and $b = 0.176$ with the novel formula in Figure 2, what is the predicted weight in kilograms for a child 3 years of age? Show your calculations.

6. Using the values $a = 7.241$ and $b = 0.176$ with the novel formula in Figure 2, what is the predicted weight in kilograms for a child 5 years of age? Show your calculations.

7. In Figure 3, some of the actual mean weights represented by the colored line with squares are above the dotted straight line for the novel formula, but others are below the straight line. Is this an expected finding? Provide a rationale for your answer.

8. In Figure 3, the novel formula is 'Weight in kilograms = $(0.331 \times$ Age in months$) - 6.868$'. What is the predicted weight in kilograms for a child 11 years old? Show your calculations.

9. Was the sample size of this study adequate for conducting simple linear regression? Provide a rationale for your answer.

10. Describe one potential clinical advantage and one potential clinical problem with using the three novel formulas presented in Figures 1, 2, and 3 in a PICU setting.

Understanding Multiple Linear Regression

STATISTICAL TECHNIQUE IN REVIEW

Simple linear regression was introduced in Exercise 14 and provides a means to estimate or predict the value of a dependent variable based on the value of an independent variable. **Multiple regression** is an extension of simple linear regression, in which more than one independent variable is entered into the analysis to predict a dependent variable (Allison, 1999; Plichta & Kelvin, 2013; Zar, 2010). The assumptions of multiple regression are as follows:

1. The independent variables are measured with minimal error.
2. Variables can be treated as interval- or ratio-level measures.
3. The residuals are not correlated.
4. Dependent variable values are normally distributed (see Exercise 26).
5. Values for the dependent variable are homoscedastic, or equally dispersed about the line of best fit (see Exercise 14).
6. y values have equal variance at each value of x; thus difference scores (residuals or error values) are random and have homogeneous variance (Kim & Mallory, 2017; Zar, 2010).

With multiple independent variables, researchers often correlate the independent variables with the dependent variable to determine which independent variables are most highly correlated with the dependent variable. The Pearson r analysis is typically computed to determine correlations for interval- and ratio-level data. To be effective predictors, independent variables need to have strong correlations with the dependent variable, but only weak correlations with the other independent variables in the equation. **Multicollinearity** occurs when the independent variables in the multiple regression equation are strongly correlated (over 0.85) with each other (Kim & Mallory, 2017). This happens in nursing studies, but it can be minimized by careful selection of independent variables that have limited correlation. Tests of multicollinearity are presented in Exercise 30.

One of the outcomes from multiple regression analysis is an R^2 value. For the addition of each independent variable to the regression formula, the change in R^2 is reported. The R^2 is used to calculate the percentage of variance that is predicted by the regression formula. For example, the independent variables of number of pack years of smoking (number of packs of cigarettes smoked per day times number of years of smoking), systolic blood pressure (SBP), and body mass index (BMI) were used to predict the incidence of myocardial infarction (MI) in older adults. The $R^2 = 0.387$, and the percentage of variance predicted is calculated by $R^2 \times 100\%$. In this example, the percentage of the variance in the dependent variable that is explained by the predictors is calculated as $0.387 \times 100\% = 38.7\%$. This means that 38.7% of the variance in the incidence of MIs in the older adult is predicted by the independent variables of pack years of smoking, SBP, and BMI. The significance of an R^2 value is tested with an analysis of variance (ANOVA; see Exercises 18 and 33). The statistic for ANOVA is F, and a significant F value indicates that the regression equation has significantly predicted the variation in the dependent variable and that the R^2 value is not a random variation. The step-by-step process for calculating multiple linear regression is presented in Exercise 30.

RESEARCH ARTICLE

Source

Franck, L. S., Wray, J., Gay, C., Dearmun, A. K., Lee, K., & Cooper, B. A. (2015). Predictors of parent post-traumatic stress symptoms after child hospitalization on general pediatric wards: A prospective cohort study. *International Journal of Nursing Studies*, *52*(1), 10–21.

Introduction

Post-traumatic stress symptoms (PTSS) are an issue for some parents of children hospitalized in intensive care settings. However, limited research has been conducted to examine either PTSS in parents of children hospitalized in nonintensive care settings or PTSS in parents after a child's hospital discharge. Franck et al. (2015) conducted a prospective cohort study for the purpose of identifying the predictors of parental PTSS following a child's hospitalization. A convenience sample of 107 parents of children hospitalized in a general (nonintensive care) ward in a United Kingdom hospital completed the initial in-hospital assessment and 3 months postdischarge follow-up. "Three months after hospital discharge, 32.7% of parents ($n = 35$) reported some degree of post-traumatic stress symptoms, and 21.5% ($n = 23$) had elevated scores (≥ 34) consistent with a probable diagnosis of post-traumatic stress disorder…Parents' hospital-related anxiety, uncertainty, and use of negative coping strategies are potentially modifiable factors that most influence post-traumatic stress symptoms" (Franck et al., 2015, p. 10). These researchers recommended future studies to assess interventions such as psychological support to address modifiable factors of PTSS identified in their study.

Relevant Study Results

"A hierarchical multiple regression analysis was conducted to determine the unique contributions of parent distress during the child's hospitalization, as well as coping strategies and resources, to subsequent PTSS, while controlling for relevant, but largely unmodifiable demographic or child health and hospitalization-related factors. Variables from Table 3 that were significantly correlated ($r \geq 0.25$, $p < 0.1$) with PTSS were entered into the model in three steps: (1) single parent status, child hospital length of stay, and the parent's rating of the child's health three months after discharge were entered first because they were non-modifiable factors in this model; (2) parent use of negative coping strategies and optimism were entered next as potentially modifiable dispositional factors; and (3) parent anxiety, depression, and uncertainty during the child's hospitalization were entered last as modifiable hospital experiential factors. Each step resulted in a significant ($p < 0.05$) increase in the model's R^2, with 5 of 8 predictors uniquely and significantly associated with PTSS: being a single parent, the parent's perception of their child's health three months after discharge, use of negative coping strategies, and parent anxiety and uncertainty during the child's hospitalization. Moderating effects were then explored and two significant two-way interactions were found, between negative coping strategies and anxiety and between negative coping strategies and depression. These findings indicate that the effect of parental use of negative coping strategies on PTSS is amplified in the context of anxiety and attenuated in the context of depression (Table 4)" (Franck et al., 2015, p. 15).

TABLE 3 CORRELATION MATRIX OF PREDICTORS OF PARENT POST-TRAUMATIC STRESS SYMPTOMS

	PTSS	1	2	3	4	5	6	7	8	9	10	11	12	13
Non-Modifiable Factors														
1. Single parent	.251													
2. Child prior hospitalization	.194	.247												
3. **Length of stay**	**.254**	−.021	−.001											
4. Child readmission	.242	−.165	.014	.281										
5. Child health	−.372	−.232	−.276	−.226	−.353									
Coping Strategies/Resources														
6. Active coping	−.074	−.123	.073	.053	−.016	.158								
7. **Negative coping**	**.350**	.207	.173	.124	−.009	−.115	−.159							
8. Social support coping	.005	−.124	.037	.009	.142	.131	.375	−.060						
9. Distraction/humor	.055	.070	.032	.034	−.141	.034	.200	.155	.122					
10. Disengagement/substance use coping	.136	.150	.058	.100	.013	−.128	−.258	.209	−.110	.106				
11. Optimism	−.265	−.271	−.261	−.053	−.051	.265	.357	−.417	.307	.052	−.119			
Parent Distress in Hospital														
12. **Anxiety**	**.488**	.032	.055	.332	.271	−.257	−.247	.417	−.125	−.116	.132	−.407		
13. **Depression**	**.273**	.023	.017	.266	.256	−.336	−.223	.323	−.182	−.180	.104	−.271	.636	
14. **Uncertainty**	**.311**	.056	.078	.136	.277	−.307	.003	.114	−.022	.041	−.023	−.274	.269	.278

Note: PTSS = post-traumatic stress symptoms as measured by the Impact of Events Scale—Revised (IES-R). PTSS was unrelated to child age or gender, chronic versus acute illness, parent relationship to child (mother versus father), parent race/ethnicity, education level, employment status, socioeconomic status, number of other children in the family, prior hospitalization of another child, prior parent hospitalization, distance or travel time from family's home to the hospital, all family environment measures, and social support during hospitalization. **Bold variables** had significant associations with PTSS ($r \geq .25$ and $p < .010$) and were included in the multivariable regression analysis. Correlations (r) > .19 are associated with $p < .05$, $r > .25$ with $p < .01$, and $r > .30$ with $p < 0.001$.

Franck, L. S., Wray, J., Gay, C., Dearman, A. K., Lee, K., & Cooper, B. A. (2015). Predictors of parent post-traumatic stress symptoms after child hospitalization on general pediatric wards: A prospective cohort study. *International Journal of Nursing Studies, 52*(1), p. 17.

TABLE 4   MULTIPLE REGRESSION ANALYSIS OF POST-TRAUMATIC STRESS SYMPTOMS (IES-R) ON PARENT COPING STRATEGIES AND DISTRESS DURING HOSPITALIZATION ($n = 105$)

Step	Predictors	B	SE B[a]	95% CI	β	p	ΔR^2
1	Relevant covariate					<.001	.217
	Single parent	8.509	3.571	1.418, 15.600	0.188	.019	
	Length of hospital stay (in days)	0.078	0.104	−0.128, 0.285	0.060	.453	
	Child health after discharge[a]	−4.440	1.580	−7.577, −1.304	−0.240	.006	
2	Parent coping strategies					.008	.073
	Negative coping (COPE)	2.763	1.339	0.104, 5.423	0.196	.042	
	Optimism (LOT-R)	0.226	0.263	−0.297, 0.749	0.077	.393	
3	Parent distress during hospitalization					<.001	.124
	Anxiety (HADS)	1.402	0.435	0.538, 2.267	0.343	.002	
	Depression (HADS)	−0.517	0.394	−1.299, 0.265	−0.132	.192	
	Uncertainty (PPUS)	0.212	0.096	0.022, 0.401	0.178	.029	
4	Interactions[b]					.001	.086
	Negative coping × depression	−1.411	0.352	−2.109, −0.713	−0.435	<.001	
	Negative coping × anxiety	0.957	0.353	0.256, 1.659	0.322	.008	
	Full model	$F(10,94) = 9.39$, $p < .001$					.500[c]

CI = confidence interval; COPE = BriefCOPE Scale; HADS = Hospital Anxiety and Depression Scale; IES-R = Impact of Events Scale–Revised; LOT-R = Life Orientation Test–Revised; PPUS = Parent Perception of Uncertainty in Illness Scale.
[a]Parent's perception of child health 3 months after discharge.
[b]Only significant two-way interactions between included variables were retained in the final model.
[c]Adjusted R^2 = .446.

Franck, L. S., Wray, J., Gay, C., Dearmun, A. K., Lee, K., & Cooper, B. A. (2015). Predictors of parent post-traumatic stress symptoms after child hospitalization on general pediatric wards: A prospective cohort study. *International Journal of Nursing Studies*, *52*(1), p. 18.

STUDY QUESTIONS

1. What is the purpose of multiple regression analysis?

2. Identify the independent and dependent variables in the Franck et al. (2015) study. What independent variables were significantly correlated to PTSS?

3. Why did Franck et al. (2015) correlate the independent and dependent variables with each other using Pearson r analysis? What results would provide the strongest study outcomes for regression analysis?

4. Which independent variable in Table 3 was most highly correlated with post-traumatic stress symptoms (PTSS)? Provide a rationale for your answer.

5. On Table 3, what correlation result is $r = -.265$? Describe in words the meaning of this correlation. Was this correlation statistically significant? Provide a rationale for your answer.

6. Were the independent variables of anxiety and depression significantly correlated with each other at 3 months post discharge? How does this affect the multiple regression results?

7. What was the percentage of variance explained by the regression analysis for the relevant covariates (single parent, length of hospital stay in days, and child health after discharge) entered in step 1 of the regression analysis presented in Table 4? Provide your calculations.

8. According to the study narrative and Table 4, "5 out of 8 predictors were uniquely and significantly associated with PTSS" (Franck et al., 2015, p. 6). What three predictors analyzed in the regression model were not significantly associated with PTSS? Provide a rationale for your answer.

9. What was the multiple regression result for PTSS during hospitalization? Was this result significant? Provide a rationale for your answer.

10. Describe one potential clinical application of the Franck et al. (2015) study results.

Answers to Study Questions

1. Multiple regression analysis is conducted to predict an outcome or dependent variable using two or more independent (predictor) variables. This analysis is an extension of simple linear regression where more than one independent variable is entered into the analysis to develop a formula for predicting the dependent variable (Gray, Grove, & Sutherland, 2017; Kim & Mallory, 2017; Plichta & Kelvin, 2013).

2. In the Franck et al. (2015) study, there were 14 independent variables (single parent, child prior hospitalization, length of stay, child readmission, child's health, active coping, negative coping, social support coping, distraction/humor, disengagement/substance use coping, optimism, anxiety, depression, and uncertainty) correlated with the dependent variable post-traumatic stress symptoms (PTSS) in Table 3. The independent variables of single parent, length of stay, child health, negative coping, optimism, anxiety, depression, and uncertainty (in bold in Table 3) were significantly correlated to PTSS.

3. With multiple independent variables, researchers often correlate the independent variables with each other and with the dependent variable. Pearson r analysis is usually conducted to determine correlations for interval- and ratio-level data. To be effective predictors, independent variables need to have strong correlations with the dependent variable but only weak (<0.30) to moderate correlations (<0.50) with the other independent variables in the equation (Kim & Mallory, 2017).

4. Anxiety in the parent distress in hospital category was the independent variable most highly correlated with the dependent variable PTSS with an $r = .488$ at 3 months post discharge. On Table 3, bolded values are significantly associated with PTSS. The farther the r value is from the zero (0) and the closer it is to $+1$ or -1, the stronger the correlation (see Exercise 13; Gray et al., 2017; Knapp, 2017).

5. The independent variable optimism was correlated with the dependent variable PTSS with $r = -.265$. This r value identifies a small, negative correlation between optimism and PTSS (see Exercise 13 for strength of correlations). The negative or inverse r value indicates the direction of the relationship, in this case increased levels of optimism are associated with decreased PTSS. The bolded r value for optimism indicates a significance at $p < 0.01$, which is less than the 0.05 level of significance set for the study (see footnote of Table 3).

6. The independent variables anxiety and depression were significantly and strongly correlated with each other at 3 months post discharge as indicated by the $r = .636$. On Table 3, anxiety is labeled number 12 and depression is labeled 13. Independent variables are stronger predictors of a dependent variable if they are not strongly correlated with each other. Since anxiety and depression were significantly correlated with each other, this probably resulted in a smaller R^2 value and percentage of variance explained for PTSS than would have been obtained

had all the independent variables had weak to moderate correlations with each other (Kim & Mallory, 2017).

7. 21.7% variance for PTSS at 3 months post discharge is explained by the relevant covariates: single parent, length of hospital stay, and child health after discharge. %variance $= R^2 \times 100\% = 0.217 \times 100\% = 21.7\%$. These demographic or nonmodifiable variables are commonly entered first in multiple regression models to control for confounding variables (Holmes, 2018).

8. Length of hospital stay (in days), optimism (LOT-R), and depression (HADS) have nonsignificant p values displayed on Table 4 of .453, .393, and .192, respectively. The p values for these three independent variables were >0.05, the level of significance or alpha, set for this study, indicating they were not statistically significant in the regression model (Grove & Gray, 2019).

9. The multiple regression result (full model) was $R^2 = .500$ for PTSS during hospitalization. The analysis of variance (ANOVA) was conducted to determine the significance of the results, and the results were statistically significant with $F = (10, 94) = 9.39$, $p < 0.001$. This result was significant as indicated by the p value that was less than alpha $= 0.05$. The footnote of Table 4 also lists the adjusted $R^2 = .446$. Unlike R^2, the adjusted R^2 accounts for the number of predictors entered into the regression model.

10. A number of potential clinical implications for this study exist, and answers may vary. Franck et al. (2015, p. 1) found that "32.7% of parents ($n = 35$) reported some degree of PTSS, and 21.5% ($n = 23$) had elevated scores (≥ 34) consistent with a probable diagnosis of posttraumatic stress disorder." This high prevalence of PTSS indicates that clinicians should assess for PTSS in parents with children hospitalized in nonintensive care settings after discharge. In addition, the multiple regression result in Table 4 was significant as indicated by $F = (10, 94) = 9.39$, $p < 0.001$, identifying the predictors of parents' PTSS during their child's hospitalization. Clinicians' awareness of the predictors of PTSS in this study could promote identification of the parents at risk of PTSS after discharge. "Parents' hospital-related anxiety, uncertainty, and use of negative coping strategies are potentially modifiable factors that most influence posttraumatic stress symptoms" (Franck et al., 2015, p. 1). Nurses have the potential to intervene to reduce parental anxiety and uncertainty while a child is hospitalized in a nonintensive care setting. The National Institute of Mental Health (NIMH) has post-traumatic stress disorder (PTSD) information and assessment tools at http://www.nimh.nih.gov/health/publications/post-traumatic-stress-disorder-ptsd/index.shtml.

Name: _____ Class: _____

Date: _____

Follow your instructor's directions to submit your answers to the following questions for grading. Your instructor may ask you to write your answers below and submit them as a hard copy for grading. Alternatively, your instructor may ask you to submit your answers online.

1. What are the assumptions for multiple linear regression?

2. Was multiple regression analysis the appropriate analysis technique to conduct in the Franck et al. (2014) study? Provide a rationale for your answer.

3. Was the independent variable length of hospital stay significantly correlated with the dependent variable parental PTSS? Provide a rationale for your answer.

4. Was the independent variable depression significantly correlated with parental PTSS in this study? Provide a rationale for your answer.

5. What is multicollinearity? Why is it important to test for multicollinearity? Is there a potential for multicollinearity in this study?

6. According to the study narrative and Table 4, "5 out of 8 predictors were uniquely and significantly associated with PTSS" (Franck et al., 2014, p. 6). Which five variables were significant predictors of PTSS in the regression model, before moderating effects and interaction terms were tested? Provide a rationale for your answer.

7. What was the percentage of variance of parental PTSS explained by the regression analysis of the independent variables parent coping strategies (negative coping and optimism) entered in step 2 of the regression analysis? Provide your calculations.

8. What was the percentage of variance for parental PTSS explained by the regression analysis for parent distress during hospitalization (anxiety, depression, and uncertainty) entered in step 3 of the regression analysis? Provide your calculations.

9. What was the percentage of variance for parental PTSS during hospitalization explained by the full regression model? Discuss the meaning of these results.

10. What additional research is needed in this area of parental PTSS after their child's hospitalization? Provide a rationale for your answer.

Understanding Independent Samples *t*-Test

STATISTICAL TECHNIQUE IN REVIEW

The **independent samples *t*-test** is a parametric statistical technique used to determine differences between the scores obtained from independent or unrelated samples or groups. For example, when subjects are randomly assigned to an intervention or control group, the groups or samples are considered independent. Because the *t*-test is considered fairly easy to calculate, researchers often use it in determining differences between two groups when variables are measured at the interval or ratio level. The *t*-test examines the differences between the means of the two groups in a study and adjusts that difference for the variability (computed by the standard error) among the data (Gray, Grove, & Sutherland, 2017; King & Eckersley, 2019). When interpreting the results of *t*-tests, the larger the calculated *t* ratio, in absolute value, the greater the difference between the two groups. The significance of a *t* ratio can be determined by comparison with the critical values in a statistical table for the *t* distribution using the degrees of freedom (*df*) for the study (see Appendix A Critical Values for Student's *t* Distribution at the back of this text). The formula for *df* for an independent *t*-test is as follows:

$$df = (\text{number of subjects in sample 1} + \text{number of subjects in sample 2}) - 2$$

$$\text{Example } df = (65 \text{ in sample 1} + 67 \text{ in sample 2}) - 2 = 132 - 2 = 130$$

The *t*-test should be conducted once to examine differences between two groups in a study, because conducting multiple *t*-tests on study data can result in an inflated Type 1 error rate. A **Type I error** occurs when the researcher rejects the null hypothesis when it is in actuality true. Researchers need to consider other statistical analysis options for their study data rather than conducting multiple *t*-tests. However, if multiple *t*-tests are conducted, researchers can perform a Bonferroni procedure or more conservative post hoc tests like Tukey's honestly significant difference (HSD), Student-Newman-Keuls, or Scheffé test to reduce the risk of a Type I error. Only the Bonferroni procedure is covered in this text; details about the other, more stringent post hoc tests can be found in Plichta and Kelvin (2013) and Zar (2010).

The Bonferroni procedure is a simple calculation in which the alpha is divided by the number of *t*-tests conducted on different aspects of the study data. The resulting number is used as the alpha or level of significance for each of the *t*-tests conducted. The Bonferroni procedure formula is as follows: alpha (α) ÷ number of *t*-tests performed on study data = more stringent study α to determine the significance of study results. For example, if a study's α was set at 0.05 and the researcher planned on conducting five *t*-tests on the study data, the α would be divided by the five *t*-tests (0.05 ÷ 5 = 0.01), with a resulting α of 0.01 to be used to determine significant differences in the study.

The *t*-test for independent samples or groups includes the following assumptions:

1. The raw scores or values in the population are normally distributed.
2. The dependent variable(s) is(are) measured at the interval or ratio levels.

3. The two groups examined for differences have equal variance, which is best achieved by a random sample and random assignment to groups.
4. All scores or observations collected within each group are independent or not related to other study scores or observations (Gray et al., 2017; Kim & Mallory, 2017).

The *t*-test is robust, meaning the results are reliable even if one of the assumptions has been violated. However, the *t*-test is not robust regarding between-samples or within-samples independence assumptions or with respect to extreme violation of the assumption of normality. Groups do not need to be of equal sizes but rather of equal variance. Groups are independent if the two sets of data were not taken from the same subjects and if the scores are not related (Gray et al., 2017; Kim & Mallory, 2017; Plichta & Kelvin, 2013). This exercise focuses on interpreting and critically appraising the *t*-tests results presented in research reports. Exercise 31 provides a step-by-step process for calculating the independent samples *t*-test.

RESEARCH ARTICLE

Source

Canbulat, N., Ayhan, F., & Inal, S. (2015). Effectiveness of external cold and vibration for procedural pain relief during peripheral intravenous cannulation in pediatric patients. *Pain Management Nursing, 16*(1), 33–39.

Introduction

Canbulat and colleagues (2015, p. 33) conducted an experimental study to determine the "effects of external cold and vibration stimulation via Buzzy on the pain and anxiety levels of children during peripheral intravenous (IV) cannulation." Buzzy is an $8 \times 5 \times 2.5$ cm battery-operated device for delivering external cold and vibration, which resembles a bee in shape and coloring and has a smiling face. A total of 176 children between the ages of 7 and 12 years who had never had an IV insertion before were recruited and randomly assigned into the equally sized intervention and control groups. During IV insertion, "the control group received no treatment. The intervention group received external cold and vibration stimulation via Buzzy…Buzzy was administered about 5 cm above the application area just before the procedure, and the vibration continued until the end of the procedure" (Canbulat et al., 2015, p. 36). Canbulat et al. (2015, pp. 37–38) concluded that "the application of external cold and vibration stimulation were effective in relieving pain and anxiety in children during peripheral IV" insertion and were "quick-acting and effective nonpharmacological measures for pain reduction." The researchers concluded that the Buzzy intervention is inexpensive and can be easily implemented in clinical practice with a pediatric population.

Relevant Study Results

The level of significance for this study was set at $\alpha = 0.05$. "There were no differences between the two groups in terms of age, sex [gender], BMI [body mass index], and pre-procedural anxiety according to the self, the parents', and the observer's reports ($p > 0.05$) (Table 1). When the pain and anxiety levels were compared with an independent samples *t* test,…the children in the external cold and vibration stimulation [intervention] group had significantly lower pain levels than the control group according to their self-reports (both WBFC [Wong Baker Faces Scale] and VAS [visual analog scale] scores; $p < 0.001$) (Table 2). The external cold and vibration stimulation group had significantly lower fear and anxiety levels than the control group, according to parents' and the observer's reports ($p < 0.001$) (Table 3)" (Canbulat et al., 2015, p. 36).

TABLE 1   COMPARISON OF GROUPS IN TERMS OF VARIABLES THAT MAY AFFECT PROCEDURAL PAIN AND ANXIETY LEVELS

Characteristic	Buzzy (*n* = 88)	Control (*n* = 88)	χ^2 *p*
Sex			
Female (%), *n*	11 (12.5)	13 (14.8)	.82
Male (%), *n*	77 (87.5)	75 (85.2)	.41

Characteristic	Buzzy (*n* = 88)	Control (*n* = 88)	*t* *p*
Age (mean ± *SD*)	8.25 ± 1.51	8.61 ± 1.69	−1.498 .136
BMI (mean ± *SD*)	25.41 ± 6.74	26.94 ± 8.68	−1.309 .192
Preprocedural anxiety			
Self-report (mean ± *SD*)	2.03 ± 1.29	2.11 ± 1.58	−0.364 .716
Parent report (mean ± *SD*)	2.11 ± 1.20	2.17 ± 1.42	−0.285 .776
Observer report (mean ± *SD*)	2.18 ± 1.17	2.24 ± 1.37	−0.295 .768

BMI, body mass index.

Canbulat, N., Ayban, F., & Inal, S. (2015). Effectiveness of external cold and vibration for procedural pain relief during peripheral intravenous cannulation in pediatric patients. *Pain Management Nursing, 16*(1), p. 36.

TABLE 2   COMPARISON OF GROUPS' PROCEDURAL PAIN LEVELS DURING PERIPHERAL IV CANNULATION

	Buzzy (*n* = 88)	Control (*n* = 88)	*t* *p*
Procedural self-reported pain with WBFS (mean ± *SD*)	2.75 ± 2.68	5.70 ± 3.31	−6.498 0.000
Procedural self-reported pain with VAS (mean ± *SD*)	1.66 ± 1.95	4.09 ± 3.21	−6.065 0.000

IV, intravenous; WBFS, Wong-Baker Faces Scale; *SD*, standard deviation; VAS, visual analog scale.

Canbulat, N., Ayban, F., & Inal, S. (2015). Effectiveness of external cold and vibration for procedural pain relief during peripheral intravenous cannulation in pediatric patients. *Pain Management Nursing, 16*(1), p. 37.

TABLE 3   COMPARISON OF GROUPS' PROCEDURAL ANXIETY LEVELS DURING PERIPHERAL IV CANNULATION

Procedural Child Anxiety	Buzzy (*n* = 88)	Control (*n* = 88)	*t* *p*
Parent reported (mean ± *SD*)	0.94 ± 1.06	2.09 ± 1.39	−6.135 0.000
Observer reported (mean ± *SD*)	0.92 ± 1.03	2.14 ± 1.34	−6.745 0.000

SD, standard deviation; IV, intravenous.

Canbulat, N., Ayban, F., & Inal, S. (2015). Effectiveness of external cold and vibration for procedural pain relief during peripheral intravenous cannulation in pediatric patients. *Pain Management Nursing, 16*(1), p. 37.

STUDY QUESTIONS

1. What type of statistical test was conducted by Canbulat et al. (2015) to examine group differences in the dependent variables of procedural pain and anxiety levels in this study? What two groups were analyzed for differences?

2. What did Canbulat et al. (2015) set the level of significance, or alpha (α), at for this study? Was this appropriate?

3. What are the *t* and *p* (probability) values for procedural self-reported pain measured with a visual analog scale (VAS)? What do these results mean?

4. What is the null hypothesis for observer-reported procedural anxiety for the two groups? Was this null hypothesis accepted or rejected in this study? Provide a rationale for your answer.

5. What is the *t*-test result for BMI? Is this result statistically significant? Provide a rationale for your answer. What does this result mean for the study?

6. What causes an increased risk for Type I errors when *t*-tests are conducted in a study? How might researchers reduce the increased risk for a Type I error in a study?

7. Assuming that the *t*-tests presented in Table 2 and Table 3 are all the *t*-tests performed by Canbulat et al. (2015) to analyze the dependent variables' data, calculate a Bonferroni procedure for this study.

8. Would the *t*-test for observer-reported procedural anxiety be significant based on the more stringent α calculated using the Bonferroni procedure in question 7? Provide a rationale for your answer.

9. The results in Table 1 indicate that the Buzzy intervention group and the control group were not significantly different for gender, age, body mass index (BMI), or preprocedural anxiety (as measured by self-report, parent report, or observer report). What do these results indicate about the equivalence of the intervention and control groups at the beginning of the study? Why are these results important?

10. Canbulat et al. (2015) conducted the χ^2 test to analyze the difference in sex or gender between the Buzzy intervention group and the control group. Would an independent samples *t*-test be appropriate to analyze the gender data in this study (review algorithm in Exercise 12)? Provide a rationale for your answer.

Answers to Study Questions

1. An independent samples *t*-test was conducted to examine group differences in the dependent variables in this study. The two groups analyzed for differences were the Buzzy experimental or intervention group and the control group.

2. The level of significance or alpha (α) was set at 0.05. Yes, $\alpha = 0.05$ is appropriate. Most nursing studies set alpha at 0.05 to decrease the risk of a Type II error of concluding there is no effect when there actually is a significant effect (Gray et al., 2017; Knapp, 2017).

3. The result was $t = -6.065$, $p = 0.000$ for procedural self-reported pain with the VAS (see Table 2). The *t* value is statistically significant as indicated by the $p = 0.000$, which is less than $\alpha = 0.05$ set for this study. The *t* result means there is a significant difference between the Buzzy intervention group and the control group in terms of the procedural self-reported pain measured with the VAS. As a point of clarification, *p* values are never zero in a study. There is always some chance of error and would be more correctly reported as $p = 0.001$ (Gray et al., 2017).

4. The null hypothesis is: *There is no difference in observer-reported procedural anxiety levels between the Buzzy intervention and the control groups for school-age children.* The $t = -6.745$ for observer-reported procedural anxiety levels, $p = 0.000$. This *p* value is significant because it is less than $\alpha = 0.05$ set for this study. Because this study result was statistically significant, the null hypothesis was rejected (Grove & Gray, 2019).

5. The $t = -1.309$ for BMI. The nonsignificant $p = .192$ for BMI is greater than $\alpha = 0.05$ set for this study. The nonsignificant result means there is no statistically significant difference between the Buzzy intervention and control groups for BMI. The two groups should be similar for demographic variables to decrease the potential for error and increase the likelihood that the results are an accurate reflection of reality (Kim & Mallory, 2017).

6. The conduct of multiple *t*-tests causes an increased risk for Type I errors. If only one *t*-test is conducted on study data, the risk of Type I error does not increase. The Bonferroni procedure and the more stringent Tukey's honestly significant difference (HSD), Student Newman-Keuls, or Scheffé test can be calculated to reduce the risk of a Type I error (Kim & Mallory, 2017; Plichta & Kelvin, 2013; Zar, 2010).

7. The Bonferroni procedure is calculated by alpha ÷ number of *t*-tests conducted on study variables' data. Note that researchers do not always report all *t*-tests conducted, especially if they were not statistically significant. The *t*-tests conducted on demographic data are not of concern. Canbulat et al. reported the results of four *t*-tests conducted to examine differences between the intervention and control groups for the dependent variables procedural self-reported pain with WBFS, procedural self-reported pain with VAS, parent-reported anxiety levels, and observer-reported anxiety levels. The Bonferroni calculation for this study: 0.05 (alpha) ÷ number of *t*-tests conducted = $0.05 \div 4 = 0.0125$. The new α set for the study is

0.0125. However, researchers have criticized the Bonferroni approach for being too conservative and reducing statistical power. Benjamini and Hochberg (1995) provide other options for adjusting alpha in a study to prevent a Type I error.

8. Based on the Bonferroni result of the more stringent alpha = 0.0125 obtained in Question 7, the $t = -6.745$, $p = 0.000$, is still significant because it is less than 0.0125 (Grove & Gray, 2019).

9. The intervention and control groups were examined for differences related to the demographic variables gender, age, and BMI and the dependent variable preprocedural anxiety that might have affected the procedural pain and anxiety posttest levels in the children 7 to 12 years old. These nonsignificant results indicate the intervention and control groups were similar or equivalent for these variables at the beginning of the study. Thus, Canbulat et al. (2015) can conclude the significant differences found between the two groups for procedural pain and anxiety levels were probably due to the effects of the intervention rather than sampling error or initial group differences (Gray et al., 2017; Kim & Mallory, 2017).

10. No, the independent samples *t*-test would not have been appropriate to analyze the differences in gender between the Buzzy intervention and control groups. The demographic variable gender is measured at the nominal level or categories of females and males. Thus, the χ^2 test is the appropriate statistic for analyzing nominal variables such as gender (see Exercise 19). In contrast, the independent samples *t*-test is appropriate for analyzing data for the demographic variables age and BMI measured at the ratio level and the dependent variable anxiety measured at the interval level. Anxiety was measured with a multiple-item Likert scale that is considered interval-level data (see Exercise 1).

Questions to Be Graded

Name: _____ Class: _____

Date: _____

Follow your instructor's directions to submit your answers to the following questions for grading. Your instructor may ask you to write your answers below and submit them as a hard copy for grading. Alternatively, your instructor may ask you to submit your answers online.

1. What do degrees of freedom (*df*) mean? Canbulat et al. (2015) did not provide the *df*s in their study. Why is it important to know the *df* for a *t* ratio? Using the *df* formula, calculate the *df* for this study.

2. What are the means and standard deviations (*SD*s) for age for the Buzzy intervention and control groups? What statistical analysis is conducted to determine the difference in means for age for the two groups? Was this an appropriate analysis technique? Provide a rationale for your answer.

3. What are the *t* value and *p* value for age? What do these results mean?

4. What are the assumptions for conducting the independent samples *t*-test?

181

5. Are the groups in this study independent or dependent? Provide a rationale for your answer.

6. What is the null hypothesis for procedural self-reported pain measured with the Wong Baker Faces Scale (WBFS) for the two groups? Was this null hypothesis accepted or rejected in this study? Provide a rationale for your answer.

7. Should a Bonferroni procedure be conducted in this study? Provide a rationale for your answer.

8. What variable has a result of $t = -6.135$, $p = 0.000$? What does the result mean?

9. In your opinion, is it an expected or unexpected finding that both *t* values on Table 2 were found to be statistically significant. Provide a rationale for your answer.

10. Describe one potential clinical benefit for pediatric patients to receive the Buzzy intervention that combined cold and vibration during IV insertion.

Understanding Paired or Dependent Samples *t*-Test

STATISTICAL TECHNIQUE IN REVIEW

The **paired or dependent samples *t*-test** is a parametric statistical procedure calculated to determine differences between two sets of repeated measures data from one group of people. The scores used in the analysis might be obtained from the same subjects under different conditions, such as the one group pretest–posttest design (Kazdin, 2017). With this type of design, a single group of subjects experiences the pretest, treatment or intervention, and posttest (Knapp, 2017). Subjects are referred to as serving as their own control during the pretest, which is then compared with the posttest scores following the treatment. Figure 17.1 presents the pretest–posttest design.

Paired scores also result from a one-group repeated measures design, where one group of participants is exposed to different levels of an intervention. For example, one group of participants might be exposed to two different doses of a medication and the outcomes for each participant for each dose of medication are measured, resulting in paired scores. The one group design is considered a weak quasi-experimental design because it is difficult to determine the effects of a treatment without a comparison to a separate control group (Gray, Grove, & Sutherland, 2017; Shadish, Cook, & Campbell, 2002). The assumptions for the paired samples *t*-test are as follows:

1. The distribution of scores is normal or approximately normal.
2. The dependent variable(s) is(are) measured at interval or ratio levels.
3. Repeated measures data are collected from one group of subjects, resulting in paired scores.
4. The differences between the paired scores are independent (Gray et al., 2017).

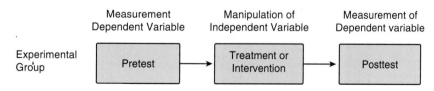

FIGURE 17-1 ■ ONE-GROUP PRETEST-POSTTEST DESIGN.

RESEARCH ARTICLE

Source

Lindseth, G. N., Coolahan, S. E., Petros, T. V., & Lindseth, P. D. (2014). Neurobehavioral effects of aspartame consumption. *Research in Nursing & Health, 37*(3), 185–193.

Introduction

Despite the widespread use of the artificial sweetener aspartame in drinks and food, there are concerns and controversy about the mixed research evidence on its neurobehavioral effects. Thus Lindseth and colleagues (2014) conducted a one-group repeated measures design to determine the neurobehavioral effects of consuming both low- and high-aspartame diets in a sample of 28 college students. "The participants served as their own controls....A random assignment of the diets was used to avoid an error of variance for possible systematic effects of order" (Lindseth et al., 2014, p. 187).

"Healthy adults who consumed a study-prepared high-aspartame diet (25 mg/kg body weight/day) for 8 days and a low-aspartame diet (10 mg/kg body weight/day) for 8 days, with a 2-week washout between the diets, were examined for within-subject differences in cognition, depression, mood, and headache. Measures included weight of foods consumed containing aspartame, mood and depression scales, and cognitive tests for working memory and spatial orientation. When consuming high-aspartame diets, participants had more irritable mood, exhibited more depression, and performed worse on spatial orientation tests. Aspartame consumption did not influence working memory. Given that the higher intake level tested here was well below the maximum acceptable daily intake level of 40–50 mg/kg body weight/day, careful consideration is warranted when consuming food products that may affect neurobehavioral health" (Lindseth et al., 2014, p. 185). Lindseth and colleagues recommend additional research to determine the safety of aspartame consumption and its implications for health, because the sample size was small and the findings were conflicting in their study.

Relevant Study Results

"The mean age of the study participants was 20.8 years (*SD* = 2.5). The average number of years of education was 13.4 (*SD* = 1.0), and the mean body mass index was 24.1 (*SD* = 3.5)....Based on Vandenberg MRT scores, spatial orientation scores were significantly better for participants after their low-aspartame intake period than after their high intake period (Table 2). Two participants had clinically significant cognitive impairment after consuming high-aspartame diets....Participants were significantly more depressed after they consumed the high-aspartame diet compared to when they consumed the low-aspartame diet (Table 2)....Only one participant reported a headache; no difference in headache incidence between high- and low-aspartame intake periods could be established" (Lindseth et al., 2014, p. 190).

Variable	M	SD	Paired *t*-Test	*p*
Spatial orientation				
High-aspartame	14.1	4.2	2.4	.03*
Low-aspartame	16.6	4.3		
Working memory				
High-aspartame	730.0	152.7	1.5	N.S.
Low-aspartame	761.1	201.6		
Mood (irritability)				
High-aspartame	33.4	9.0	3.4	.002**
Low-aspartame	30.5	7.3		
Depression				
High-aspartame	36.8	7.0	3.8	.001**
Low-aspartame	34.4	6.2		

TABLE 2 WITHIN-SUBJECT DIFFERENCES IN NEUROBEHAVIOR SCORES AFTER HIGH AND LOW ASPARTAME INTAKE (*N* = 28)

*p < .05.
**p < .01.
M = Mean; *SD* = Standard deviation; N.S. = Nonsignificant.

Lindseth, G. N., Coolahan, S. E., Petros, T. V., & Lindseth, P. D. (2014). Neurobehavioral effects of aspartame consumption. *Research in Nursing & Health, 37*(3), p. 190.

STUDY QUESTIONS

1. Are independent or dependent (paired) scores examined in this study? Provide a rationale for your answer.

2. What independent (intervention) and dependent (outcome) variables were included in this study?

3. What inferential statistical technique was calculated to examine differences in the participants when they received the high-aspartame diet intervention versus the low-aspartame diet? Is this technique appropriate? Provide a rationale for your answer.

4. What statistical techniques were calculated to describe spatial orientation for the participants consuming low- and high-aspartame diets? Were these techniques appropriate? Provide a rationale for your answer.

5. What was the dispersion of the scores for spatial orientation for the high- and low-aspartame diets? Is the dispersion of these scores similar or different? Provide a rationale for your answer.

6. What is the paired *t*-test value for spatial orientation between the participants' consumption of high- and low-aspartame diets? Are these results significant? Provide a rationale for your answer.

7. State the null hypothesis for spatial orientation for this study. Was this hypothesis accepted or rejected? Provide a rationale for your answer.

8. Discuss the meaning of the results regarding spatial orientation for this study. What is the clinical importance of this result? Document your answer.

9. Was there a significant difference in the participants' reported headaches between the high- and low-aspartame intake periods? What does the result indicate?

10. What additional research is needed to determine the neurobehavioral effects of aspartame consumption?

Answers to Study Questions

1. This study was conducted using one group of 28 college students who consumed both high- and low- aspartame diets and differences in their neurobehavioral responses to these two diets (interventions) were examined. Lindseth et al. (2014, p. 187) stated that "the participants served as their own controls" in this study. The scores from the one group are paired with their responses to the different levels of aspartame in their diet. In Table 2, the *t*-tests are identified as paired *t*-tests, which are conducted on dependent or paired samples (Gray et al., 2017).

2. The interventions were high-aspartame diet (25 mg/kg body weight/day) and low-aspartame diet (10 mg/kg body weight/day). The dependent or outcome variables were spatial orientation, working memory, mood (irritability), depression, and headaches (see Table 2 and the study narrative of results).

3. Differences were examined with the paired *t*-test (see Table 2). This statistical technique is appropriate since the study included one group and the participants' scores obtained following the two levels of aspartame diet are compared (paired scores) (Knapp, 2017; Plichta & Kelvin, 2013). The dependent variables were measured at least at the interval level for each subject following their consumption of high- and low-aspartame diets and were then examined for differences to determine the effects of the two aspartame diets.

4. Means and standard deviations (*SD*s) were used to describe spatial orientation for high- and low-aspartame diets. The data in the study were considered at least interval level, so means and *SD*s are the appropriate analysis techniques for describing the study dependent variables (Grove & Gray, 2019).

5. Standard deviation (*SD*) is a measure of dispersion that was reported in this study. Spatial orientation following a high-aspartame diet had an *SD* = 4.2 and an *SD* = 4.3 for a low-aspartame diet. These *SD*s are very similar, indicating similar dispersions or spread of spatial orientation scores following the two aspartame diets.

6. Paired *t*-test = 2.4 for spatial orientation, which is a statistically significant result since *p* = .03*. The single asterisk (*) directs the reader to the footnote at the bottom of the table, which identifies * *p* < .05. Because the study result of *p* = .03 is less than α = .05 set for this study, this result is statistically significant (Grove & Gray, 2019).

7. Null hypothesis: *There is no difference in spatial orientation scores for participants following consumption of a low-aspartame diet versus a high-aspartame diet*. The null hypothesis was rejected because of the significant difference found for spatial orientation (see the answer to Question 6). Significant results cause the rejection of the null hypothesis and lend support to the research hypothesis that the levels of aspartame do significantly effect spatial orientation (Gray et al., 2017).

8. The researchers reported, "Based on Vandenberg MRT scores, spatial orientation scores were significantly better for participants after their low-aspartame intake period than after their high intake period (Table 2)" (Lindseth et al., 2014, p. 190). This result is clinically important since the high-aspartame diet significantly reduced the participants' spatial orientation. Healthcare providers need to be aware of this finding, since it is consistent with previous research, and encourage people to consume fewer diet drinks and foods with aspartame. The American Heart Association (search their website at http://www.heart.org/HEARTORG/ for aspartame effects) and the American Diabetic Association (search their website at http://www.diabetes.org for aspartame effects) have provided statements about the negative effects of aspartame.

9. There was no significant difference in reported headaches based on the level (high or low) of aspartame diet consumed. Additional research is needed to determine if this result is an accurate reflection of reality or is due to design weaknesses, sampling or data collection errors, or chance (Gray et al., 2017).

10. Additional studies, such as randomized controlled trials, are needed with larger samples to determine the effects of aspartame in the diet. The sample size for this was small at $N = 28$, which increased the potential for a Type II error. Diets higher in aspartame (40–50 mg/kg body weight/day) should be examined for neurobehavioral effects. Longitudinal studies to examine the effects of aspartame over more than 8 days are needed. Future research needs to examine the length of washout period needed between the different levels of aspartame diets. Researchers also need to examine the measurement methods to ensure they have strong validity and reliability (Waltz, Strickland, & Lenz, 2017). Could a more reliable and valid test of working memory be used in future research?

Questions to Be Graded

Name: _____ Class: _____

Date: _____

Follow your instructor's directions to submit your answers to the following questions for grading. Your instructor may ask you to write your answers below and submit them as a hard copy for grading. Alternatively, your instructor may ask you to submit your answers online.

1. What are the assumptions for conducting a paired or dependent samples *t*-test in a study? Which of these assumptions do you think were met by the Lindseth et al. (2014) study?

2. In the introduction, Lindseth et al. (2014, p. 187) described a "2-week washout between diets." What does this mean? Why is this important?

3. What is the paired *t*-test value for mood (irritability) between the participants' consumption of high- versus low-aspartame diets? Is this result statistically significant? Provide a rationale for your answer.

4. State the null hypothesis for mood (irritability) that was tested in this study. Was this hypothesis accepted or rejected? Provide a rationale for your answer.

5. Which *t* value in Table 2 represents the greatest relative or standardized difference between the high- and low-aspartame diets? Is this *t* value statistically significant? Provide a rationale for your answer.

6. Discuss why the larger *t* values are more likely to be statistically significant.

7. Discuss the meaning of the results regarding depression for this study. What is the clinical importance of this result?

8. What is the smallest, paired *t*-test value in Table 2? Why do you think the smaller *t* values are not statistically significant?

9. Discuss the clinical importance of these study results about the consumption of aspartame. Document your answer with a relevant source.

10. Are these study findings related to the consumption of high- and low-aspartame diets ready for implementation in practice? Provide a rationale for your answer.

Understanding Analysis of Variance (ANOVA) and Post Hoc Analyses

STATISTICAL TECHNIQUE IN REVIEW

Analysis of variance (ANOVA) is a parametric statistical technique conducted to determine whether a statistically significant difference exists among the means of three or more groups. There are different types of ANOVAs, with the most basic being the **one-way ANOVA**, which is conducted to analyze data on a variable that is normally distributed and measured at the interval or ratio level (Plichta & Kelvin, 2013). More details on the types of ANOVAs can be found in your research textbook and statistical texts (Gray, Grove, & Sutherland, 2017; Kim & Mallory, 2017; Plichta & Kelvin, 2013). The outcome of ANOVA is a numerical value for the F statistic. The calculated F-ratio from ANOVA indicates the extent to which group means differ, taking into account the variability within the groups. Assuming the null hypothesis of no differences among the groups studied is true; the probability of obtaining an F-ratio as large as the obtained value in a given sample is determined by the calculated p value. If the p value is greater than the level of significance, or alpha (α), set for the study, then the study results are nonsignificant and the F-ratio will be less than the critical values for F in the statistical table (see Appendix C, Critical Values of F for $\alpha = 0.05$ and $\alpha = 0.01$ at the back of this text). With nonsignificant results, researchers will accept the null hypothesis of no significant differences among the groups. In a study, if $p = 0.01$, this value is less than $\alpha = 0.05$, which indicates the groups are significantly different and the null hypothesis is rejected. However, there is always a possibility that this decision is in error, and the probability of committing this Type I error is determined by α. When $\alpha = 0.05$, there are 5 chances in 100 the results are a Type I error, or concluding something is significant when it is not.

ANOVA is similar to the t-test because the null hypothesis (no differences between groups) is rejected when the analysis yields a smaller p value, such as $p \leq 0.05$, than the α set for the study. *Assumptions* for the ANOVA statistical technique include the following:

1. The populations from which the samples were drawn or the random samples are normally distributed.
2. The groups should be mutually exclusive.
3. The groups should have equal variance, also known as homogeneity of variance.
4. The observations are independent.
5. The dependent variable is measured at the interval or ratio level (Plichta & Kelvin, 2013; Zar, 2010).

Researchers who perform ANOVA on their data report their results in an ANOVA summary table or in the text of a research article. An example of how an ANOVA result is commonly expressed is as follows:

$$F(2, 120) = 4.79, p = 0.01$$

where:

- F is the statistic.
- 2 is the group degrees of freedom (df) calculated by $k - 1$, where k = number of groups in the study. In this example, $k - 1 = 3 - 1 = 2$.
- 120 is the error degrees of freedom (df) that is calculated based upon the number of participants, or $N - k$. In this example, 123 subjects − 3 groups = 120 error df.
- 4.79 is the F-ratio or value.
- p indicates the significance of the F-ratio in this study or $p = 0.01$.

The simplest ANOVA is the one-way ANOVA, but many of the studies in the literature include more complex ANOVA statistical techniques. A commonly used ANOVA technique is the **repeated-measures analysis of variance**, which is used to analyze data from studies where the same variable(s) is(are) repeatedly measured over time on a group or groups of subjects. The intent is to determine the change that occurs over time in the dependent variable(s) with exposure to the independent or intervention variable(s) (Gray et al., 2017; Kim & Mallory, 2017).

Post Hoc Analyses Following ANOVA

When a significant F value is obtained from the conduct of ANOVA, additional analyses are needed to determine the specific location of the differences in a study with more than two groups. **Post hoc analyses** were developed to determine where the differences lie, because some of the groups might be different and others might be similar. For example, a study might include three groups, an experimental group (receiving an intervention), placebo group (receiving a pseudo or false treatment such as a sugar pill in a drug study), and a comparison group (receiving standard care). The ANOVA resulted in a significant F-ratio or value, but post hoc analyses are needed to determine the exact location of the differences. With post hoc analyses, researchers might find that the experimental group is significantly different from both the placebo and comparison groups but that the placebo and comparison groups were not significantly different from each other. One could conduct three t-tests to determine differences among the three groups, but that would inflate the Type I error. A Type I error occurs when the results indicate that two groups are significantly different when, in actuality, the groups are not different (Grove & Gray, 2019). Thus post hoc analyses were developed to detect the differences following ANOVA in studies with more than two groups to prevent an inflation of a Type I error. The frequently used post hoc analyses include the Newman-Keuls test, the Tukey Honestly Significant Difference (HSD) test, the Scheffé test, and the Dunnett test (Plichta & Kelvin, 2013).

With many post hoc analyses, the α level is reduced in proportion to the number of additional tests required to locate the statistically significant differences. As the α level is decreased, reaching the level of significance becomes increasingly more difficult. The Newman-Keuls test compares all possible pairs of means and is the most liberal of the post hoc tests discussed here. "Liberal" indicates that the α is not as severely decreased. The Tukey HSD test computes one value with which all means within the data set are compared. It is considered more stringent than the Newman-Keuls test and requires approximately equal sample sizes in each group. The Scheffé is one of the more conservative post hoc tests, but with the decrease in Type I error there is an increase in Type II error, which is concluding something is not significant when it is. The Dunnett test requires a control group, and the experimental groups are compared with the control group without a decrease in α. Exercise 33 provides the step-by-step process for calculating ANOVA and post hoc analyses.

RESEARCH ARTICLE

Source

Mayland, C. R., Williams, E. M., Addington-Hall, J., Cox, T. F., & Ellershaw, J. E. (2014). Assessing the quality of care for dying patients from the bereaved relatives' perspective: Further validation of "Evaluating Care and Health Outcomes—for the Dying." *Journal of Pain and Symptom Management, 47*(4), 687–696.

Introduction

The Liverpool Care Pathway (LCP) for the Dying Patient was created to address the need for better end of life care for both patients and families, which had been identified as an issue in the United Kingdom at the national level. "LCP is an integrated care pathway used in the last days and hours of life that aims to transfer the hospice principles of best practice into the acute hospital and other settings" (Mayland et al., 2014, p. 688). "Evaluating Care and Health Outcomes—for the Dying (ECHO-D) is a post-bereavement questionnaire that assesses quality of care for the dying and is linked with the Liverpool Care Pathway for the Dying Patient (LCP)" (Mayland et al., 2014, p. 687).

The purpose of this comparative descriptive study was to assess the internal consistency reliability, test-retest reliability, and construct validity of the key composite subscales of the ECHO-D scale. The study's convenience sample consisted of 255 next-of-kin or close family members of the patients with an anticipated death from cancer at either the selected hospice or hospital in Liverpool, United Kingdom. The sample consisted of three groups of family members based on where the patients received end of life care; the hospice, which used LCP; the hospital group that also used LCP; and another group from the same hospital that did not use LCP. The ECHO-D questionnaire was completed by all 255 study participants and a subset of self-selected participants completed a second ECHO-D 1 month after the completion of the first ECHO-D. Mayland and colleagues (2014) concluded their study provided additional evidence of reliability and validity for ECHO-D in the assessment of end of life care.

Relevant Study Results

"Overall, hospice participants had the highest scores for all composite scales, and 'hospital without LCP' participants had the lowest scores (Tables 2 and 3). The scores for the 'hospital with LCP' participants were between these two levels" (Mayland et al., 2014, p. 693). The level of significance was set at $\alpha = 0.05$ for the study. One-way analysis of variance was calculated to assess differences among the hospice, hospital with LCP, and hospital without LCP groups. Post hoc testing was conducted with the Tukey HSD test. ANOVA and post hoc results are displayed in Tables 2 and 3.

TABLE 2   COMPARISON OF HOSPICE AND HOSPITAL PARTICIPANTS' SCORES FOR COMPOSITE SCALES WITHIN THE ECHO-D QUESTIONNAIRE

Composite Scale	Mean (SD) Range					Post Hoc Comparisons Using Tukey HSD Test[b]		
	All Participants (n = 255)	Hospice (n = 109)	Hospital with LCP (n = 78)	Hospital without LCP (n = 68)	ANOVA (p)[a]	Hospice vs. Hospital with LCP	Hospice vs. Hospital without LCP	Hospital with LCP vs. Hospital without LCP
Ward environment	7.3 (2.7) 0−10	9.1 (1.2) 5−10	6.4 (2.6) 0−10	5.4 (2.7) 0−10	60.4 (<0.0001)	<0.0001	<0.0001	0.01
Facilities	7.3 (4.8) 0−18	10.5 (4.0) 2−18	4.5 (3.8) 0−18	4.1 (2.7) 0−18	76.7 (<0.0001)	<0.0001	<0.0001	0.85
Care	18.4 (6.4) 0−25	22.0 (3.75) 7−25	16.8 (0.66) 3−25	14.6 (7.33) 0−25	35.9 (<0.0001)	<0.0001	<0.0001	0.05
Communication	9.8 (3.7) 0−14	11.2 (3.2) 0−14	9.4 (3.5) 0−14	8.2 (3.8) 0−14	16.6 (<0.0001)	0.002	<0.0001	0.86

ECHO-D = Evaluating Care and Health Outcomes for the Dying; *ANOVA* = analysis of variance; *HSD* = honestly significant difference; *LCP* = Liverpool Care Pathway for the Dying Patient.
[a]One-way ANOVA (between-groups ANOVA with planned comparisons).
[b]Post hoc comparisons allow further exploration of the differences between individual groups using the Tukey HSD test, which assumes equal variances for the groups.

Mayland, C. R., Williams, E. M., Addington-Hall, J., Cox, T. F., & Ellershaw, J. E. (2014). Assessing the quality of care for dying patients from the bereaved relatives' perspective: Further validation of "Evaluating Care and Health Outcomes-for the Dying." *Journal of Pain and Symptom Management, 47*(4), p. 691.

TABLE 3   COMPARISON OF HOSPICE AND HOSPITAL PARTICIPANTS' SCORES FOR COMPOSITE VARIABLES WITHIN THE ECHO-D QUESTIONNAIRE

Composite Variable	Mean (Range)				ANOVA (p)	Post Hoc Comparisons Using Tukey HSD Test		
	All Participants (n = 255)	Hospice (n = 109)	Hospital with LCP (n = 78)	Hospital without LCP (n = 68)		Hospice vs. Hospital with LCP	Hospice vs. Hospital without LCP	Hospital with LCP vs. Hospital without LCP
Symptom Control Degree of affliction from symptoms commonly associated with dying patients: pain, restlessness, respiratory tract secretions, nausea and/or vomiting, and breathlessness. Scores range from 0 (all five symptoms present all of the time) to 10 (no symptoms present).	6.8 (0–10)	7.0 (0–10)	7.0 (2–10)	6.1 (1–10)	4.4 (0.01)	0.99	0.02	0.03
Symptom Management Reflecting whether more should have been done by staff to control symptoms. Scores range from 0 (not enough done by staff to control symptoms) to 6 (staff did all they could to control symptoms).	4.8 (0–6)	5.2 (2–6)	4.8 (0–6)	4.2 (0–6)	10.6 (<0.0001)	0.17	<0.0001	0.02
Spiritual Need—Patient Reflecting whether patients' spiritual and religious needs were met. Scores range from 0 (where need was not met at all) to 6 (where needs were extremely well met).	3.0 (1.9)	3.9 (0–6)	2.9 (0–6)	1.6 (0–6)	38.1 (<0.0001)	0.0001	0.0001	0.0001
Spiritual Need—Next-of-Kin Reflecting whether relatives' religious and spiritual needs were met. Scores range from 0 (where need was not met at all) to 7 (where needs were extremely well met).	2.7 (0–7)	3.5 (0–7)	2.6 (0–7)	1.5 (0–7)	22.6 (<0.0001)	0.006	0.0001	0.002

ECHO-D = Evaluating Care and Health Outcomes for the Dying; ANOVA = analysis of variance; HSD = Honestly Significant Difference; LCP = Liverpool Care Pathway for the Dying Patient.

Mayland, C. R., Williams, E. M., Addington-Hall, J., Cox, T. F., & Ellershaw, J. E. (2014). Assessing the quality of care for dying patients from the bereaved relatives' perspective: Further validation of "Evaluating Care and Health Outcomes-for the Dying." *Journal of Pain and Symptom Management, 47*(4), p. 692.

STUDY QUESTIONS

1. What type of analysis was conducted in this study to examine group differences? What three groups were analyzed for differences?

2. What did the researcher set the level of significance, or alpha (α), at for this study? What is the potential for Type I error with this level of alpha?

3. State the null hypothesis for communication for the three groups. Should this null hypothesis be accepted or rejected? Provide a rationale for your answer.

4. What is the purpose of conducting post hoc analysis? What type of post hoc test was conducted in the Mayland et al. (2014) study?

5. Identify the post hoc results for communication on Table 2. Which results are statistically significant? What do these results mean?

6. What variable on Table 2 has the result $F = 60.4$ ($p < 0.0001$)? What does this result mean?

7. Mayland et al. (2014) reported means, standard deviations, and range on Table 2 and Table 3. In your opinion, is this information helpful? Provide a rationale for your answer with documentation.

8. What is the F for spiritual need—next-of-kin? Is this result statistically significant? Provide a rationale for your answer.

9. What are the post hoc results for spiritual need—next-of-kin? Which results are statistically significant? What do the results mean?

10. Mayland et al. (2014) chose the dying patients' next-of-kin rather than the patients themselves as study participants to assess end of life care. In your opinion, was this an appropriate choice?

Answers to Study Questions

1. One-way analysis of variance (ANOVA) was used to analyze the differences among the three groups in the Mayland et al. (2014) study. The three groups analyzed were hospice with Liverpool care pathway for the dying patient (LCP), hospital with LCP, and hospital without LCP. Although not identified in Tables 2 and 3 in this study, the hospice setting did include the LCP. For consistency, the following answers will refer to just hospice as in the Tables 2 and 3.

2. The level of significance or alpha (α) for this study was set at 0.05. The potential for a Type I error is 5 chances in 100 (Grove & Gray, 2019).

3. The null hypothesis is: *The three care groups of hospice, hospital with LCP, and hospital without LCP have no difference in communication scores for the next-of-kin of patients who had died of cancer.* According to Table 2, $F = 16.6$, $p < 0.0001$, for composite scale communication. This F value is statistically significant because the p value is less than $\alpha = 0.05$ that was set for this study. The significant result means that there was a statistically significant difference among the three groups for communication; therefore, the null hypothesis was rejected (Gray et al., 2017).

4. A statistically significant F value for ANOVA indicates that a difference is present among the groups analyzed but post hoc testing is necessary to identify the location(s) of the differences when a study has more than two groups. Mayland et al. (2014, p. 691) explains the purpose of post hoc testing in the footnote of Table 2 as "Post hoc comparisons allow further exploration of the differences between individual groups." The post hoc test conducted in this study was the Tukey honestly significant difference (HSD) test.

5. The post hoc results for communication are: $p = 0.002$ for hospice versus hospital with LCP and $p = 0.0001$ for hospice versus hospital without LCP. These results identify statistically significant differences for communication among these identified groups since the p values are less than $\alpha = 0.05$. The post hoc result of $p = 0.86$ for hospital with LCP versus hospital without LCP is >0.05 and is not statistically significant. This result means there is no significant difference between the hospital with LCP and the hospital without LCP groups in terms of communication.

6. Ward environment is the variable on Table 2 that has the result $F = 60.4$ ($p < 0.0001$). This statistically significant result means there is a significant difference among the three groups of hospice, hospital with LCP, and hospital without LCP in terms of the ward environment.

7. Yes, these results are helpful. The means, standard deviations, and ranges are important for describing the variables in this study. The results from these analyses provide more information about the central tendencies and dispersion of data for the study variables (Gray et al., 2017; Kim & Mallory, 2017). Additionally, means and standard deviations are essential for conducting power analyses to determine sample sizes for future studies and are important for conducting meta-analyses used to summarize the results from multiple studies to facilitate evidence-based practice (Cohen, 1988; Melnyk & Fineout-Overholt, 2019).

8. The ANOVA statistic for spiritual need—next-of-kin is $F = 22.6$, $p < 0.0001$. Since $\alpha = 0.05$ in this study, any results with a p (probability) of ≤ 0.05 is considered statistically significant; therefore, $p < 0.0001$ is statistically significant (Grove & Gray, 2019). This result means there is a statistically significant difference among the three groups of hospice, hospital with LCP, and hospital without LCP in terms of spiritual need—next-of-kin.

9. The post hoc results for spiritual need—next-of-kin were $p = 0.006$ for hospice versus hospital with LCP, $p = 0.0001$ for hospice versus hospital without LCP, and $p = 0.002$ for hospital with LCP versus hospital without LCP. All three groups are significantly different since the p values are less than $\alpha = 0.05$ set for this study. These results mean there are statistically significant differences between the hospice and hospital with LCP groups, between the hospice and hospital without LCP, and between the hospital with LCP and hospital without LCP in terms of spiritual need—next-of-kin.

10. Answers may vary. End of life care extends beyond the patient and includes next-of-kin or patients' family members. Mayland et al. (2014) described the need to improve end of life care for both patients and family. With end of life care, "one recognized method of evaluation involves the use of bereaved relatives as 'proxy' measures to assess the quality of care" (Mayland et al., 2014, p. 688). For additional resources on end of life care, hospice care, and grief process, you might search the American Cancer Society website at http://www.cancer.org.

Questions to Be Graded

Name: _____ Class: _____

Date: _____

Follow your instructor's directions to submit your answers to the following questions for grading. Your instructor may ask you to write your answers below and submit them as a hard copy for grading. Alternatively, your instructor may ask you to submit your answers online.

1. Mayland et al. (2014) do not provide the degrees of freedom (df) in their study. Use the degrees of freedom formulas provided at the beginning of this exercise to calculate the group df and the error df.

2. What is the F value and p value for spiritual need—patient? What do these results mean?

3. What is the post hoc result for facilities for the hospital with LCP vs. the hospital without LCP (see Table 2)? Is this result statistically significant? In your opinion, is this an expected finding?

4. What are the assumptions for use of ANOVA?

5. What variable on Table 3 has the result $F = 10.6$, $p < 0.0001$? What does the result mean?

6. ANOVA was used for analysis by Mayland et al. (2014). Would t-tests have also been appropriate? Provide a rationale for your answer.

7. Which group had the largest mean for the care variable? Identify the mean, standard deviation, and range for this group and discuss what these results mean.

8. State the null hypothesis for care for the three study groups (see Table 2). Should the null hypothesis be accepted or rejected? Provide a rationale for your answer.

9. What are the post hoc results for care? Which results are statistically significant? What do the results mean? Document your answer.

10. In your opinion, do the study findings presented in Tables 2 and 3 have implications for end of life care in the United States? Provide a rationale for your answer. Document your answer.

Understanding Pearson Chi-Square

STATISTICAL TECHNIQUE IN REVIEW

The **Pearson Chi-square (χ^2)** is an inferential statistical test calculated to examine differences among groups with variables measured at the nominal level. There are different types of χ^2 tests and the Pearson chi-square is commonly reported in nursing studies. The Pearson χ^2 test compares the frequencies that are observed with the frequencies that were expected. The *assumptions* for the χ^2 test are as follows:

1. The data are nominal-level or frequency data.
2. The sample size is adequate.
3. The measures are independent of each other or that a subject's data only fit into one category (Pett, 2016; Plichta & Kelvin, 2013).

The χ^2 values calculated are compared with the critical values in the χ^2 table (see Appendix D, Critical Values of the χ^2 Distribution). If the result is greater than or equal to the value in the table, significant differences exist. If the values are statistically significant, the null hypothesis is rejected (Gray, Grove, & Sutherland, 2017). These results indicate that the differences are probably an actual reflection of reality and not due to random sampling error or chance.

In addition to the χ^2 value, researchers often report the degrees of freedom (df). This statistical concept is important for calculating and determining levels of significance. The standard formula for df is sample size (N) minus 1, or $df = N - 1$; however, this formula is adjusted based on the analysis technique performed (Pett, 2016; Plichta & Kelvin, 2013). The df formula for the χ^2 test varies based on the number of categories examined in the analysis. The formula for df for the two-way χ^2 test is $df = (R - 1)(C - 1)$, where R is number of rows and C is the number of columns in a χ^2 table. For example, in a 2×2 χ^2 table, $df = (2 - 1)(2 - 1) = 1$. Therefore, the df is equal to 1. Table 19-1 includes a 2×2 chi-square contingency table based on the findings of An et al. (2014) study. In Table 19-1, the rows represent the two nominal categories of alcohol use and alcohol nonuse and the

TABLE 19-1 CONTINGENCY TABLE BASED ON THE RESULTS OF AN ET AL. (2014) STUDY

	Nonsmokers *n* = 742	Smokers *n* = 57*
No alcohol use	551	14
Alcohol use[†]	191	43

*Smokers defined as "smoking at least 1 cigarette daily during the past month."
[†]Alcohol use "defined as at least 1 alcoholic beverage per month during the past year."
An, F. R., Xiang, Y. T., Yu., L., Ding, Y. M., Ungvari, G. S., Chan, S. W. C., et al. (2014). Prevalence of nurses' smoking habits in psychiatric and general hospitals in China. *Archives of Psychiatric Nursing, 28*(2), 120.

two columns represent the two nominal categories of smokers and nonsmokers. The $df = (2 − 1) (2 − 1) = (1) (1) = 1$, and the study results were as follows: χ^2 (1, $N = 799$) = 63.1; $p < 0.0001$. It is important to note that the df can also be reported without the sample size, as in $\chi^2(1) = 63.1$, $p < 0.0001$. Among nurses in China, the rates of alcohol use are significantly higher among smokers. Alternatively, the rates of smoking are significantly higher among alcohol users (An et al., 2014).

If more than two groups are being examined, χ^2 does not determine where the differences lie; it only determines that a statistically significant difference exists. A post hoc analysis will determine the location of the difference. χ^2 is one of the weaker statistical tests conducted, and the results are usually only reported if statistically significant values are found (Pett, 2016). The step-by-step process for calculating the Pearson chi-square test is presented in Exercise 35.

RESEARCH ARTICLE

Source

Darling-Fisher, C. S., Salerno, J., Dahlem, C. H. Y., & Martyn, K. K. (2014). The Rapid Assessment for Adolescent Preventive Services (RAAPS): Providers' assessment of its usefulness in their clinical practice settings. *Journal of Pediatric Health Care, 28*(3), 217–226.

Introduction

Darling-Fisher and colleagues (2014, p. 219) conducted a mixed-methods descriptive study (Creswell & Clark, 2018) to evaluate the clinical usefulness of the Rapid Assessment for Adolescent Preventative Services (RAAPS) screening tool "by surveying healthcare providers from a wide variety of clinical settings and geographic locations." The study participants were recruited from the RAAPS website to complete an online survey. The RAAPS risk-screening tool "was developed to identify the high-risk behaviors contributing most to adolescent morbidity, mortality, and social problems, and to provide a more streamlined assessment to help providers address key adolescent risk behaviors in a time-efficient and user-friendly format" (Darling-Fisher et al., 2014, p. 218). The RAAPS is an established 21-item questionnaire with evidence of reliability and validity that can be completed by adolescents in 5–7 minutes.

"Quantitative and qualitative analyses indicated the RAAPS facilitated identification of risk behaviors and risk discussions and provided efficient and consistent assessments; 86% of providers believed that the RAAPS positively influenced their practice" (Darling-Fisher et al., 2014, p. 217). The researchers concluded the use of RAAPS by healthcare providers could improve the assessment and identification of adolescents at risk and lead to the delivery of more effective adolescent preventive services.

Relevant Study Results

In the Darling-Fisher et al. (2014, p. 220) study, "The provider survey was distributed to 567 providers, of whom 201 responded, for a response rate of 35%. Responses came from providers from 26 U.S. states and three foreign countries (Canada, Korea, and Ireland)." More than half of the participants ($n = 111$; 55%) reported they were using the RAAPS in their clinical practices. "When asked if they would recommend the RAAPS to other providers, 86 responded, and 98% ($n = 84$) stated they would recommend RAAPS. The two most common reasons cited for their recommendation were for screening ($n = 76$, 92%) and identification of risk behaviors ($n = 75$, 90%). Improved communication ($n = 52$, 63%)

and improved documentation ($n = 46$, 55%) and increased patient understanding of their risk behaviors ($n = 48$, 58%) were also cited by respondents as reasons to recommend the RAAPS" (Darling-Fisher et al., 2014, p. 222).

"Respondents who were not using the RAAPS ($n = 90$; 45%), had a variety of reasons for not using it. Most reasons were related to constraints of their health system or practice site; other reasons were satisfaction with their current method of assessment…and that they were interested in the RAAPS for academic or research purposes rather than clinical use" (Darling-Fisher et al., 2014, p. 220).

Chi-square analysis was calculated to determine if any statistically significant differences existed between the characteristics of the RAAPS users and nonusers. Darling-Fisher et al. (2014) did not provide a level of significance or α for their study, but many nursing studies use $\alpha = 0.05$. "Statistically significant differences were noted between RAAPS users and nonusers with respect to provider types, practice setting, percent of adolescent patients, years in practice, and practice region. No statistically significant demographic differences were found between RAAPS users and nonusers with respect to race, age" (Darling-Fisher et al., 2014, p. 221). The χ^2 results are presented in Table 2. Three of the p values in this table were recorded as $< .00$, which is not accurate because a p value is never zero. The values would have been more accurately expressed as $p < 0.001$ (Gray et al., 2017).

TABLE 2 DEMOGRAPHIC COMPARISONS BETWEEN RAPID ASSESSMENT FOR ADOLESCENT PREVENTIVE SERVICE USERS AND NONUSERS

Current user	Yes (%)	No (%)	χ^2	p
Provider type ($n = 161$)			12.7652, $df = 2$	$< .00$
Health care provider	64 (75.3)	55 (72.4)		
Mental health provider	13 (15.3)	2 (2.6)		
Other	8 (9.4)	19 (25.0)		
Practice setting ($n = 152$)			12.7652, $df = 1$	$< .00$
Outpatient health clinic	20 (24.1)	36 (52.2)		
School-based health clinic	63 (75.9)	33 (47.8)		
% Adolescent patients ($n = 154$)			7.3780, $df = 1$	.01
≤50%	26 (30.6)	36 (52.2)		
>50%	59 (69.4)	33 (47.8)		
Years in practice ($n = 157$)			6.2597, $df = 1$	.01
≤5 years	44 (51.8)	23 (31.9)		
>5 years	41 (48.2)	49 (68.1)		
U.S. practice region ($n = 151$)			29.68, $df = 3$	$< .00$
Northeastern United States	13 (15.3)	15 (22.7)		
Southern United States	11 (12.9)	22 (33.3)		
Midwestern United States	57 (67.1)	16 (24.2)		
Western United States	4 (4.7)	13 (19.7)		
Race ($n = 201$)			1.2865, $df = 2$	.53
Black/African American	11 (9.9)	5 (5.6)		
White/Caucasian	66 (59.5)	56 (62.2)		
Other	34 (30.6)	29 (32.2)		
Provider age in years ($n = 145$)			4.00, $df = 2$	.14
20–39 years	21 (25.6)	8 (12.7)		
40–49 years	24 (29.3)	19 (30.2)		
50+ years	37 (45.1)	36 (57.1)		

χ^2, Chi-square statistic.
df, degrees of freedom.

Darling-Fisher, C. S., Salerno, J., Dahlem, C. H. Y., & Martyn, K. K. (2014). The Rapid Assessment for Adolescent Preventive Services (RAAPS): Providers' assessment of its usefulness in their clinical practice settings. *Journal of Pediatric Health Care, 28*(3), p. 221.

STUDY QUESTIONS

1. What is the sample size for the Darling-Fisher et al. (2014) study? How many study participants (percentage) are RAAPS users and how many are RAAPS nonusers? Was this sample size adequate for this study?

2. State the null hypothesis for the provider type in the Darling-Fisher et al. (2014) study. What is the chi-square (χ^2) value and degrees of freedom (*df*) for provider type?

3. What is the *p* value for provider type? Is the χ^2 value for provider type statistically significant? Was the null hypothesis accepted or rejected? Provide rationales for your answers.

4. Does a statistically significant χ^2 value provide evidence of causation between the variables? Provide a rationale for your answer.

5. What is the χ^2 value for race? Is the χ^2 value statistically significant? Provide a rationale for your answer.

6. Is there a statistically significant difference between RAAPS users and RAAPS nonusers with regard to percentage of adolescent patients? In your own opinion is this an expected finding? Document your answer.

7. What is the *df* for U.S. practice region? Complete the *df* formula for U.S. practice region to visualize how Darling-Fisher et al. (2014) determined the appropriate *df* for that region.

8. State the null hypothesis for the years in practice variable for RAAPS users and RAAPS nonusers.

9. Should the null hypothesis for years in practice developed for Question 8 be accepted or rejected? Provide a rationale for your answer.

10. Bhatta, Champion, Young, and Loika (2018, p. 8) conducted a study to determine "outcomes of depression screening among adolescents accessing school-based pediatric primary care clinic services." These researchers reported "Female adolescents were more likely to report sleep problems (χ^2 = 9.147, p = 0.002) and tiredness . . . (χ^2 = 6.165, p = 0.013) than male adolescents" (Bhatta et al., 2018, p. 11). Were these results statistically significant? Were these results clinically important? Provide rationales for your answers. The Bhatta et al. (2018) article is available in the Article Library for this text.

Answers to Study Questions

1. The sample size is $N = 201$ with $n = 111$ (55%) RAAPS users and $n = 90$ (45%) RAAPS nonusers as indicated in the narrative results. Answers might vary because the sample size is limited for an online survey with only 35% of the providers responding. However, many of the chi-square values were significant, indicating a decreased potential for a Type II error. In addition, the group sizes were fairly equal, which is a study strength (Gray et al., 2017).

2. The null hypothesis is: *There is no difference in provider type for the users and nonusers of the RAAPS screening tool.* The $\chi^2 = 12.7652$ and $df = 2$ for provider type as presented in Table 2.

3. The $p = < .00$ for the provider type. Yes, the $\chi^2 = 12.7652$ for provider type is statistically significant as indicated by the p value presented in Table 2. The specific χ^2 value obtained could be compared against the critical value in a χ^2 table (see Appendix D) to determine the significance for the specific degrees of freedom (df), but readers of research reports usually rely on the p value provided by the researcher(s) to determine significance. Many nurse researchers set the level of significance or alpha (α) = 0.05 (Grove & Gray, 2019). Since the p value is less than alpha, the result is statistically significant. The null hypothesis is rejected when study results are statistically significant (Gray et al., 2017; Pett, 2016). You need to note that p values never equal zero as they appear in this study. The p values would not be zero if carried out more decimal places.

4. No, a statistically significant χ^2 value does not provide evidence of causation. A statistically significant χ^2 value indicates a significant difference between groups exists but does not provide a causal link (Grove & Gray, 2019; Shadish, Cook, & Campbell, 2002).

5. The $\chi^2 = 1.2865$ for race. Since $p = .53$ for race, the χ^2 value is not statistically significant. The level of significance is set at $\alpha = 0.05$ and the p value is larger than alpha, so the result is nonsignificant (Grove & Gray, 2019; Pett, 2016).

6. Yes, there is a statistically significant difference between RAAPS users and RAAPS nonusers with regard to percentage of adolescent patients. The chi-square value = 7.3780 with a $p = .01$, which is less than alpha = 0.05. You might expect that nurses caring for more adolescents might have higher RAAPS use as indicated in Table 2. However, nurses need to be knowledgeable of assessment and care needs of populations and subpopulations in their practice even if not frequently encountered. Two valuable sources for adolescent care include the Centers for Disease Control and Prevention (CDC) Adolescent and School Health at http://www.cdc.gov/HealthyYouth/ and the World Health Organization (WHO) adolescent health at http://www.who.int/topics/adolescent_health/en/.

7. The $df = 3$ for U.S. practice region is provided in Table 2. The df formula, $df = (R - 1)(C - 1)$ is used (Kim & Mallory, 2017; Pett, 2016). There are four "R" rows, Northeastern United States, Southern United States, Midwestern United States, and Western United States. There are two "C" columns, RAAPS users and RAAPS nonusers. $df = (4 - 1)(2 - 1) = (3)(1) = 3$.

8. The null hypothesis: *There is no difference between RAAPS users and RAAPS nonusers for providers with ≤5 years of practice and those with >5 years of practice.*

9. The null hypothesis for years in practice stated in Questions 8 should be rejected. The $\chi^2 = 6.2597$ for years in practice is statistically significant, $p = .01$. A statistically significant χ^2 indicates a significant difference exists between the users and nonusers of RAAPS for years in practice; therefore the null hypothesis should be rejected (Kim & Mallory, 2017).

10. The Bhatta et al. (2018) results were statistically significant with female adolescents reporting significantly more sleep problems ($\chi^2 = 9.147$, $p = 0.002$) and tiredness ($\chi^2 = 6.165$, $p = 0.013$) than male adolescents. The results are statistically significant because the p values are less than alpha set at 0.05. The results are clinically important because the sleep and tiredness outcomes vary based on gender and additional screening and interventions are needed to manage these health problems in females.

Questions to Be Graded

Name: _____ Class: _____

Date: _____

Follow your instructor's directions to submit your answers to the following questions for grading. Your instructor may ask you to write your answers below and submit them as a hard copy for grading. Alternatively, your instructor may ask you to submit your answers online.

1. According to the relevant study results section of the Darling-Fisher et al. (2014) study, what variables are reported to be statistically significant?

2. What level of measurement is appropriate for calculating the χ^2 statistic? Give two examples from Table 2 of demographic variables measured at the level appropriate for χ^2.

3. What is the χ^2 for U.S. practice region? Is the χ^2 value statistically significant? Is the p value accurately expressed for this variable? Provide a rationale for your answer.

4. What is the df for provider type? Provide a rationale for why the df for provider type presented in Table 2 is correct.

5. Is there a statistically significant difference for practice setting between the Rapid Assessment for Adolescent Preventive Services (RAAPS) users and nonusers? Provide a rationale for your answer.

6. State the null hypothesis for provider age in years for RAAPS users and RAAPS nonusers.

7. Should the null hypothesis for provider age in years developed for Question 6 be accepted or rejected? Provide a rationale for your answer.

8. Describe at least one clinical advantage and one clinical challenge of using RAAPS as described by Darling-Fisher et al. (2014).

9. How many null hypotheses are rejected in the Darling-Fisher et al. (2014) study for the results presented in Table 2? How many null hypotheses were accepted? Provide rationales for your answers.

10. A statistically significant difference is present between RAAPS users and RAAPS nonusers for U.S. practice region, $\chi^2 = 29.68$. Does the χ^2 result provide the location of the difference? Provide a rationale for your answer.

Understanding Spearman Rank-Order Correlation Coefficient

STATISTICAL TECHNIQUE IN REVIEW

The **Spearman rank-order correlation coefficient**, or **Spearman *rho***, is a nonparametric test conducted to identify relationships or associations between two variables. The Spearman analysis technique is an adaptation of the Pearson product-moment correlation (see Exercises 13 and 28) and is calculated when the assumptions of the Pearson analysis cannot be met. Thus, the Spearman *rho* statistical technique is conducted to analyze data that are ordinal level of measurement or variables measured at the interval or ratio levels with values that are skewed or not normally distributed (Pett, 2016).

Each subject included in the analysis must have a score (or value) on each of two variables, variable *x* and variable *y*. The values for both variables must be ranked to conduct this analysis. The values on each variable are ranked separately (Pett, 2016; Plichta & Kelvin, 2013). Calculation of Spearman *rho* is based on **difference scores** between a subject's ranking on the first (variable *x*) and second (variable *y*) sets of values. The formula for difference scores is $D = x - y$. Because results with negative values cancel out positive values, results are squared for use in the analysis. The formula for calculation of Spearman *rho* is:

$$rho = 1 - \frac{6 \sum D^2}{N^3 - N}$$

where:

rho = Statistic for the Spearman correlation coefficient
D = Difference between the rankings of a subject's score or value on both variables *x* and *y*
N = Number of paired ranked scores (Daniel, 2000)

The Spearman rank-order correlation coefficient values range from −1 to +1, where a positive value indicates a positive relationship and a negative value indicates a negative or inverse relationship. Numbers closest to +1 or −1 indicate the strongest relationships. In comparison to the Pearson correlation coefficient (*r*), the Spearman *rho* has a statistical power of 91%, which means the Spearman *rho* has a 9% smaller probability of detecting a relationship or association if one exists. If the study sample size is greater than 50 participants, the power of the Spearman *rho* is approximately equal to the Pearson *r* in detecting a relationship in a study. The strength of *rho* values are as follows: < 0.3 or < −0.3 are weak relationships, 0.3 to 0.5 or −0.3 to −0.5 are moderate relationships, and > 0.5 or > −0.5 are strong relationships. A Spearman *rho* of 0 indicates no relationship between the two variables; the closer the *rho* value is to 0, the weaker the relationship (Gray, Grove, & Sutherland, 2017; Pett, 2016). The significance of *rho* is determined by comparing the calculated value with the critical value in a Spearman *rho* table. The computer output for Spearman *rho* includes one- and two-tailed *t*-test results and *p* values to determine significance (see Appendix A for the one- and two-tailed *t*-test values).

The Spearman *rho* is calculated using the following hypothetical example, where five students' intramuscular (IM) injection techniques were ranked by two instructors from a high score of 1 to a low score of 5. The data or rankings for this example are ordinal and presented in Table 20-1. The purpose of this example is to examine the relationship between the two instructors' rankings of the five students' IM injection techniques. The null hypothesis is: *The rankings of students' IM injection technique by instructors A and B are not associated or related.*

TABLE 20-1   RELATIONSHIP OF INSTRUCTORS' RANKING WITH STUDENTS' INTRAMUSCULAR INJECTIONS TECHNIQUES

Student	Instructor A	Instructor B	D	D^2
Amy	1	1	0	0
Jeff	3	2	1	1
John	5	4	1	1
Julie	2	3	−1	1
Mary	4	5	−1	1
Sum				4

Calculations:

$$rho = 1 - \frac{6 \sum D^2}{N^3 - N} \quad rho = 1 - \frac{6(4)}{125 - 5} = 1 - \frac{24}{120} = 1 - 0.2 = 0.80$$

In this example, a strong positive correlation or relationship (*rho* = 0.80) was found between the two instructors' ranking of students on IM injection techniques. This value for *rho* when compared with the critical value in a Spearman correlation coefficient table of 0.80 for *n* = 5 for a one-tailed test is statistically significant because it is equal to the critical value (see Appendix K in Plichta & Kelvin, 2013, pp 543–544). Because the *rho* value is statistically significant, the null hypothesis is rejected. The Spearman *rho* is usually calculated with a larger sample and using a statistical computer package, such as the Statistical Package for the Social Sciences (SPSS), that determines the *rho* value and its significance (Pett, 2016).

RESEARCH ARTICLE

Source

Li, H., Jiang, Y. F., & Lin, C. C. (2014). Factors associated with self-management by people undergoing hemodialysis: A descriptive study. *International Journal of Nursing Studies, 51*(2), 208–216.

Introduction

Li, Jiang, and Lin (2014) conducted a descriptive correlational study to determine the factors associated with self-management in people undergoing hemodialysis. A convenience sampling method was used to recruit 216 hemodialysis patients from three Beijing hospitals; 198 of these patients completed the data collection process. Data were collected using the 20-item Hemodialysis Self-Management Instrument (HDSMI), which is organized into four subscales of problem-solving, emotional management, self-care, and partnership. Each item on the HDSMI is measured using a four-point scale, with scores ranging from 0 to 80 with "the higher scores indicating higher levels of self-management" (Li et al., 2014, p. 210). The total HDSMI score for the sample had a mean = 56.01 (SD = 10.75).

Li and colleagues (2014) concluded that self-management was suboptimal among study participants. Key self-management factors for participants were knowledge, self-efficacy, the availability of social support, and depression. Future research is needed to explore self-efficacy training or other interventions aimed at increasing self-management in hemodialysis patients.

Relevant Study Results

The statistical analyses in this study included descriptive statistics and the inferential statistics of Spearman correlation, chi square (χ^2) (see Exercise 19), and multiple linear regression (see Exercise 15). The level of significance, or α, was set at 0.05. "The relationship between self-management and the influencing factors were all linear. Knowledge, self-efficacy, objective support, and availability of social support positively correlated with overall self-management as well as the subscales ($p < 0.05$) (Table 3). Anxiety and depression were negatively correlated with overall self-management and all of the subscales ($p < 0.01$). Subjective support was positively correlated with self-management and the subscales: partnership; emotional management; and problem-solving ($p < 0.05$)....Age and number of complications were negatively correlated with problem-solving ($p < 0.05$)" (Li et al., 2014, p. 212).

TABLE 3   CORRELATION MATRIX FOR SELF-MANAGEMENT AND INFLUENCING FACTORS (N = 198)

Variables	Partnership	Emotional Management	Problem Solving	Self-Care	Total
Age	−	−	−0.225**	−	−
Number of complications	−	−	−0.146*	−	−
Knowledge	0.388**	0.284**	0.314**	0.338**	0.432**
Self-efficacy	0.413**	0.349**	0.300**	0.380**	0.471**
Anxiety	−0.340**	−0.279**	−0.282**	−0.230**	−0.334**
Depression	−0.429**	−0.375**	−0.382**	−0.360**	−0.488**
Subjective support	0.181*	0.242**	0.157*	−	0.217**
Objective support	0.225**	0.211**	0.171*	0.153*	0.239**
Availability of social support	0.215**	0.440**	0.281**	0.260**	0.368**

Spearman correlation coefficient (rho): *p < 0.05; **p < 0.01.

Li, H., Jiang, Y. F., & Lin, C. C. (2014). Factors associated with self-management by people undergoing hemodialysis: A descriptive study. *International Journal of Nursing Studies, 51*(2), p. 212.

STUDY QUESTIONS

1. What is the Spearman *rho* value for the relationship or association between anxiety and self-care?

2. Describe the strength and direction of the relationship between anxiety and self-care. Is this relationship statistically significant? Provide a rationale for your answer.

3. What does the relationship between anxiety and self-care described in Question 2 mean for the patient?

4. What relationship is described on Table 3 with Spearman *rho* = 0.153, $p < 0.05$?

5. What was the relationship between age and emotional management?

6. Is there a stronger correlation between objective support and problem solving or depression and problem solving? Provide a rationale for your answer.

7. Describe the strength and direction of the relationship between knowledge and total self-management. Is this relationship statistically significant? Provide a rationale for your answer.

8. What does the relationship between knowledge and total self-management described in Question 7 mean for the patient?

9. How many relationships presented on Table 3 are statistically significant at $p < 0.01$?

10. The nonparametric Spearman rank-order correlation coefficient was used to examine the relationships in this study. Was this analysis appropriate? Provide a rationale for your answer. What is the preferred parametric analysis for identifying relationships between variables (review Exercise 13)?

Answers to Study Questions

1. The Spearman *rho* = −0.230 for the relationship between anxiety and self-care.

2. *rho* = −0.230** represents a weak, negative or inverse relationship between the variables anxiety and self-care. This relationship is statistically significant at $p < 0.01$ as indicated by the ** in the footnote of Table 3. Li et al. (2014), like most nurse researchers, set their level of significance or alpha (α) = 0.05. Since $p < 0.01$ is smaller than α, the relationship is statistically significant (Pett, 2016).

3. The relationship between anxiety and self-care is *rho* = −0.230 ($p < 0.01$). This correlation indicates as patient anxiety increases, patient self-care decreases. This is a significant correlation but it is still a small association ($< −0.30$, closer to zero) between anxiety and self-care (Kim & Mallory, 2017; Pett, 2016).

4. The relationship described on Table 3 with *rho* = 0.153, $p < 0.05$ is the weak, positive relationship between objective support and self-care.

5. There is a nonsignificant (*ns*) relationship between age and emotional management, and no value was provided. Nurse researchers sometimes do not present the specific results for nonsignificant findings (Gray et al., 2017). However, any journal that requires American Psychological Association (APA, 2010) or American Medical Association (AMA) formatting dictates that the exact p value be reported, unless the p value is less than 0.001.

6. The stronger correlation is between depression and problem solving with *rho* = −0.382 ($p < 0.01$), which is a moderate relationship. The relationship between objective support and problem solving is a weak relationship with *rho* = 0.171 ($p < 0.05$) and is weaker, or closer to 0, than the relationship between depression and problem solving. The closer the *rho* value is to +1 or −1, the stronger the correlation or relationship between variables. Note that the negative sign in *rho* = −0.382 indicates the direction of the relationship and not the strength of the relationship (Gray et al., 2017; Pett, 2016).

7. The relationship between knowledge and total self-care management is moderate, positive, and significant with *rho* = 0.432** ($p < 0.01$). The $p < 0.01$ is less than $\alpha = 0.05$, indicating a statistically significant result (Grove & Gray, 2019).

8. The relationship between knowledge and total self-care management described in Question 7 indicates as patient knowledge increases total self-care management also increases. Clinically, improving a patient's knowledge may help improve their overall self-care management. The National Kidney Foundation http://www.kidney.org offers patient and provider information on kidney disease and dialysis including hemodialysis.

9. A total of 31 relationships identified on Table 3 are statistically significant at $p < 0.01$ as indicated by the ** beside the *rho* value and described in the footnote of Table 3.

10. Spearman *rho* was used to examine the relationships in this study and was the appropriate choice because some of the study data were considered at the ordinal level of measurement by the researchers. Pearson product-moment correlation is the parametric and the preferred analysis technique to identify relationships between two variables when the assumptions for this test are met, which includes the study variables being measured at the interval or ratio level (see Exercise 13). The Pearson *r* is preferred because it is more powerful in identifying significant relationships than the Spearman *rho*.

Name: _____ Class: _____

Date: _____

Follow your instructor's directions to submit your answers to the following questions for grading. Your instructor may ask you to write your answers below and submit them as a hard copy for grading. Alternatively, your instructor may ask you to submit your answers online.

1. How many of the relationships presented in Table 3 of the Li et al. (2014) study are statistically significant at $p < 0.05$? Provide a rationale for your answer.

2. What two variables from Table 3 have the strongest positive correlation? Provide a rationale for your answer.

3. What do the results in Question 2 mean? How might this information be used clinically in caring for patients on hemodialysis?

4. What two variables from Table 3 have the strongest negative relationship?

5. What do the results in Question 4 mean? How might this information be used clinically in caring for patients on hemodialysis?

6. Is the relationship between age and total self-management significant? Provide a rationale for your answer.

7. Is there a stronger relationship between depression and partnership or subjective support and partnership? Provide a rationale for your answer.

8. Describe the relationship between availability of social support and emotional management. What is the strength of the relationship, is it positive or negative, and is it statistically significant?

9. Identify one relationship in Table 3 for which the direction of the relationship (positive or negative) with total self-management in your opinion makes sense clinically. Provide a rationale for your answer.

10. Calculate the Spearman *rho* value for the evaluations of four nurses' patient care by two managers, with 1 indicating the highest quality of care and 4 indicating the lowest quality of care. Discuss the meaning of the result. State the null hypothesis, and was the null hypothesis accepted or rejected?

Nurses	Manager #1 Rankings	Manager #2 Rankings
M. Jones	3	4
C. Smith	2	3
T. Robert	1	1
S. Hart	4	2

Understanding Mann-Whitney *U* Test

STATISTICAL TECHNIQUE IN REVIEW

The **Mann-Whitney *U* test** is a nonparametric statistical technique conducted to detect differences between two independent samples. This statistical technique is the most powerful of the nonparametric tests, with 95% of the power of the *t*-test. If the assumptions for the *t*-test cannot be satisfied, i.e., ordinal-level data are collected or the distribution of scores or values is not normal or is skewed, then the Mann-Whitney *U* is often computed. Exercise 12 provides an algorithm that will assist you in determining if the Mann-Whitney *U* was the appropriate statistical technique included in a published study (Gray, Grove, & Sutherland, 2017; Kim & Mallory, 2017).

The Mann-Whitney *U* tests the null hypothesis: *There is no difference between two independent samples for a selected variable.* For example, *there is no difference between the education intervention group and control group regarding their self-care activities following surgery.* In this example, self-care activities data need to be measured at least at the ordinal level. When reporting the Mann-Whitney *U* test results, researchers should identify the sample size for each of the independent groups and the medians for the groups so readers will know how the sample statistics differ. For example, the education intervention group included 11 post-surgical patients (median = 16.55) and the control group include 9 post-surgical patients (median = 8.75). The value of the *U* statistic and its associated *p* value should also be reported, such as $U = 19.60$, $p = 0.006$ for this example. The *p* value is based on the *z* score for one- or two-tailed test (Kim & Mallory, 2017; Plichta & Kelvin, 2013).

To calculate the value of *U*, scores of both samples are combined, and each score is assigned a rank. The lowest score is ranked 1, the next score is ranked 2, and so forth until all scores are ranked, regardless from which sample the score was obtained. The idea is that if two distributions came from the same population, the average of the ranks of their scores would be equal as well. Kim and Mallory (2017, pp. 324–329) and Plichta and Kelvin (2013, pp. 111–117) provide the details for calculating the Mann-Whitney *U* test. When reporting the Mann-Whitney *U* test results, researchers should identify the sample size of each of the independent groups, the value of the *U* statistic and its associated *p* value, as well as the medians for the groups so readers will know how the sample statistics are different from the population (Kim & Mallory, 2017).

RESEARCH ARTICLE

Source

Eckerblad, J., Tödt, K., Jakobsson, P., Unosson, M., Skargren, E., Kentsson, M., & Theander, K. (2014). Symptom burden in stable COPD patients with moderate or severe airflow limitation. *Heart & Lung, 43*(4), 351–357.

Introduction

Eckerblad and colleagues (2014, p. 351) conducted a comparative descriptive study to describe the symptoms of "patients with stable chronic obstructive pulmonary disease (COPD) and determine whether symptom experience differed between patients with moderate or severe airflow limitations." Table 1 from this study is included in Exercise 6 and provides a description of the sample characteristics. The Memorial Symptom Assessment Scale (MSAS) was used to measure the physical and psychological symptoms of 42 outpatients with moderate airflow limitations and 49 patients with severe airflow limitations. The results indicate that the mean number of symptoms was 7.9 (±4.3) for the sample of 91 patients with COPD. The Mann-Whitney *U* analysis technique was conducted to determine physical and psychological symptom differences between the moderate and severe airflow limitation groups. The researchers concluded that patients with moderate and severe airflow limitations experienced multiple severe symptoms that caused high levels of distress. Quality assessment of COPD patients' physical and psychological symptoms should be a high priority in the care of these patients in order to improve the management of their symptoms and to reduce symptom burden progression.

Relevant Study Results

"MSAS evaluates a multidimensional symptom profile, including the prevalence of 32 symptoms and the symptom experience of 26 physical and six psychological symptoms during the previous week. Symptom prevalence was recorded as yes = 1 or no = 0. Whenever a symptom was present, the symptom experience was assessed by the dimensions of frequency (1 = rarely to 4 = almost constantly) for 24 symptoms, severity (1 = slight to 4 = very severe), and distress (0.8 = not at all to 4.0 = very much) associated with all 32 symptoms during the preceding week. Higher scores indicate greater frequency, severity, and distress. A score for each symptom, defined as an MSAS symptom burden score, was calculated by averaging the scores for frequency, severity and distress dimensions" (Eckerblad et al., 2014, p. 352).

"The six symptoms rated with the highest MSAS symptom burden score, mean (±SD), in the whole sample were shortness of breath, 2.4 (±1.0); dry mouth, 1.6 (±1.4); cough, 1.4 (±1.1); sleep problems, 1.4 (±1.4); lack of energy, 1.3 (±1.3); and pain, 1.2 (±1.4). The mean (±SD) MSAS symptom burden scores for moderate and severe airflow limitations are presented in Table 3. Patients with moderate airflow limitation had significantly lower MSAS symptom burden scores for shortness of breath than patients with severe airflow limitation (Table 3)" (Eckerblad et al., 2014, p. 353).

TABLE 3	COMPARISON OF PHYSICAL AND PSYCHOLOGICAL MSAS SYMPTOM BURDEN SCORE BETWEEN PATIENTS WITH MODERATE AND SEVERE AIRFLOW LIMITATION		
	MSAS Symptom Burden Score		
	Moderate *n* = 42 Mean (*SD*)	Severe *n* = 49 Mean (*SD*)	*p* Value
Physical Symptoms			
Shortness of breath	2.12 ± (1.09)	2.58 ± (0.90)	0.02
Cough	1.56 ± (1.16)	1.24 ± (1.06)	0.22
Dry mouth	1.38 ± (1.42)	1.81 ± (1.27)	0.17
Lack of energy	1.01 ± (1.22)	1.53 ± (1.37)	0.10
Feeling drowsy	0.82 ± (1.04)	1.07 ± (1.12)	0.32
Pain	1.35 ± (1.46)	0.99 ± (1.31)	0.20
Numbness/tingling in hands/feet	0.91 ± (1.16)	0.53 ± (1.03)	0.07
Feeling bloated	0.56 ± (1.22)	0.49 ± (1.17)	0.78
Dizziness	0.49 ± (0.88)	0.74 ± (1.20)	0.43
Sweats	0.47 ± (0.96)	0.65 ± (1.06)	0.38
Psychological Symptoms			
Difficulty sleeping	1.26 ± (1.44)	1.44 ± (1.43)	0.54
Worrying	0.73 ± (0.99)	0.71 ± (1.17)	0.68
Feeling irritable	0.55 ± (1.00)	0.52 ± (0.94)	0.88

The MSAS symptom burden score is the average of the frequency, severity, and distress associated with each symptom. Analyses performed with the Mann-Whitney *U*-test. Only symptoms reported by ≥25% of the patients are included in this table.

Eckerblad, J., Tödt, K., Jakobsson, P, Unosson, M., Skargren, E., Kentsson, M., & Theander, K. (2014). Symptom burden in stable COPD patients with moderate or severe airflow limitation. *Heart & Lung, 43*(4), p. 354.

The MSAS is a Likert-type scale that measured symptom frequency and severity on scales of 1 to 4 (with 1 being low and 4 being high) and distress on a scale of 0.8 = not at all to 4.0 = very much (see previous discussion of the scale). The frequency, severity, and distress scores were summed to obtain the MSAS symptom burden scores. Likert scale data are often considered interval-level data, especially if the data are summed to obtain total scores. These summed scores are analyzed with parametric analysis techniques if the scores are normally distributed, not skewed. However, Eckerblad et al. (2014, p. 353) indicated that the "MSAS symptom scores are presented as the mean (*SD*) for comparison with previous research, although the data are skewed." Since the data collected with the MSAS are skewed or not normally distributed, the nonparametric Mann-Whitney *U* test was calculated to determine differences between the moderate and severe airflow limitation groups for reported physical and psychological symptoms (see Table 3), using a significance level of *p* ≤ 0.05 (Kim & Mallory, 2017; Pett, 2016).

STUDY QUESTIONS

1. What is the purpose of the Mann-Whitney *U* statistical technique? Document your response.

2. Mann-Whitney *U* is the appropriate statistical test to use in which of the following situations:

   a. Correlation or relationship between two variables is being examined in a descriptive correlational study.
   b. Interval/ratio-level data with a non-normal distribution of scores for a study variable.
   c. The difference between two dependent or paired groups is being examined in a quasi-experimental study.
   d. The data collected on study variables are at the nominal level of measurement.
   Provide a rationale for your answer.

3. In a quasi-experimental study, data were collected from an intervention group of 100 individuals who were randomly assigned to receive cognitive behavioral counseling for their depression and a comparison group of 100 patients receiving standard care. The data were collected using the Center for Epidemiologic Studies Depression Scale (CES-D scale) and found to be normally distributed. What analysis technique needs to be conducted to determine differences in depression between the intervention and comparison groups? Provide a rationale for your answer.

4. State the null hypothesis for the Eckerblad et al. (2014) study regarding psychological symptoms experienced by the moderate and severe airflow limitation groups.

5. Was the null hypothesis in Question 4 accepted or rejected? Provide a rationale for your answer.

6. What was the total number of the research participants for this study? Could this sample size have contributed to the nonsignificant findings? Provide a rationale for your answer.

7. What was the mean (*SD*) for the total sample for lack of energy? Describe the meaning of these results.

8. Was there a significant difference between the moderate and severe airflow limitation groups for lack of energy? Provide a rationale for your response.

9. What psychological symptom had the highest MSAS symptom burden scores for both the moderate and severe airflow limitation groups? Provide results that support your answer.

10. What is the clinical importance of knowing the psychological symptom that had the highest MSAS symptom burden score for both the moderate and severe airflow limitation groups? Document your response.

Answers to Study Questions

1. The Mann-Whitney U test is a nonparametric statistical technique used to detect differences between two independent samples (Kim & Mallory, 2017; Knapp, 2017; Plichta & Kelvin, 2013). You might use a variety of statistical sources for documenting your answer.

2. b. Interval/ratio-level data with a non-normal distribution of scores on a study variable is correct. The Mann-Whitney U test is appropriate for analyzing interval/ratio-level data when the requirements for conducting a parametric test cannot be satisfied, i.e., when the collected data have a non-normal or skewed distribution. The Mann-Whitney U test is designed to determine differences between groups and not test for relationships between variables. The Mann-Whitney U test is to be used with independent and not dependent or paired groups and is for at least ordinal-level data and not nominal-level data (Pett, 2016).

3. The t-test for independent groups is the most appropriate analysis technique. The CES-D Scale is a Likert scale, and the data from these scales are considered interval level (see Exercise 1; Gray et al., 2017; Kim & Mallory, 2017). Since the data were normally distributed and at the interval level of measurement, parametric analyses can be conducted on the data. The two groups are independent because the study participants were randomly assigned to the intervention and comparison groups (Kazdin, 2017). The focus of the analysis is difference between two groups so the most appropriate analysis technique is the t-test for independent groups (see the algorithm in Exercise 12).

4. The null hypothesis: *There are no differences between the moderate and severe airflow limitation groups for reported psychological symptoms.*

5. The null hypothesis was accepted because no significant differences were found between the moderate and severe airflow limitation groups for psychological symptoms. Eckerblad et al. (2014) indicated in their study that the significance level was set at $p \leq 0.05$. Review the p values in Table 3 for the psychological symptoms. All the p values are > 0.05, indicating no statistically significant differences between the groups for psychological symptoms.

6. Sample size $N = 91$ for the study. The sample size might have been too small to detect small differences between the moderate and severe airflow limitation groups for the physical and psychological symptoms. The Eckerblad et al. (2014) study did not include power analysis results to identify the appropriate sample size. Descriptive studies require larger samples when several variables are being examined as in this study. Thus, the study would have been stronger if power analysis results were included and the study was conducted with a larger sample (Aberson, 2019; Cohen, 1988).

7. The lack of energy for the total sample had mean = 1.3 and $SD \pm 1.3$. Answer is in the narrative results for the study. Lack of energy was one of six symptoms that had high MSAS symptom burden score. However, shortness of breath, dry mouth, cough, and sleep problems had higher MSAS symptom burden scores than lack of energy.

236

8. There was no significant difference between the moderate and severe airflow limitation groups for lack of energy as indicated by $p = 0.10$ (see Table 3). This result is not statistically significant since it is greater than the level of significance for this study that was set at $p \leq 0.05$.

9. Difficulty sleeping was the psychological symptom that had the highest burden scores as indicated by mean = 1.26 for the moderate airflow limitation group and a mean = 1.44 for the severe airflow limitation group. Difficulty sleeping had the highest means in both groups, and the higher the mean the greater the burden scores for the participants in these groups (Grove & Gray, 2019).

10. The clinical importance is that patients with COPD who have either moderate or severe airflow limitations have identified difficulty sleeping as their number one psychological symptom. Management of these patients requires assessment, diagnosis, and management of sleeping disorders. The Global Initiative for Chronic Obstructive Lung Disease website is an excellent resource for evidence-based guidelines at http://www.goldcopd.org/Guidelines/guidelines-resources.html. Cochrane Library in England has a large collection of systematic reviews and evidence-based guidelines and includes several resources on COPD (see http://www.cochrane.org and search for COPD). You might document with other websites, research articles, or textbooks that focus on generation of research evidence for practice (Melnyk & Fineout-Overholt, 2019).

Questions to Be Graded

Name: _____ Class: _____

Date: _____

Follow your instructor's directions to submit your answers to the following questions for grading. Your instructor may ask you to write your answers below and submit them as a hard copy for grading. Alternatively, your instructor may ask you to submit your answers online.

1. What type of measurement method is the Memorial Symptom Assessment Scale (MSAS) that was used to collect data in the Eckerblad et al. (2014) study? The data collected with this scale are at what level of measurement? Provide a rationale for your answer.

2. What statistical technique was computed to determine differences between the moderate and severe airflow limitation groups for physical and psychological symptom burden scores? What was the rationale for using this technique?

3. What statistics were used to describe the physical and psychological symptoms presented in Table 3? Were these statistics appropriate for describing the MSAS symptom burden scores? Provide a rationale for your answer.

4. What statistics were more appropriate to describe the physical and psychological symptoms in Table 3? Provide a rationale for your answer.

5. State the null hypothesis for the Eckerblad et al. (2014) study focused on examining the differences in shortness of breath between the moderate and severe airflow limitation groups.

6. Was the null hypothesis in Question 5 accepted or rejected? Provide a rationale for your answer.

7. Was there a significant difference between the moderate and severe airflow limitation groups for cough? Provide a rationale for your response.

8. Provide at least three possible reasons for the nonsignificant results in Table 3.

9. What physical symptom had the highest MSAS symptom burden score for the whole sample? Provide the results that support your answer.

10. Discuss the clinical importance of the results about shortness of breath experienced by both the moderate and severe airflow limitation groups. Document your response.

Understanding Wilcoxon Signed-Rank Test

STATISTICAL TECHNIQUE IN REVIEW

The **Wilcoxon signed-rank test** is a nonparametric test conducted to examine differences or changes that occur between the first and second observations, such as "pretest or posttest measures for a single sample or subjects who have been matched on certain criteria" (Pett, 2016, p. 111). The Wilcoxon signed-rank test is an appropriate alternative to the paired-samples *t*-test when the assumptions for the *t*-test are not met. For example, the Wilcoxon signed-rank test would be calculated when the data were interval or ratio level but were not normally distributed. This nonparametric test is powerful in the sense that it not only examines the direction of the change but also the degree of the change. The Wilcoxon signed-rank test requires a calculation of a difference score for each pair of scores. The greater the amount of change, the more weight the pair is given, and when no change occurs, the pair is omitted and the sample size is decreased (Daniel, 2000). This test is especially effective when the sample size is small (Pett, 2016). In summary, the Wilcoxon signed-rank test is a strong statistical technique used to examine differences for related groups when the data are ordinal level or when the data are interval/ratio level but not normally distributed (Daniel, 2000; Kim & Mallory, 2017; Pett, 2016).

RESEARCH ARTICLE

Source

Dal'Ava, N., Bahamondes, L., Bahamondes, M. V., Bottura, B. F., & Monteiro, I. (2014). Body weight and body composition of depot medroxyprogesterone acetate users. *Contraception, 90*(2), 182–187.

Introduction

According to Dal'Ava and colleagues (2014), obesity is a global public health concern. Depot medroxyprogesterone acetate (DMPA), a progestin-only contraceptive, has previously been associated with an increase in weight among users, resulting in subsequent discontinuation of the contraceptive by some users. Dal'Ava et al. (2014, p. 182) conducted a prospective cohort study for the purpose of comparing "body weight (BW) and body composition (BC) in DMPA and copper intrauterine device (IUD) users at baseline and after one year of use." Ninety-seven adult women who self-selected to use DMPA or the TCu 380A IUD at selected sites in Brazil were recruited, and 26 matched pairs completed the study.

A power analysis was conducted prior to the initiation of the study with a power of 80% and a significance level of 0.05. This analysis indicated the group sizes should include a minimum of 20 cases. "The new DMPA users were matched by age ($\pm$2 years) and weight ($\pm$2 kg) to new IUD users at the beginning of the study. The exclusion criteria consisted of: breastfeeding; the use of DMPA in the previous 6 months; any disease that affects body mass such as diabetes mellitus, pituitary disorders, liver and kidney disorders, and cancer; the use of corticosteroids, diuretics, thyroid hormones, growth hormone therapy; and eating disorders, such as bulimia and anorexia" (Dal'Ava et al., 2014, p. 183). Matched samples' data are analyzed using paired samples t-test (see Exercise 17) for interval/ratio-level data or Wilcoxon signed-rank test for ordinal level data or non-normally distributed interval/ratio-level data. At baseline, the DMPA and IUD groups had no significant differences for the variables age, body mass index (BMI), parity, race (% White), coffee consumption, alcohol use, smoking, previous breastfeeding, or physical activity. At baseline, the BMI means for the DMPA and TCu 380A IUD groups were 25.3 and 26.2, respectively; both BMI means are categorized as overweight.

"An increase of 1.9 kg occurred in BW ($p = 0.02$) in DMPA users at 12 months of use, resulting from an increase in fat mass of 1.6 kg ($p = 0.03$). Weight remained stable in IUD users; however, there was an increase in lean mass at 12 months of use ($p = 0.001$). The number of women practicing physical activity increased in the TCu 380A IUD group" (Dal'Ava et al., 2014, p. 182). In this study, nutrition was not assessed and physical activity was measured as a dichotomous variable of $\geq$150 minutes a week of specific physical activities. Dal'Ava et al. (2014, p. 187) recommends future research "evaluate caloric intake and energy expenditure" to assess the role of DMPA in weight gain and "to evaluate whether body composition can be modified by caloric intake and physical activity during DMPA use."

Relevant Study Results

"After 12 months' use of the contraceptive method, DMPA users experienced a mean increase in weight of 1.9 ± 3.5 kg ($p = 0.02$), whereas weight remained stable in the women in the IUD group (1.1 ± 3.2 kg, $p = 0.15$). Nevertheless, there was no significant difference in weight between the two groups ($p = 0.38$). The DMPA group gained a mean of 1.6 ± 3.4 kg ($p = 0.03$) of fat mass, while women in the IUD group gained a mean of 1.3 ± 2.3 kg of lean mass ($p = 0.001$). After 12 months of use, fat mass distribution (the percent variation in central fat and in peripheral fat) did not change significantly within each group. Nevertheless, there was a significant increase of 5.0% in the percentage of overall fat mass in the DMPA group compared to a reduction of 2.2% in the IUD users ($p = 0.03$). Additionally, an increase of 4.6% was found in the central-to-peripheral fat ratio in the women in the DMPA group ($p = 0.04$); however, a slight reduction of 3.7% was also found in the women in the IUD group ($p = 0.03$) (Table 2)" (Dal'Ava et al., 2014, p. 185).

TABLE 2   VARIATION IN BODY COMPOSITION OVER 12 MONTHS ACCORDING TO THE CONTRACEPTIVE METHOD USED

Body Composition	DMPA (n = 26) Mean (±SD)	TCu 380A IUD (n = 26) Mean (±SD)	p Value
Baseline weight (kg)	65.0 (±12.8)	65.1 (±13.2)	0.98[a]
Weight at 12 months (kg)	66.9 (±13.7)	66.2 (±15.2)	0.80[a]
Δ weight gain (kg)	1.9 (±3.5)	1.1 (±3.2)	0.38[a]
p Value	0.02[b]	0.15[b]	
Fat mass at baseline (kg)	25.5 (±9.1)	28.5 (±9.3)	0.27[a]
Fat mass at 12 months (kg)	27.1 (±9.1)	27.7 (±10.8)	0.88[a]
Variation in fat mass (kg)	1.6 (±3.4)	−0.9 (±7.2)	0.14[b]
p Value	0.03[b]	0.71[b]	
Lean mass at baseline (kg)	37.8 (±4.8)	34.6 (±6.1)	0.19[a]
Lean mass at 12 months (kg)	37.2 (±5.4)	35.9 (±5.4)	0.43[a]
Variation in lean mass (kg)	0.3 (±1.8)	1.2 (±2.3)	0.11[b]
p Value	0.62[b]	0.001[b]	
Central-to-peripheral fat ratio at baseline	0.89 (±0.17)	0.88 (±0.13)	0.48[a]
Central-to-peripheral fat ratio at 12 months	0.87 (±0.19)	0.85 (±0.14)	0.31[a]
p Value	0.96[b]	0.03[b]	
Variation in central fat (%)	4.56 (±14.1)	−3.69 (±10.9)	0.04[a]
p Value	0.25[a]	0.08[a]	
Variation in peripheral fat (%)	1.80 (±9.17)	−0.7 (±4.49)	12[a]
p Value	0.22[a]	0.28[a]	

[a]Student's t-test paired.
[b]Wilcoxon paired test.

Dal'Ava, N., Bahamondes, L., Bahamondes, M. V., Bottura, B. F., & Monteiro, I. (2014). Body weight and body composition of depot medroxyprogesterone acetate users. *Contraception, 90*(2), p. 185.

STUDY QUESTIONS

1. What was the sample size for this study? Were the number of subjects in the depot-medroxyprogesterone acetate (DMPA) and copper intrauterine device (TCu 380A IUD) groups adequate? Provide a rationale for your answer.

2. What two types of analyses (displayed in Table 2) were conducted by Dal'Ava et al. (2014) to examine differences in matched samples?

3. What are the mean value and standard deviation (SD) for baseline weight (kg) for the DMPA group? What was the mean value and standard deviation (SD) for weight (kg) at 12 months for the DMPA group? What is the mean value and standard deviation (SD) for change weight gain (kg) for the DMPA group?

4. What was the p value for the Wilcoxon signed-rank test for change in weight gain (kg) for the DMPA group? Is this p value statistically significant? Provide a rationale for your answer.

5. What was the p value for the Wilcoxon signed-rank test for change in weight gain for the TCu 380A IUD group? Is this p value statistically significant? Provide a rationale for your answer.

6. State the null hypothesis for variation in fat mass from baseline to 12 months for the DMPA group. Should this null hypothesis be accepted or rejected? Provide a rationale for your answer.

7. State the null hypothesis for variation in central-to-peripheral fat ratio from baseline to 12 months for the DMPA group. Should this null hypothesis be accepted or rejected? Provide a rationale for your answer.

8. What Wilcoxon signed-rank test result on Table 2 is $p = 0.14$? Is this p value statistically significant? Provide a rationale for your answer.

9. Describe one potential clinical application of the Dal'Ava et al. (2014) study results.

10. Moore, Finch, Mac Arthur, and Ward (2018) implemented a clinical simulation intervention to cross-train staff and enhance perceptions of teamwork when hospital units are merged for budget reasons. The Wilcoxon signed-ranks test result was $p = 0.012$ for the perceptions of teamwork. Discuss the meaning of this result. This article can be found in the Resource Library for this text.

Answers to Study Questions

1. The sample size was 26 matched pairs consisting of 52 women, $n = 26$ depot-medroxyprogesterone acetate (DMPA) and $n = 26$ copper intrauterine device (TCu 380A IUD), as indicated by the study narrative and Table 2. Yes, the number of subjects in each group was adequate based on the power analysis recommendation of a minimum of 20 subjects per group (Aberson, 2019; Gray, Grove, & Sutherland, 2017). The groups were of equal size, which is another study strength (Grove & Gray, 2019).

2. According to Table 2 and the study narrative, both parametric paired samples t-test (Student's t-test paired) and nonparametric Wilcoxon signed-rank test were conducted to examine differences in these paired samples. On Table 2, t-test results are labeled with an "a" and Wilcoxon results are labeled with a "b." Two types of pairs were examined: differences in baseline measurements and 12 months measurements (pretest and posttest measures) as well as differences between DMPA and TCu 380A IUD matched pairs. Wilcoxon signed-rank test p values for differences from baseline to 12 months for the DMPA group are reported in the DMPA column in Table 2 and differences from baseline to 12 months for the TCu 380A IUD group are reported in the TCu 380A IUD column in Table 2. Wilcoxon signed-rank test p values for differences between the DMPA group and TCu 380 IUD are reported in the p value column in Table 2.

3. The mean value for baseline weight is 65.0 kg with a standard deviation (SD) ± 12.8, and the mean value for weight at 12 months is 66.9 kg with an SD ± 13.7 for the DMPA group. The mean change in weight gain was 1.9 kg with an SD ± 3.5 for the DMPA group.

4. For the DMPA group, the Wilcoxon signed-rank test resulted in $p = 0.02$ for the change in weight gain from baseline to 12 months, meaning weight (kg) was significantly greater 12 months after initiating DMPA use when compared with baseline weight. The value for statistical significance for this study was set at $\alpha = 0.05$. Thus, the results for the change in weight gain for the DMPA sample is statistically significant because $p = 0.02$ is less than $\alpha = 0.05$ (Grove & Gray, 2019).

5. For the TCu 380A IUD group, the Wilcoxon signed-rank test resulted in $p = 0.15$ for the change in weight gain, meaning weight (kg) was not significantly changed 12 months after initiating the TCu 380A IUD when compared with baseline weight. The value of $p = 0.15$ is not statistically significant because this p value is greater than $\alpha = 0.05$ set for this study (Pett, 2016).

6. Null hypothesis: *There is no variation in fat mass from baseline to 12 months for the DMPA group.* The Wilcoxon signed-rank test resulted in $p = 0.03$ for variation in fat mass from baseline to 12 months for the DMPA group, which is significant because it is less than $\alpha = 0.05$. When the results are significant, the null hypothesis is rejected (Grove & Gray, 2019).

7. Null hypothesis: *There is no variation in central-to-peripheral fat ratio from baseline to 12 months for the DMPA group.* The Wilcoxon signed-rank test resulted in $p = 0.96$ for variation in central-to-peripheral fat ratio from baseline to 12 months for the DMPA group. Because this p value is greater than $\alpha = 0.05$, the result was nonsignificant and the null hypothesis was accepted (Pett, 2016).

8. The Wilcoxon signed-rank test result for variation in fat mass (kg) for DMPA and TCu 380A IUD group in Table 2 is $p = 0.14$. This p value is greater than $\alpha = 0.05$ set for this study so this result is not statistically significant.

9. Answers may vary. Clinical implications may include patient education on the potential risk of weight gain for DMPA users or the potential benefit of exercise in maintaining weight for TCu 380A users. The Centers for Disease Control and Prevention (CDC) has contraception information for consumers and healthcare providers at http://www.cdc.gov/reproductivehealth/UnintendedPregnancy/Contraception.htm and obesity, weight, and healthy lifestyle information at http://www.cdc.gov/obesity/index.html.

   The National Institutes of Health (NIH) has a healthy weight resource that contains family and provider information including BMI calculator at http://www.nhlbi.nih.gov/health/education/lose_wt/index.htm.

10. The Moore et al. (2018) study result of $p = 0.012$ for perceptions of teamwork indicated that the clinical simulation intervention was significantly effective in promoting the nursing staff's perceptions of teamwork. The result was significant because $p = 0.012$ is less than alpha set a 0.05 for this study.

Questions to Be Graded

Name: _____ Class: _____

Date: _____

Follow your instructor's directions to submit your answers to the following questions for grading. Your instructor may ask you to write your answers below and submit them as a hard copy for grading. Alternatively, your instructor may ask you to submit your answers online.

1. What are the mean and standard deviation (*SD*) for central-to-peripheral fat ratio at baseline for the depot-medroxyprogesterone acetate (DMPA) user group in the Dal'Ava et al. (2014) study? What are the mean and standard deviation (*SD*) for central-to-peripheral fat ratio at baseline for the TCu 380A intrauterine device (IUD) user group?

2. What criteria were used to match the pairs of subjects from the DMPA and TCu 380A IUD groups? What were the study exclusion criteria? What is the purpose of the study exclusion criteria?

3. According to the study narrative, at baseline there were no statistically significant differences between the DMPA and TCu 380A IUD groups for what nine variables? What do these results indicate?

4. Dal'Ava et al. (2014) took steps such as matching criteria and assessing relevant variables at baseline to help ensure the matched pairs from the two groups (DMPA and TCu 380A IUD) were equivalent. In your opinion, do you believe these steps were sufficient to create equivalent matched pairs and groups? Provide a rationale for your answer.

5. What was the p value for the Wilcoxon signed-rank test for variation in lean mass (kg) between the DMPA and TCu 380A IUD groups? Is this p value statistically significant? Provide a rationale for your answer.

6. State the null hypothesis for variation in central-to-peripheral fat ratio (kg) from baseline to 12 months for the TCu 380A IUD group. Should the null hypothesis be accepted or rejected? Provide a rationale for your answer.

7. What Wilcoxon signed-rank test result in Table 2 is $p = 0.001$? Is this p value statistically significant? Is this result clinically important? Provide rationales for your answers.

8. What was the p value for the Wilcoxon signed-rank test for variation in fat mass from baseline to 12 months for the TCu 380A IUD group? Is this p value statistically significant? Provide a rationales for your answer.

9. Dal'Ava et al. (2014) reports a statistically significant ($p = 0.02$) weight change of 1.9 kg from baseline to 12 months for the DMPA group. In your own opinion, is this result clinically important? Provide a rationale for your answer.

10. Are the Dal'Ava et al. (2014) findings ready for use in practice? Provide a rationale for your answer.

PART 2

Conducting and Interpreting Statistical Analyses

Selecting Appropriate Analysis Techniques for Studies

Multiple factors are involved in determining the suitability of a statistical procedure for a particular study. Some of these factors are related to the nature of the study, some to the nature of the researcher, and others to the nature of statistical theory. Specific factors include the following: (1) purpose of the study; (2) study hypotheses, questions, or objectives; (3) study design; (4) level of measurement of variables in a study; (5) previous experience in statistical analysis; (6) statistical knowledge level; (7) availability of statistical consultation; (8) financial resources; and (9) access and knowledge of statistical software. Use items 1 to 4 to identify statistical procedures that meet the requirements of a particular study, and then further narrow your options through the process of elimination based on items 5 through 9.

The most important factor to examine when choosing a statistical procedure is the study hypothesis or primary research question. The hypothesis that is clearly stated indicates the statistic(s) needed to test it. An example of a clearly developed hypothesis is, *There is a difference in employment rates between veterans who receive vocational rehabilitation and veterans who are on a wait-list control.* This statement tells the researcher that a statistic to determine differences between two groups is appropriate to address this hypothesis. This statement also informs the researcher that the dependent variable is a rate, which is dichotomous: employed or unemployed.

One approach to selecting an appropriate statistical procedure or judging the appropriateness of an analysis technique is to use an algorithm or decision tree. A statistical algorithm directs your choices by gradually narrowing your options through the decisions you make. A statistical algorithm developed by Cipher (2019) that can be helpful in selecting statistical procedures is presented in Figure 23-1. This is the same algorithm presented and reviewed in Exercise 12 for determining the appropriateness of the statistical tests and results presented in research reports.

One disadvantage of statistical algorithm is that if you make an incorrect or uninformed decision (guess), you can be led down a path in which you might select an inappropriate statistical procedure for your study. Algorithms are often constrained by space and therefore do not include all the information needed to make an appropriate selection of a statistical procedure for a study. The following examples of questions are designed to guide the selection or evaluation of statistical procedures that are reflected in Figure 23-1. Each question confronts you with a decision, and the decision you make narrows the field of available statistical procedures.

1. Is the research question/hypothesis descriptive, associational (correlational), or difference-oriented?
2. How many variables are involved?
3. What is the measurement scale (see Exercise 1) of the independent and dependent variable(s)?

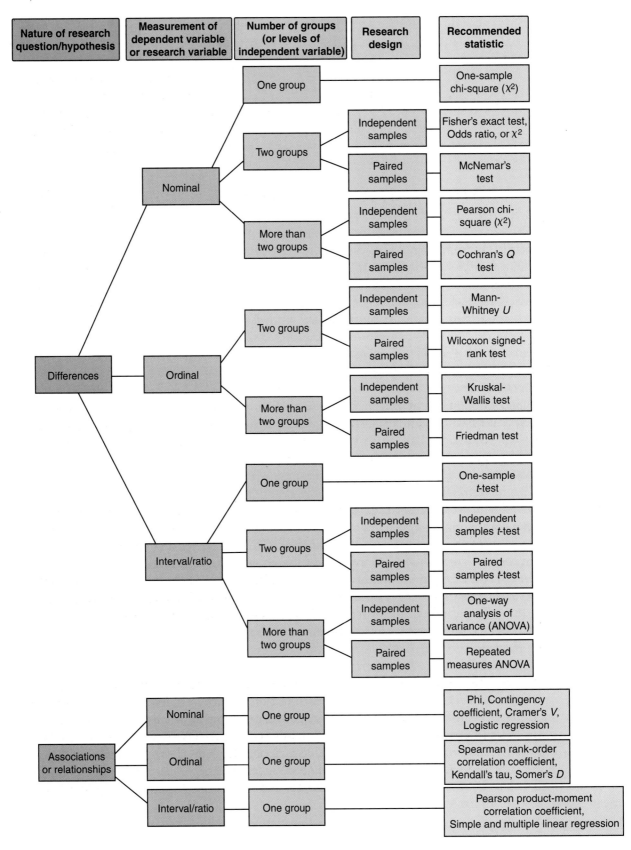

FIGURE 23-1 ■ **STATISTICAL SELECTION ALGORITHM.**

4. What is the distribution of the dependent variables (normal, non-normal)?
5. Do the data meet the assumptions for a parametric statistic?

As you can see, selecting and evaluating statistical procedures requires that you make a number of judgments regarding the nature of the data and what you want to know. Knowledge of the statistical procedures and their assumptions is necessary for selecting appropriate procedures. You must weigh the advantages and disadvantages of various statistical options. Access to a statistician can be invaluable in selecting the appropriate procedures.

STATISTICS TO ADDRESS BASIC DIFFERENCE RESEARCH QUESTIONS AND HYPOTHESES

The following statistics address research questions or hypotheses that involve differences between groups or assessments. This list is by no means exhaustive, but it represents the most common parametric and nonparametric inferential statistics involving differences. Exercise 12 discusses the concepts of parametric versus nonparametric statistics and inferential versus descriptive statistics.

t-Test for Independent Samples

One of the most common statistical tests chosen to investigate differences between two independent samples is the independent samples t-test, which is a parametric inferential statistic. The independent samples t-test only compares two groups at a time, and the dependent variable must be continuous and normally distributed (Zar, 2010). The independent samples t-test is reviewed in Exercise 16, and the process for conducting the independent samples t-test is in Exercise 31.

t-Test for Paired Samples

A paired samples t-test (also referred to as a dependent samples t-test) is a statistical procedure that compares two sets of data from one group of people (or naturally occurring pairs, such as siblings or spouses). This t-test is a parametric inferential statistical test. The dependent variable in a paired samples t-test must be continuous and normally distributed (Zar, 2010). The term *paired samples* refers to a research design that repeatedly assesses the same group of people, an approach commonly referred to as *repeated measures*. The t-test for paired samples is reviewed in Exercise 17, and the process for conducting the paired samples t-test is in Exercise 32.

One-Way Analysis of Variance (ANOVA)

The one-way analysis of variance (ANOVA) is a parametric inferential statistical procedure that compares data between two or more groups or conditions to investigate the presence of differences between those groups on some continuous, normally distributed dependent variable (see Figure 23-1). There are many types of ANOVAs. The one-way ANOVA involves testing one independent variable and one dependent variable (as opposed to other types of ANOVAs, such as factorial ANOVAs, that incorporate multiple independent variables). ANOVA is reviewed in Exercise 18, and the process for conducting ANOVA is presented in Exercise 33.

Repeated-Measures ANOVA

A repeated-measures ANOVA is a statistical procedure that compares multiple sets of data from one group of people. The dependent variable in a repeated-measures ANOVA must be continuous and normally distributed. The term *repeated measures* refers to a research design that repeatedly assesses the same group of people over time. Repeated measures can also refer to naturally occurring pairs, such as siblings or spouses (Gliner, Morgan, & Leech, 2009).

Mann-Whitney *U*

The Mann-Whitney *U* test is the nonparametric alternative to an independent samples *t*-test. Like the independent samples *t*-test, the Mann-Whitney *U* test is a statistical procedure that compares differences between two independent samples. However, the Mann-Whitney *U* is the preferred test over the independent samples *t*-test when the distribution of the dependent variable significantly deviates from normality, or the dependent variable is ordinal and cannot be treated as an interval/ratio scaled variable. The Mann-Whitney *U* is reviewed in Exercise 21.

Kruskal-Wallis Test

The Kruskal-Wallis test is the nonparametric alternative to the one-way ANOVA. Like the one-way ANOVA, the Kruskal-Wallis test is a statistical procedure that compares differences between two or more groups. However, the Kruskal-Wallis test is the preferred test over the ANOVA when the distribution of the dependent variable significantly deviates from normality, or the dependent variable is ordinal and cannot be treated as an interval/ratio scaled variable (Holmes, 2018; Kim & Mallory, 2017; Pett, 2016).

Friedman Test

The Friedman test is the nonparametric alternative to a repeated-measures ANOVA. Like the repeated-measures ANOVA, the Friedman test is a statistical procedure that compares multiple sets of data from one group of people. However, the Friedman test is the preferred test over the repeated-measures ANOVA when the dependent variable data significantly deviate from a normal distribution, or the dependent variable is ordinal and cannot be treated as an interval/ratio scaled variable (Pett, 2016).

Wilcoxon Signed-Rank Test

The Wilcoxon signed-rank test is the nonparametric alternative to the paired samples *t*-test. Like the paired samples *t*-test, the Wilcoxon signed-rank test is a statistical procedure that compares two sets of data from one group of people. However, the Wilcoxon signed-rank test is the preferred test over the paired samples *t*-test when the dependent variable data significantly deviate from a normal distribution, or the dependent variable is ordinal and cannot be treated as an interval/ratio scaled variable (Pett, 2016). The Wilcoxon signed-rank test is reviewed in Exercise 22.

Pearson Chi-Square Test

The Pearson chi-square test (χ^2) is a nonparametric inferential statistical test that compares differences between groups on variables measured at the nominal level. The χ^2 compares the frequencies that are observed with the frequencies that are expected. When a study requires that researchers compare proportions (percentages) in one category versus another category, the χ^2 is a statistic that will reveal if the difference in proportion is statistically improbable. A one-way χ^2 is a statistic that compares different levels of one variable only. A two-way χ^2 is a statistic that tests whether proportions in levels of one nominal variable are significantly different from proportions of the second nominal variable. The Pearson χ^2 test is reviewed in Exercise 19, and Exercise 35 provides the steps for conducting this test.

STATISTICS TO ADDRESS BASIC ASSOCIATIONAL/CORRELATIONAL RESEARCH QUESTIONS AND HYPOTHESES

The following statistics address research questions or hypotheses that involve associations or correlations between variables. This list is by no means exhaustive, but it represents the most common parametric and nonparametric inferential statistics involving associations.

Pearson Product-Moment Correlation Coefficient (r)

The Pearson product-moment correlation coefficient is a parametric inferential statistic computed between two continuous, normally distributed variables (see Figure 23-1). The Pearson correlation is represented by the statistic r, and the value of the r is always between –1.00 and +1.00. A value of zero indicates absolutely no relationship between the two variables; a positive correlation indicates that higher values of x are associated with higher values of y; and a negative, or inverse, correlation indicates that higher values of x are associated with lower values of y. The Pearson r is reviewed in Exercise 13, and Exercise 28 provides steps for conducting this analysis.

Spearman Rank-Order Correlation Coefficient

The Spearman rank-order correlation coefficient is the nonparametric alternative to the Pearson r. Like the Pearson correlation, the Spearman rank-order correlation is a statistical procedure that examines the association between two continuous variables. However, the Spearman rank-order correlation is the preferred test over the Pearson r when one or both of the variables of data significantly deviate from a normal distribution, or the variables are ordinal and cannot be treated as an interval/ratio scaled variable. The Spearman rank-order correlation is reviewed in Exercise 20.

Phi/Cramer's V

The phi (Φ) coefficient is the nonparametric alternative to the Pearson r when the two variables being correlated are both dichotomous. Like the Pearson r and Spearman rank-order correlation coefficient, the phi yields a value between –1.0 and 1.0, where a zero represents no association between the variables. The Cramer's V is the nonparametric alternative to the Pearson r when the two variables being correlated are both nominal. The Cramer's V yields a value between 0 and 1, where a zero represents no association between the variables and a 1 represents a perfect association between the variables.

Odds Ratio

When both the predictor and the dependent variables are dichotomous (variables that have only two values), the odds ratio is a commonly used statistic to obtain an indication of association. The odds ratio (OR) is defined as the ratio of the odds of an event occurring in one group to the odds of it occurring in another group. The OR can also be computed when the dependent variable is dichotomous and the predictor is continuous and would be computed by performing logistic regression analysis. Logistic regression analysis tests a predictor (or set of predictors) with a dichotomous dependent variable. Whether the predictor is dichotomous or continuous, an OR of 1.0 indicates that the predictor does not affect the odds of the outcome. An OR of >1.0 indicates that the predictor is associated with a higher odds of the outcome, and an OR of <1.0 indicates that predictor is associated with a lower odds of the outcome (Gordis, 2014). The steps for conducting the odds ratio are presented in Exercise 36.

Simple and Multiple Linear Regression

Linear regression is a procedure that provides an estimate of the value of a dependent variable based on the value of an independent variable or set of independent variables, also referred to as predictors. Knowing that estimate with some degree of accuracy, we can use regression analysis to predict the value of one variable if we know the value of the other variable. The regression equation is a mathematical expression of the influence that a predictor (or set of predictors) has on a dependent variable, based on a theoretical framework. A regression equation can be generated with a data set containing subjects' x and y values. The score on variable y (dependent variable, or outcome) is predicted from the same subject's known score on variable x (independent variable, or predictor) (King & Eckersley, 2019). Simple linear regression is reviewed in Exercise 14, and Exercise 29 provides the steps for conducting this analysis. Multiple linear regression is reviewed in Exercise 15, and Exercise 30 provides steps for conducting this analysis.

APPLYING INFERENTIAL STATISTICS TO POPULATION DATA

Secondary data analyses of large state and national data sets can be an economically feasible and time-efficient way for nurse researchers to address important health, epidemiological, and clinical research questions. However, data that were collected on a national level using complex sampling procedures, such as those survey data made available to researchers by the Centers for Disease Control and Prevention or the Centers for Medicare and Medicaid Services, require specific weighting procedures prior to computing inferential statistics. Aponte (2010) conducted a thorough review of publicly available population data sets with nurse researchers in mind and elaborated on the advantages and disadvantages of using population survey data.

When the researcher is analyzing secondary population-based data sets, much attention must be given to the quality of the data, the extent of missing data, and the manner in which the data were sampled. Analyses of secondary population data involve much data cleaning, which can include recoding, missing data imputation, and weighting for complex sampling approaches. *Point and click* software programs such as SPSS Statistics Base (*IBM SPSS Statistics for Windows, Version 22.0.* Armonk, NY: IBM Corp.) can be used by the researcher for data cleaning; however, they cannot be used to adjust the data for complex sampling. There are only a handful of statistical software programs that can address the adjustments for sampling required by population survey data (Aday & Cornelius, 2006; Aponte, 2010). When such data are analyzed without adjusting for sampling, the results are at risk for Type I error and are generally considered invalid (Aday & Cornelius, 2006). In this text, the exercises focused on calculating statistical analyses (Exercises 28–36) involve data from samples and not data from populations.

STUDY QUESTIONS

1. What statistic would be appropriate for an associational research question or hypothesis involving the correlation between two normally distributed continuous variables?

2. What statistic would be appropriate for a difference research question involving the comparison of two repeated assessments from one group of participants, where the dependent variable is measured at the interval/ratio level or is continuous and the data are normally distributed?

3. A nurse educator is interested in the difference between traditional clinical instruction in pediatrics and simulated pediatrics instruction in a BSN (Bachelor's of Science in Nursing) program. She randomizes students to receiving 50 hours of either traditional clinical rotations in a pediatrics department or 50 hours of simulated instruction in pediatrics. At the end of the 50 hours, the students are assessed for clinical competency in pediatrics using a standardized instrument that yields a continuous score, where higher values represent higher levels of competency. Her research question is: *Is there a difference between the traditional clinical group and the simulation group on clinical competency?* What is the appropriate statistic to address the research question, if the scores are normally distributed?

4. What is the appropriate statistic to address the research question in Question 3 above if the scores are *NOT* normally distributed?

5. What statistic would be appropriate for a difference research question involving the comparison of two groups on a dichotomous dependent variable?

6. A diabetes educator wants to track diabetic patients' progress throughout an educational program for glycemic control. She collects each of her patients' HbA1c levels at baseline, again halfway through the educational program, and once again at the end of the program (a total of three HbA1c values). Her research question is: *Did the patients' glycemic control (as measured by HbA1c values) change over the course of the program, from baseline to end of program?* What is the appropriate statistic to address the research question, if the HbA1c values are normally distributed?

7. What is the appropriate statistic to address the research question in Question 6 above if the scores are *NOT* normally distributed?

8. In the scenario presented in Question 6 above, the researcher also collected data on the participants, such as gender, duration of disease, age, and depression levels. Her research question is: *Do gender, duration of disease, age, and depression levels predict baseline HbA1c levels?* What is the appropriate statistic to address the research question, if the baseline HbA1c levels are normally distributed?

9. What statistic would be appropriate for a difference research question involving the comparison of three independent groups on a normally distributed continuous dependent variable?

10. What statistic would be appropriate for a difference research question involving the comparison of three independent groups on a non-normally distributed, skewed, continuous dependent variable?

Answers to Study Questions

1. A Pearson r is an appropriate statistic to test an association between two normally distributed continuous variables or variables measured at the interval or ratio level.

2. A paired samples t-test is an appropriate statistic to compare two repeated assessments from one group of participants, where the dependent variable is continuous or measured at the interval/ratio level and the data are normally distributed (see Figure 23-1).

3. An independent samples t-test is an appropriate statistic to compare two groups on a normally distributed continuous dependent variable (clinical competency scores).

4. Mann-Whitney U is an appropriate statistic to compare two independent groups on a non-normally distributed continuous dependent variable.

5. A Pearson chi-square test is an appropriate statistic to compare two groups on a dichotomous dependent variable.

6. A repeated-measures ANOVA is an appropriate statistic to compare three or more repeated assessments of the HbA1C from one group of diabetic patients, where the dependent variable is normally distributed (see Figure 23-1).

7. A Friedman test is an appropriate statistic to compare three or more repeated assessments from one group of participants, where the dependent variable is not normally distributed.

8. Multiple linear regression is the appropriate statistical procedure that tests the extent to which a set of variables predicts a normally distributed dependent variable.

9. A one-way ANOVA is an appropriate statistic to compare three independent groups on a normally distributed continuous dependent variable.

10. A Kruskal-Wallis test is an appropriate statistic to compare three independent groups on a non-normally, skewed continuous dependent variable (see Figure 23-1).

Questions to Be Graded

Name: _____ Class: _____

Date: _____ _____

Follow your instructor's directions to submit your answers to the following questions for grading. Your instructor may ask you to write your answers below and submit them as a hard copy for grading. Alternatively, your instructor may ask you to submit your answers online.

1. A researcher surveyed two groups of professionals, nurse practitioners and physicians, and asked them whether or not they supported expanding the role of nurse practitioners' (NPs) prescribing privileges, answered as either "yes" or "no." Her research question is: *Is there a difference between NPs and physicians on proportions of support for expanded prescription privileges?* What is the appropriate statistic to address the research question?

2. What statistic would be appropriate for an associational research question involving the correlation between two non-normally distributed, skewed continuous variables?

3. A researcher is interested in the extent to which years of practice among NPs predicts level of support for expanded prescription privileges, measured on a 10-point Likert scale. She finds that both variables, years of practice and level of support, are normally distributed. Her research question is: *Does years of practice among NPs predict level of support for expanded prescription privileges?* What is the appropriate statistic to address the research question?

4. What statistic would be appropriate for a difference research question involving the comparison of two independent groups on a normally distributed continuous dependent variable?

5. A statistics professor tests her students' level of knowledge at the beginning of the semester and administers the same test at the end of the semester. She compares the two sets of continuous scores. Her research question is: *Is there a difference in statistics knowledge from the beginning to the end of the semester?* What is the appropriate statistic to address the research question, if the scores are normally distributed?

6. What is the appropriate statistic to address the research question in Question 5 if the scores are *NOT* normally distributed?

7. What is the appropriate statistic to identify the association between two dichotomous variables, where the researcher is interested in identifying the odds of an outcome occurring?

8. What statistic would be appropriate for a difference research question involving the comparison of two independent groups on a non-normally distributed, skewed continuous dependent variable?

9. A nurse educator is interested in the difference between traditional clinical instruction in pediatrics and simulated pediatrics instruction in a BSN (Bachelor's of Science in Nursing) program. She randomizes students to receiving 50 hours of either traditional clinical rotations in a pediatrics department or 50 hours of simulated instruction in pediatrics. At the end of the 50 hours, the students are assessed for clinical competency in pediatrics using a standardized instrument that yields a pass/fail result. Her research question is: *Is there a difference in between the traditional clinical group and the simulation group on rates of passing the competency assessment?* What is the appropriate statistic to address the research question?

10. What statistic would be appropriate for an associational research question involving the extent to which a set of variables predict a continuous, normally distributed dependent variable?

EXERCISE 24

Describing the Elements of Power Analysis: Power, Effect Size, Alpha, and Sample Size

The deciding factor in determining an adequate sample size for descriptive, correlational, quasi-experimental, and experimental studies is power. **Power** is the probability that a statistical test will detect an effect when it actually exists. Therefore, power is the inverse of Type II error and is calculated as $1 - \beta$. Type II error is the probability of retaining the null hypothesis when it is in fact false. When the researcher sets Type II error at the conventional value of 0.20 prior to conducting a study, this means that the power of the planned statistic has been set to 0.80. In other words, the statistic will have an 80% chance of detecting an effect if an effect actually exists.

Power analysis can address the number of participants required for a study or, conversely, the extent of the power of a statistical test. A power analysis performed prior to the study beginning to determine the required number of participants needed to identify an effect is termed an **a priori power analysis**. A power analysis performed after the study ends to determine the power of the statistical result is termed a **post hoc power analysis**. Optimally, the power analysis is performed prior to the study beginning so that the researcher can plan to include an adequate number of participants. Otherwise, the researcher risks conducting a study with an inadequate number of participants and putting the study at risk for Type II error (Taylor & Spurlock, 2018). The four factors involved in a power analysis are as follows:

1. Level of significance (α, or alpha level), usually 0.05.
2. Probability of obtaining a significant result (power desired, or $1 - \beta$), usually 0.80.
3. The hypothesized or actual effect (association among variables or difference between your groups).
4. Sample size.

Knowing any of the three factors listed above allows researchers to compute the fourth (Cohen, 1988; Hayat, 2013). Significance (α) level and sample size are fairly straightforward. **Effect size** is "the degree to which the phenomenon is present in the population, or the degree to which the null hypothesis is false" (Cohen, 1988, pp. 9–10). For example, suppose you were measuring changes in anxiety levels, measured first when the patient is at home and then just before surgery. The effect size would be large if you expected a great change in anxiety. If you expected only a small change in the level of anxiety, the effect size would be small.

Small effect sizes require larger samples to detect these small differences. If the power is too low, it may not be worthwhile conducting the study unless a sample large enough to detect an effect can be obtained. Deciding to conduct a study in these circumstances is costly in terms of time and money, minimally adds to the body of nursing knowledge,

270

and can actually lead to false conclusions (Taylor & Spurlock, 2018). Power analysis can be conducted via hand calculations, computer software, or online calculators and should be performed to determine the sample size necessary for a particular study (Aberson, 2019). For example, a power analysis can be calculated by using the free power analysis software G*Power (Faul, Erdfelder, Lang, & Buchner, 2009) or statistical software such as NCSS, SAS, and SPSS. Moreover, there are many free sample size calculators online that are easy to use and understand.

The notion of whether researchers should conduct a post hoc power analysis after a study fails to reject the null hypothesis has been greatly debated (Hayat, 2013). This is because there is a strong association between the p value of the finding and the post hoc power; the lower the p value, the higher the power, and vice versa. Therefore any finding that fails to yield statistical significance will inevitably be associated with low power (Levine & Ensom, 2001). Because of this phenomenon, reporting a post hoc power analysis may be considered redundant. On the other hand, if power was high, the post hoc power analysis may strengthen the meaning of the findings. Many researchers advocate the reporting of effect sizes and confidence intervals in the results of research articles in addition to or instead of post hoc power analyses (Hayat, 2013; Levine & Ensom, 2001).

One appropriate context for a post hoc power analysis might be an exploratory pilot study, when a researcher analyzes the study data and reports the obtained effect size on which to base a future study (Hayat, 2013). For any study that results in low statistical power, the researcher needs to address this issue in the discussion of limitations and implications of the study findings. Modifications in the research methodology that resulted from the use of power analysis also need to be reported. Therefore, the researcher must evaluate the elements of the methodology that affect the required sample size, which include the following:

1. Statistical power corresponds to one type of statistical test at a time. If the researcher is planning to compute different categories of statistical tests, in order to adequately power the study one must perform a power analysis for each planned statistical procedure (Hayat, 2013). For example, if the researcher is planning an ANOVA to address the first research question, and a χ^2 to address the second research question, the study will not be adequately powered unless both statistical tests are addressed with power analyses. In this example, the researcher would need to perform two power analyses, one for each research objective or hypothesis.
2. The more stringent the α (e.g., 0.001 vs. 0.05), the greater the necessary sample size due to the reduced probability of a Type I error. With $\alpha = 0.001$, the probability of Type I error is 1 chance in 1000; with $\alpha = 0.05$, there are 5 chances for error in 100 analyses conducted.
3. Two-tailed statistical tests require larger sample sizes than one-tailed tests because two-tailed tests require a larger critical statistical value to yield significance than a one-tailed test (Plichta & Kelvin, 2013; Zar, 2010).
4. The smaller the effect size, the larger the necessary sample size because the effect size indicates how strong the relationship is between variables and the strength of the differences between groups (Taylor & Spurlock, 2018).
5. The larger the power required, the larger the necessary sample size. For example, a power set at 0.90 requires a larger sample size than the standard power set at 0.80.
6. The smaller the sample size, the smaller the power of the study (Cohen, 1988).

EFFECT SIZE

Cohen (1965) defined effect size as "a measure of the degree of difference or association deemed large enough to be of practical significance" (Cohen, 1962). There are many different types of effect size measures, and each corresponds to the type of statistic computed. A decision tree developed by Cipher that can be helpful in selecting statistical procedures is presented in Figure 23-1 of Exercise 23 in this text. The researcher needs to have identified the statistic(s) required to address the research question or hypothesis prior to conducting the power analysis. For example, if we were planning to compute an independent samples t-test, then the effect size in the power analysis would be a Cohen's d (Cohen, 1988). If we were planning to compute one-way ANOVA, then the effect size in the power analysis would be a Cohen's f. A Pearson correlation coefficient (r) serves as its own effect size, as does the odds ratio. Table 24-1 is a compilation of seven of the most common effect sizes used in power analyses. This table was created by extracting the information presented in the seminal text on power analysis by Cohen (1988) and provides three magnitudes of effects: small, moderate, and large.

TABLE 24-1   MAGNITUDE RANGES OF SEVEN COMMON EFFECT SIZES

Effect Size	Cohen's d	Cohen's d_z	Cohen's f	r	R^2	OR	d
Small	0.20	0.20	0.10	0.10	0.02	1.5	0.05
Moderate	0.50	0.50	0.25	0.30	0.13	2.5	0.15
Large	0.80	0.80	0.40	0.50	0.26	4.3	0.25

Cohen's d = difference between two groups in standard deviation units
Cohen's d_z = difference between two paired assessments when the correlation between the pairs is $r = 0.50$
Cohen's f = difference between more than two groups
r = Pearson r
R^2 = variance explained in linear regression model
OR = odds ratio.
d = difference between proportions when one of the two groups' rates = 50%

Cohen's d

The most common effect size measure for a two-sample design (that is, a two-group comparison) is Cohen's d. Cohen's d is calculated as follows:

$$d = \frac{\bar{X}_1 - \bar{X}_2}{SD}$$

where $\bar{X}_1$ and $\bar{X}_2$ are the means for Groups 1 and 2, respectively, and the SD would be the standard deviation of either group, considering that both groups are assumed to have approximately equal SDs.

The resulting d value represents the difference between the means of Groups 1 and 2, in SD units. Thus, a value of 1.0 means that the two groups differed exactly 1 SD unit from one another. One can still compute the Cohen's d even if the design has more than two groups, but the Cohen's d is calculated one pair at a time. However, the more appropriate effect size for comparing three or more groups, such as a one-way ANOVA, is the f.

Cohen's d_z

Cohen's d_z is almost identical to Cohen's d above, except the d_z applies to paired samples instead of independent samples. Like Cohen's d, Cohen's d_z also represents the difference between two means in SD units. However, Cohen's d_z is computed with two means of paired values. These paired values are most often from one group of people, but they can also be comprised of paired data from naturally occurring pairs, such as siblings or spouses.

When the correlation (r) between the paired values is approximately $r = 0.50$, then the ranges of the magnitude of effect in terms of small, moderate, and large are the same as that of Cohen's d, where small = 0.20, moderate = 0.50, and large = 0.80 or greater. However, when the correlation between the paired values is smaller, then the resulting magnitude of effect is smaller. Likewise, when the correlation between the paired values is larger, the resulting magnitude of effect is larger. For example, if there is a 0.50 mean difference between two paired samples, with a high r of the paired values at $r = 0.80$, the $d_z = 0.79$ (a large effect). On the other hand, if there is a 0.50 mean difference between two paired samples, with a low r of the paired values at $r = 0.20$, the $d_z = 0.40$ (a small to moderate effect). Therefore the magnitude of the association between the pairs has a direct impact on the magnitude of the d_z value (Cohen, 1988).

Cohen's f

Like Cohen's d, Cohen's f also expresses effect size in standard deviation units but does so for two or more groups. When planning a one-way ANOVA, Cohen's f can be computed to determine the differences between the groups. Like the ANOVA, the Cohen's f will identify the magnitude of the differences among all of the groups, but it will not explain differences between specific groups. For two groups, $f = 1/2d$. Conversely, $d = 2f$ (Cohen, 1988).

Pearson r

The Pearson product-moment correlation coefficient was the first of the correlation measures developed and is computed on two continuous, approximately normally distributed variables (see Exercise 28). This coefficient (statistic) is represented by the letter r, and the value of the r is always between -1.00 and $+1.00$. A value of zero indicates absolutely no relationship between the two variables; a positive correlation indicates that higher values of x are associated with higher values of y; and a negative, or inverse, correlation indicates that higher values of x are associated with lower values of y and vice versa. The r value is indicative of the slope of the line (called a regression line) that can be drawn through a standard scatterplot of the two variables. The strengths of different relationships are identified in Table 24-1.

R^2

The R^2, also referred to as the **coefficient of determination,** is the effect size for linear regression. The R^2 represents the percentage of variance explained in y by the predictor (see Exercise 29). Simple linear regression provides a means to estimate the value of a dependent variable based on the value of an independent variable. Multiple regression analysis is an extension of simple linear regression in which more than one independent variable is entered into the analysis to predict a dependent variable (see Exercise 30).

Odds Ratio

When both the predictor and the dependent variable are dichotomous, the odds ratio (OR) is a commonly used statistic to obtain an indication of association (see Exercise 36). The odds ratio is defined as the ratio of the odds of an event occurring in one group to the odds of it occurring in another group (Gordis, 2014). Put simply, the OR is a way of comparing whether the odds of a certain event is the same for two groups. The OR can also be computed when the dependent variable is dichotomous and the predictor is continuous, and would be computed by performing logistic regression analysis. Logistic regression analysis tests a predictor (or set of predictors) with a dichotomous dependent variable. The output yields an adjusted OR, meaning that each predictor's OR represents the relationship between that predictor and y, after adjusting for the presence of the other predictors in the model (Tabachnick & Fidell, 2013).

d

For a two-sample comparative design where the dependent variable is dichotomous, the d is the effect size used in the power analysis. The letter "d" represents the difference in percentages in Group 1 versus Group 2. One example might be to compare employment rates in an intervention and control groups. We have evidence that our control group will have a 50% employment rate, and the intervention will be 15% higher, at 65%. Thus, our anticipated d would be 65% − 50% = 15%. In Exercise 25, we will present a power analysis using each of the effect sizes described in this exercise.

STUDY QUESTIONS

1. Define statistical power.

2. List the four components of a power analysis.

3. Define power and beta and discuss the importance of power and beta in a study.

4. What is the difference between Cohen's d and Cohen's d_z?

5. Using the values in Table 24-1, what would be considered a large Pearson r? How would this value affect sample size for a study?

6. Prior to conducting a power analysis, a researcher reviewed the literature and discovered that a study similar to hers reported an OR value of 1.2. According to Table 24-1, how would you characterize the magnitude of that effect?

7. Prior to conducting a power analysis, a researcher reviewed the literature and discovered a similar study reported an R^2 value of 0.35, or 35%. According to Table 24-1, how would you characterize the magnitude of that effect?

8. Prior to performing the power analysis, a researcher debates whether to set the study α at 0.05 or 0.01. Which α level will require more study participants? Provide a rationale for your answer.

9. Prior to performing the power analysis, a researcher debates whether to set the study beta (β) at 0.15 or 0.20. Which beta level will require more study participants? Provide a rationale for your answer.

10. What is the difference between Cohen's d and d?

Answers to Study Questions

1. Power is the probability that a statistical test will detect an effect (that is, a difference between groups or a relationship between variables) when it actually exists.

2. The four components of a power analysis are alpha, power, effect size, and sample size (Aberson, 2019).

3. Beta (β) is the probability of making a Type II error, and power is the inverse of beta, or $1 - \beta$. Because of the inverse association between beta and power, lower values of beta allow for a larger likelihood of finding an effect when one is present (power).

4. Cohen's d is the effect size for a two-sample design for a continuous, normally distributed dependent variable, whereas Cohen's d_z is the effect size for a one-sample design for a continuous, normally distributed dependent variable. Both Cohen's d and Cohen's d_z represent the difference between two means in SD units. However, Cohen's d is computed with two independent means, and Cohen's d_z is computed with two means of paired values.

5. A large Pearson r would be any value of 0.50 or greater, and would result in a lower required sample size because a large effect size requires a lower critical statistical value to yield significance (Cohen, 1988; Taylor & Spurlock, 2018).

6. An OR value of 1.2 would be considered a small effect size.

7. An R^2 value of 35% would be considered a large effect size.

8. Setting the alpha at 0.01 will require more study participants. A smaller alpha requires a larger sample size because the statistical test will require a larger critical statistical value to yield significance (Gray, Grove, & Sutherland, 2017).

9. Setting the beta at 0.15 will require more study participants since there is less potential for error than with beta set at 0.20. With beta set at 0.15, the power is stronger (85%) than with beta set at 0.20 (80%) (Cohen, 1988).

10. Cohen's d is the effect size for a two-sample design for a continuous, normally distributed dependent variable, whereas d is the effect size for a two-sample design for a dichotomous dependent variable (Aberson, 2019; Cohen, 1988).

Questions to Be Graded

Name: _____ Class: _____

Date: _____

Follow your instructor's directions to submit your answers to the following questions for grading. Your instructor may ask you to write your answers below and submit them as a hard copy for grading. Alternatively, your instructor may ask you to submit your answers online.

1. When is the optimal time to perform a power analysis—before the beginning of the study or after the study ends? Provide a rationale for your answer.

2. Define *effect size*.

3. A researcher is planning to compute a Pearson *r*. What effect size measure should be used in the power analysis? Provide a rationale for your answer.

4. A researcher is planning to compute a one-way ANOVA. What effect size measure should be used in the power analysis? Provide a rationale for your answer.

5. A researcher is planning to compute an independent samples *t*-test. What effect size measure should be used in the power analysis?

6. A researcher is planning to perform paired samples *t*-test. What effect size measure should be used in the power analysis?

7. A study reported an *OR* of 1.70, which was not significant. The authors note that their power analysis was based on a large effect size. Can they accept the null hypothesis?

8. Before conducting a power analysis, you reviewed the literature and discovered that two similar studies reported Cohens *d* values of 0.50 and 0.75. Which effect will require more study participants? Provide a rationale for your answer.

9. Before conducting a power analysis, a researcher reviews the literature and discovered a similar study comparing differences between groups. The authors reported a d value of 27%. How would you characterize the magnitude of that effect?

10. A researcher plans a study whereby she will compute three statistical tests: a Pearson *r*, a paired samples *t*-test, and multiple regression. She performs a power analysis based on an anticipated R^2 and enrolls the required number of participants based on the results of that power analysis, states that the study has adequate statistical power, and begins the study. Is the researcher correct? Provide a rationale for your answer.

Conducting Power Analysis

EXERCISE

25

Exercise 24 described the components of a power analysis: α, power (1 − β), hypothesized effect, and sample size (N). Seven common effect sizes were presented: r, R^2, Cohen's d, Cohen's d_z, Cohen's f, d, and OR (Table 25-1). For an *a priori* power analysis, the researcher has already stated the research problem and the corresponding research question or hypothesis. Because the size of the effect in a power analysis is directly linked to the required sample size, it is crucial that the hypothesized effect be accurate. Sometimes, prior reports of a similar study or studies exist in the literature to determine the magnitude of the hypothesized effect chosen for the power analysis. Other times, a paucity of published studies hinders the researcher's ability to find effect size information. Effect size information includes any values in the study that allow the reader to directly or indirectly calculate an effect size. For example, reporting means and SDs would allow the reader to calculate a Cohen's d. A table of percentages for different groups would allow the reader to compute a d value (difference between rates).

It is very important to conduct an extensive search of the literature to yield the most accurate effect size information possible (Taylor & Spurlock, 2018). Sometimes, effect sizes found in the literature differ in magnitude. For example, a researcher may be investigating effects for an association between two variables of interest, and finds studies reporting Pearson r values of varying sizes. The process of deciding which effect size to use in one's own power analysis can be very difficult. The researcher must take into account the sample sizes of each study, the quality of the methodology, the quality of the measurement, and the similarity of the population to which the researcher plans to investigate. A study with a larger sample size using a sample with characteristics similar to the researcher's own target population is likely to yield the highest generalizability.

If the literature review does not produce any helpful effect size information, then the researcher may consider contacting other investigators in the field to obtain guidance (Hulley, Cummings, Browner, Grady, & Newman, 2013). A small pilot study could be conducted to obtain effect size information, although the typically smaller sample sizes used in pilot studies yield less stable or reliable effect size estimates because sample size affects power. If these options are not available, then the planned study should be considered a pilot study, because it has been established that it is the first of its kind to address the research question. Pilot studies, by and large, are by definition underpowered studies. Therefore, although a pilot study can provide useful information about the presence of an effect, the researcher should take caution in relying solely on this information when conducting a power analysis (Hayat, 2013). Ultimately, effects from prior published empirical studies are the preferred method to obtaining effect sizes for a *priori* power analyses.

G*Power 3.1 is a free power analysis software available for download (Faul, Erdfelder, Buchner, & Lang, 2009). The download is available at http://www.gpower.hhu.de/en.html. Exercise 25 presents seven power analyses using G*Power 3.1, one for each of the effect sizes presented in Exercise 24. Each of the seven power analyses present hypothetical effect sizes in the small, moderate, or large ranges, in order to provide the reader with the opportunity to perform power analyses using G*Power.

TABLE 25-1	MAGNITUDE RANGES OF SEVEN COMMON EFFECT SIZES						
Effect Size	**Cohen's d**	**Cohen's d_z**	**Cohen's f**	**r**	**R^2**	**OR**	**d**
Small	0.20	0.20	0.10	0.10	0.02	1.5	0.05
Moderate	0.50	0.50	0.25	0.30	0.13	2.5	0.15
Large	0.80	0.80	0.40	0.50	0.26	4.3	0.25

Cohen's d = difference between two groups in standard deviation units
Cohen's d_z = difference between two paired assessments when the correlation between the pairs is $r = 0.50$
Cohen's f = difference between more than two groups
r = Pearson r
R^2 = variance explained in linear regression model
OR = Odds ratio.
d = difference between proportions when one of the two groups' rates = 50%

POWER ANALYSIS 1: COHEN'S *d*

Cohen's *d* is an effect that represents the magnitude of the difference between two groups expressed in standard deviation units. The following instructions outline the steps required to perform a hypothetical power analysis with a *moderate* anticipated effect size of Cohen's *d* = 0.50 (see Table 25-1), α = 0.05, and power = 0.80.

Step 1: Open G*Power 3.1.

Step 2: Select "t-tests" from the pull-down menu labeled "Test family."

Step 3: Select "Means: Differences between two independent means (two groups)" from the pull-down menu labeled "Statistical test."

Step 4: Make sure that the type of power analysis listed is "A priori: Compute required sample size—given α, power, and effect size." This is the default setting.

Step 5: In the "Input parameters" section, select a two-tailed test.

Step 6: Enter the hypothesized effect next to "Effect size d." For our example, it will be 0.50.

Step 7: Enter the α next to "α err prob." For our example, it will be 0.05.

Step 8: Enter the desired power next to "Power (1 − β err prob)." For our example, it will be 0.80.

Step 9: Leave "Allocation ratio N2/N1" at 1 unless there is a specific reason to anticipate unequal sample sizes.

Step 10: Click Calculate. The window should look like the screen shot in Figure 25-1.

As can be observed in Figure 25-1, 128 total participants are required (64 in each group) to test a study hypothesis using an independent samples *t*-test, based on a *moderate* Cohen's *d* of 0.50, α = 0.05, and power = 0.80.

POWER ANALYSIS 2: COHEN'S *f*

When planning a one-way ANOVA, Cohen's *f* can be computed to determine the differences between the groups. Like the ANOVA, Cohen's *f* will identify the magnitude of the differences among the groups, but it will not explain differences between specific groups.

The following instructions outline the steps required to perform a hypothetical power analysis for a three-group design with a *small* anticipated effect size of $f = 0.10$ (see Table 25-1), $\alpha = 0.05$, and power = 0.80.

Step 1: Open G*Power 3.1.

Step 2: Select "F-tests" from the pull-down menu labeled "Test family."

Step 3: Select "ANOVA: Fixed effects, omnibus, one-way" from the pull-down menu labeled "Statistical test."

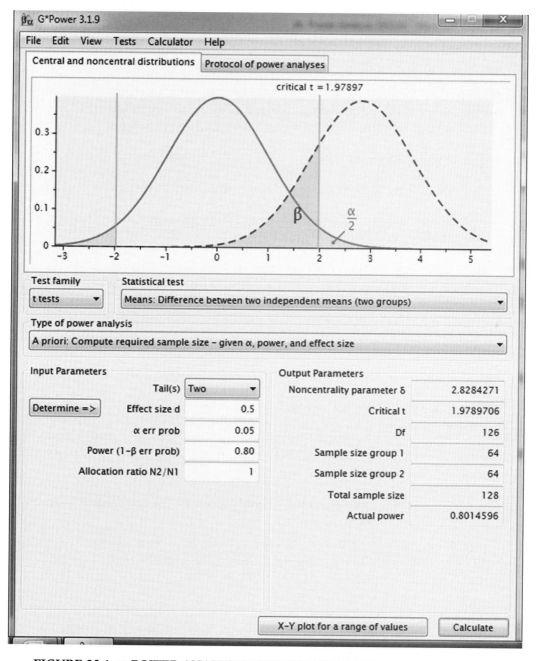

FIGURE 25-1 ■ **POWER ANALYSIS RESULTS OF A MODERATE HYPOTHESIZED COHEN'S *d*, $\alpha = 0.05$, AND POWER = 0.80.**

Step 4: Make sure that the type of power analysis listed is "A priori: Compute required sample size—given α, power, and effect size." This is the default setting.

Step 5: In the "Input parameters" section, select a two-tailed test.

Step 6: Enter the hypothesized effect next to "Effect size f." For our example, it will be 0.10.

Step 7: Enter the α next to "α err prob." For our example, it will be 0.05.

Step 8: Enter the desired power next to "Power (1 − β err prob)." For our example, it will be 0.80.

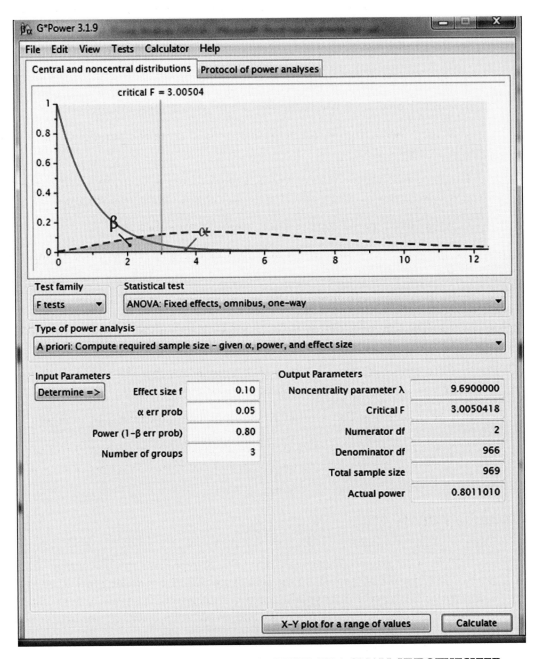

FIGURE 25-2 ■ **POWER ANALYSIS RESULTS OF A SMALL HYPOTHESIZED COHEN'S f, α = 0.05, AND POWER = 0.80, WITH THREE GROUPS.**

Step 9: Enter 3 next to "Number of groups."

Step 10: Click Calculate. The window should look like the screen shot in Figure 25-2.

As can be observed in Figure 25-2, 969 total participants are required (323 in each group) to test a study hypothesis using a three-group one-way ANOVA based on a Cohen's f of 0.10, $\alpha = 0.05$, and power $= 0.80$.

POWER ANALYSIS 3: PEARSON *r*

The Pearson product-moment correlation is always between -1.00 and $+1.00$, where a value of zero indicates absolutely no relationship between the two variables (see Exercises 13 and 28). The following instructions outline the steps required to perform a power analysis with a *large* anticipated effect size of $r = 0.50$ (see Table 25-1), $\alpha = 0.05$, and power $= 0.80$.

Step 1: Open G*Power 3.1.

Step 2: Select "Exact" from the pull-down menu labeled "Test family."

Step 3: Select "Correlation: Bivariate normal model" from the pull-down menu labeled "Statistical test."

Step 4: Make sure that the type of power analysis listed is "A priori: Compute required sample size—given α, power, and effect size." This is the default setting.

Step 5: In the "Input parameters" section, choose a two-tailed test.

Step 6: Enter the hypothesized effect next to "Correlation ρ H1." For our example, it will be 0.50.

Step 7: Enter the α next to "α err prob." For our example, it will be 0.05.

Step 8: Enter the desired power next to "Power (1 − β err prob)." For our example, it will be 0.80.

Step 9: Enter 0 next to "Correlation ρ H0." This means that the null hypothesis states that there is no correlation between the two variables ($r = 0.0$).

Step 10: Click Calculate. The window should look like the screen shot in Figure 25-3.

As can be observed in Figure 25-3, 29 total participants are required to test a study hypothesis using a Pearson correlation coefficient, based on a Pearson r of 0.50, $\alpha = 0.05$, and power $= 0.80$.

POWER ANALYSIS 4: R^2

The R^2 is the effect size for linear regression. The R^2 represents the percentage of variance explained in y by the predictor (see Exercises 14 and 29). The following instructions outline the steps required to perform a hypothetical power analysis with a *moderate* anticipated effect size of $R^2 = 0.15$ (see Table 25-1), $\alpha = 0.05$, and power $= 0.80$, with a three-predictor model.

Step 1: Open G*Power 3.1.

Step 2: Select "F-Tests" from the pull-down menu labeled "Test family."

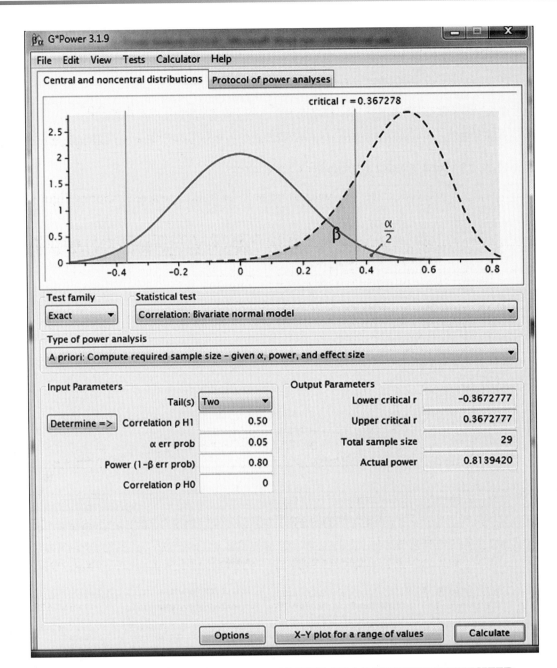

FIGURE 25-3 ■ **POWER ANALYSIS RESULTS OF A LARGE HYPOTHESIZED PEARSON *r*, α = 0.05, AND POWER = 0.80.**

Step 3: Select "Linear multiple regression: Fixed model, R^2 deviation from zero" from the pull-down menu labeled "Statistical test."

Step 4: Make sure that the type of power analysis listed is "A priori: Compute required sample size—given α, power, and effect size." This is the default setting.

Step 5: Underneath the phrase "Input parameters," click "Determine." A window will slide out to the right of your screen. This is so you can convert your hypothesized R^2 value to an f^2 value, which is what G*Power uses to perform a power analysis for multiple regression.

Step 6: Enter the hypothesized effect next to "Squared multiple correlation ρ^2." For our example, it will be 0.15.

Step 7: Click "Calculate and transfer to main window."

Step 8: Enter the α next to "α err prob." For our example, it will be 0.05.

Step 9: Enter the desired power next to "Power $(1 - \beta$ err prob)." For our example, it will be 0.80.

Step 10: Enter 3 next to "Number of predictors."

Step 11: Click Calculate. The window should look like the screen shot in Figure 25-4.

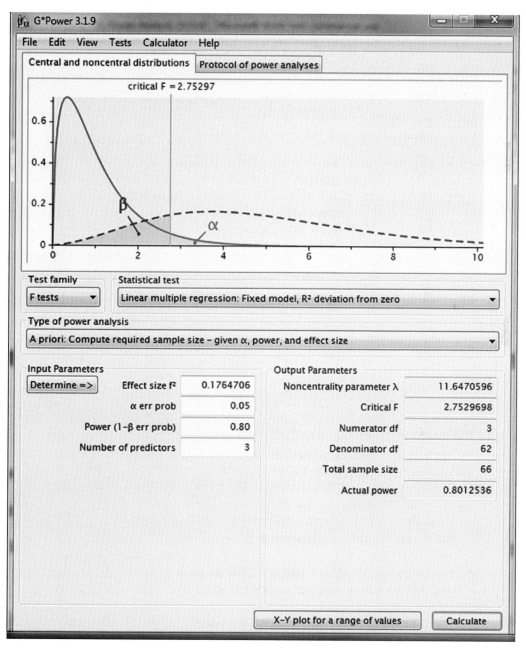

FIGURE 25-4 ▪ **POWER ANALYSIS RESULTS OF A MODERATE HYPOTHESIZED R^2, $\alpha = 0.05$, AND POWER = 0.80.**

As can be observed in Figure 25-4, 66 total participants are required to test a study hypothesis using a three-predictor multiple regression model, based on an R^2 of 0.15, $\alpha = 0.05$, and power $= 0.80$.

POWER ANALYSIS 5: ODDS RATIO

An *OR* is computed when the dependent variable is dichotomous and the predictor is either continuous or dichotomous. With multiple predictors, *OR*s are computed by performing logistic regression analysis. Logistic regression analysis tests a predictor (or set of predictors) with a dichotomous dependent variable (Tabachnick & Fidell, 2013). Because an *OR* in a power analysis is often being planned within the context of logistic regression, the following example uses the logistic regression feature of G*Power. The following instructions outline the steps required to perform a hypothetical power analysis with a *small* anticipated effect size of *OR* $= 1.5$ (see Table 25-1), $\alpha = 0.05$, and power $= 0.80$.

Step 1: Open G*Power 3.1.

Step 2: Select "z-tests" from the pull-down menu labeled "Test family."

Step 3: Select "Logistic regression" from the pull-down menu labeled "Statistical test."

Step 4: Make sure that the type of power analysis listed is "A priori: Compute required sample size—given α, power, and effect size." This is the default setting.

Step 5: In the "Input parameters" section, choose a two-tailed test.

Step 6: Enter the hypothesized effect next to "Odds ratio." For our example, it will be 1.5.

Step 7: Enter 0.30 next to "Pr(Y=1|X=1) H0."

Step 8: Enter the α next to "α err prob." For our example, it will be 0.05.

Step 9: Enter the desired power next to "Power (1 − β err prob)." For our example, it will be 0.80.

Step 10: Leave the default value of 0 next to "R^2 other predictors."

Step 11: Select "Binomial" from the pull-down menu next to "X distribution."

Step 12: Click Calculate. The window should look like the screen shot in Figure 25-5.

As can be observed in Figure 25-5, 853 total participants are required to test a study hypothesis using an unadjusted odds ratio, based on an *OR* of 1.5, $\alpha = 0.05$, and power $= 0.80$.

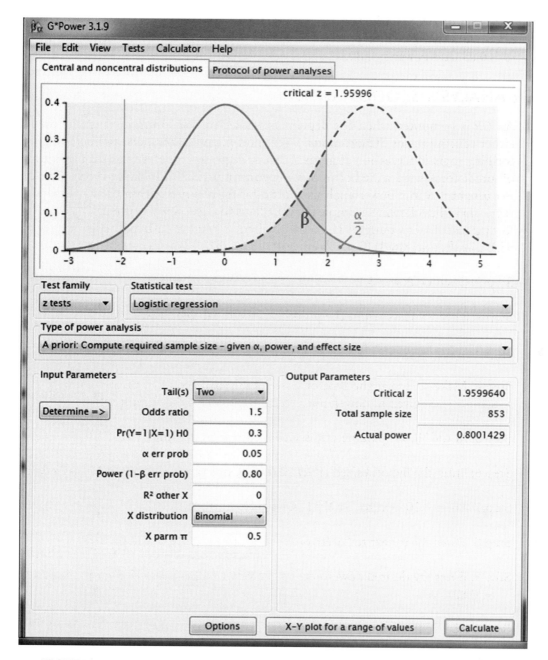

FIGURE 25-5 ■ **POWER ANALYSIS RESULTS OF A SMALL HYPOTHESIZED OR, α = 0.05, AND POWER = 0.80.**

POWER ANALYSIS 6: d

When both the predictor and the dependent variable are dichotomous, you may use either the *OR* or the d as the effect size in a power analysis. However, the d is the preferred effect size in a power analysis for a two-sample comparative design where the dependent variable is dichotomous. Recall that the letter "d" represents the difference in percentages in Group 1 versus Group 2. A power analysis based on the effect size d can involve any two pairs of proportions. However, in this exercise, for ease of understanding one proportion will always be 0.50, or 50%. This is because the ranges of effect size magnitudes in Table 25-1 for d only apply when one group's proportion is 50% (Cohen, 1988). The following instructions outline the steps required to perform a hypothetical power analysis with a *large* anticipated effect size of d = 0.25, α = 0.05, and power = 0.80.

Step 1: Open G*Power 3.1.

Step 2: Select "Exact" from the pull-down menu labeled "Test family."

Step 3: Select "Proportions: Inequality, two independent groups (Fisher's exact test)" from the pull-down menu labeled "Statistical test."

Step 4: Make sure that the type of power analysis listed is "A priori: Compute required sample size—given α, power, and effect size." This is the default setting.

Step 5: In the "Input parameters" section, choose a two-tailed test.

Step 6: Enter the hypothesized proportions next to "Proportion p1 and Proportion p2." For our example, it will be 0.50 and 0.25 to represent a 25% difference. It does not matter which proportion, p1 or p2, is 0.25 and 0.50. Thus, 0.25 and 0.50 can be entered in p1 and p2, or vice versa.

Step 7: Enter the α next to "α err prob." For our example, it will be 0.05.

Step 8: Enter the desired power next to "Power (1 − β err prob)." For our example, it will be 0.80.

Step 9: Leave "Allocation ratio N2/N1" at 1 unless there is a specific reason to anticipate unequal sample sizes.

Step 10: Click Calculate. The window should look like the screen shot in Figure 25-6.

As can be observed in Figure 25-6, 128 total participants are required (64 in each group) to test a study hypothesis using a Fisher's exact test, based on a large d of 0.25, α = 0.05, and power = 0.80.

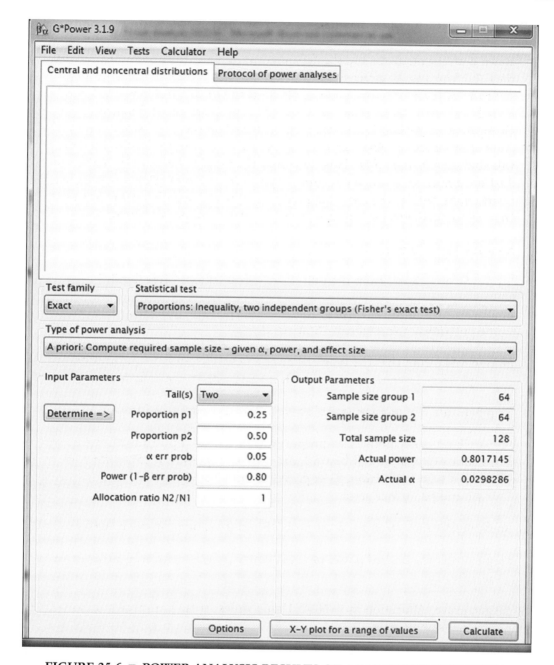

FIGURE 25-6 ▦ **POWER ANALYSIS RESULTS OF A LARGE HYPOTHESIZED d, α = 0.05, AND POWER = 0.80.**

POWER ANALYSIS 7: COHEN'S d_z

Cohen's d_z is an effect that represents the magnitude of the difference between two sets of paired data expressed in standard deviation units. The following instructions outline the steps required to perform a hypothetical power analysis with a *small* anticipated effect size of Cohen's $d_z = 0.20$ (see Table 25-1), α = 0.05, and power = 0.80.

Step 1: Open G*Power 3.1.

Step 2: Select "t-tests" from the pull-down menu labeled "Test family."

Step 3: Select "Means: Differences between two dependent means (matched pairs)" from the pull-down menu labeled "Statistical test."

Step 4: Make sure that the type of power analysis listed is "A priori: Compute required sample size—given α, power, and effect size." This is the default setting.

Step 5: In the "Input parameters" section, select a two-tailed test.

Step 6: Enter the hypothesized effect next to "Effect size d_z." For our example, it will be 0.20.

Step 7: Enter the α next to "α err prob." For our example, it will be 0.05.

Step 8: Enter the desired power next to "Power ($1 - \beta$ err prob)." For our example, it will be 0.80.

Step 9: Click Calculate. The window should look like the screen shot in Figure 25-7.

As can be observed in Figure 25-7, 199 total participants are required to test a study hypothesis using a paired samples *t*-test, based on a *small* Cohen's d_z of 0.20, α = 0.05, and power = 0.80.

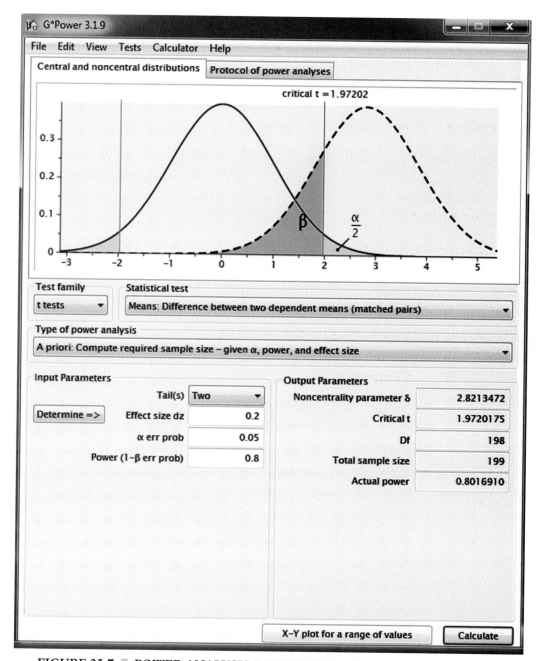

FIGURE 25-7 ▪ POWER ANALYSIS RESULTS OF A SMALL HYPOTHESIZED COHEN'S d_z, α = 0.05, AND POWER = 0.80.

STUDY QUESTIONS

1. Perform a power analysis based on a small hypothesized Cohen's d_z, $\alpha = 0.05$ and power $= 0.80$, two-tailed test, using G*Power. What is the required N?

2. Perform a power analysis based on a large hypothesized R^2 with four predictors in the model, $\alpha = 0.05$, and power $= 0.80$ using G*Power. What is the required N?

3. Perform a power analysis based on a large hypothesized three-group Cohen's f, $\alpha = 0.05$, and power $= 0.80$ using G*Power. What is the required N?

4. Redo your power analysis from Question 3 using a moderate hypothesized Cohen's f. How many more participants are required? Provide a rationale for the difference in the sample size.

5. Perform a power analysis based on a moderate hypothesized d where Group 1 $= 50\%$ and Group 2 $= 65\%$, $\alpha = 0.05$, and power $= 0.80$, two-tailed test, using G*Power. What is the required N?

6. Redo your power analysis from Question 5, using an α of 0.01. How many more participants are required? Provide a rationale for your difference in sample size.

7. Prior to conducting a power analysis, a researcher reviewed the literature and discovered that a study similar to hers reported a Cohen's *d* of 0.15. According to Table 25-1, how would you characterize the magnitude of that effect?

8. Perform a power analysis based on a moderate Pearson *r*, $\alpha = 0.05$, and power $= 0.80$, two-tailed test, using G*Power. What is the required *N*?

9. Redo your power analysis from Question 8, using a power of 85% instead of 80%. How many more participants are required? Provide a rationale for the change in sample size.

10. Prior to conducting a power analysis, a researcher reviewed the literature and discovered a similar study reported a Pearson *r* of 0.104. According to Table 25-1, how would you characterize the magnitude of that effect?

Answers to Study Questions

1. The required N would be 199.

Input Parameters		Output Parameters	
Tail(s) Two		Noncentrality parameter δ	2.8213472
Determine => Effect size dz	0.2	Critical t	1.9720175
α err prob	0.05	Df	198
Power (1–β err prob)	0.8	Total sample size	199
		Actual power	0.8016910

2. The required N would be 40.

Input Parameters		Output Parameters	
Determine => Effect size f²	0.3513514	Noncentrality parameter λ	14.0540560
α err prob	0.05	Critical F	2.6414652
Power (1–β err prob)	0.8	Numerator df	4
Number of predictors	4	Denominator df	35
		Total sample size	40
		Actual power	0.8127117

3. The required N would be 66.

Input Parameters		Output Parameters	
Determine => Effect size f	0.4	Noncentrality parameter λ	10.5600000
α err prob	0.05	Critical F	3.1428085
Power (1–β err prob)	0.8	Numerator df	2
Number of groups	3	Denominator df	63
		Total sample size	66
		Actual power	0.8180744

4. The required N would be 159, which would be 93 more participants than would be needed in Question 3. This example demonstrates that the smaller the anticipated effect size, the larger the sample size required to conduct the study.

Input Parameters		Output Parameters	
Determine => Effect size f	0.25	Noncentrality parameter λ	9.9375000
α err prob	0.05	Critical F	3.0540042
Power (1–β err prob)	0.8	Numerator df	2
Number of groups	3	Denominator df	156
		Total sample size	159
		Actual power	0.8048873

5. The required *N* would be 366.

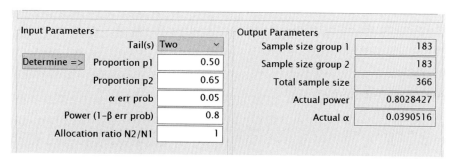

6. The required *N* would be 534, which would be 168 more participants than would be needed in Question 5. This example demonstrates that the smaller the alpha, the larger the sample size required to conduct the study.

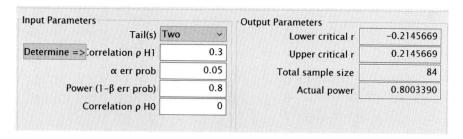

7. A Cohen's *d* of 0.15 would be considered a small effect according to Table 25-1.

8. The required *N* would be 84.

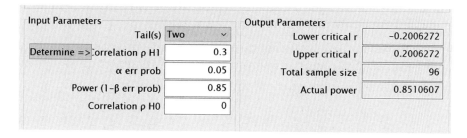

9. The required *N* would be 96, which would be 12 more participants than would be needed in Question 8. This example demonstrates that the larger the desired statistical power, the larger the sample size required to conduct the study.

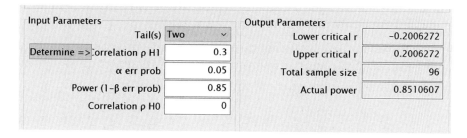

10. A Pearson *r* of 0.104 would be considered a small effect, because it is so close to .10 (a small effect according to Table 25-1).

Questions to Be Graded

Name: _____ Class: _____

Date: _____

Follow your instructor's directions to submit your answers to the following questions for grading. Your instructor may ask you to write your answers below and submit them as a hard copy for grading. Alternatively, your instructor may ask you to submit your answers online.

1. What is one approach a researcher can take when there is a lack of information in the literature concerning effect sizes that can be used as a basis for her power analysis?

2. Perform a power analysis based on a small hypothesized Cohen's d, $\alpha = 0.05$, and power $= 0.80$, two-tailed test, with two groups of equal size using G*Power. What is the required N?

3. Redo your power analysis from Question 2 using a power of 85% instead of 80%. How many more participants are required? Provide a rationale for the difference in sample size.

4. Perform a power analysis based on a moderate hypothesized Cohen's f with a four-group design, $\alpha = 0.05$, and power $= 0.80$ using G*Power. What is the required N?

5. Redo your power analysis from Question 4 using an α of 0.01. How many more participants are required? Provide a rationale for the difference in sample size.

6. Perform a power analysis based on a small hypothesized R^2 with two predictors in the model, $\alpha = 0.05$, and power $= 0.80$ using G*Power. What is the required N?

7. Redo your power analysis from Question 6 using four predictors instead of two. How many more participants are required? Provide a rationale for the difference in sample size.

8. Perform a power analysis based on a small hypothesized d where group 1 $= 45\%$ and group 2 $= 50\%$, $\alpha = 0.05$, and power $= 0.80$, two-tailed test, using G*Power. What is the required N?

9. Redo your power analysis from Question 8 using a one-tailed test. How many fewer participants are required? Provide a rationale for the difference in sample size.

10. Perform a power analysis based on a small Pearson r, $\alpha = 0.01$, and power $= 0.80$, two-tailed test, using G*Power. What is the required N?

Determining the Normality of a Distribution

Most parametric statistics require that the variables being studied are normally distributed. The normal curve has a symmetrical or equal distribution of scores around the mean with a small number of outliers in the two tails. The first step to determining normality is to create a frequency distribution of the variable(s) being studied. A frequency distribution can be displayed in a table or figure. A line graph figure can be created whereby the x axis consists of the possible values of that variable, and the y axis is the tally of each value. The frequency distributions presented in this Exercise focus on values of continuous variables. With a continuous variable, higher numbers represent more of that variable and the lower numbers represent less of that variable, or vice versa. Common examples of continuous variables are age, income, blood pressure, weight, height, pain levels, and health status (see Exercise 1; Waltz, Strickland, & Lenz, 2017).

The frequency distribution of a variable can be presented in a **frequency table,** which is a way of organizing the data by listing every possible value in the first column of numbers, and the frequency (tally) of each value as the second column of numbers. For example, consider the following hypothetical age data for patients from a primary care clinic. The ages of 20 patients were: 45, 26, 59, 51, 42, 28, 26, 32, 31, 55, 43, 47, 67, 39, 52, 48, 36, 42, 61, and 57.

First, we must sort the patients' ages from lowest to highest values:

26
26
28
31
32
36
39
42
42
43
45
47
48
51
52
55
57
59
61
67

Next, each age value is tallied to create the frequency. This is an example of an ungrouped frequency distribution. In an **ungrouped frequency distribution**, researchers list all categories of the variable on which they have data and tally each datum on the listing. In this example, all the different ages of the 20 patients are listed and then tallied for each age.

Age	Frequency
26	2
28	1
31	1
32	1
36	1
39	1
42	2
43	1
45	1
47	1
48	1
51	1
52	1
55	1
57	1
59	1
61	1
67	1

Because most of the ages in this dataset have frequencies of "1," it is better to group the ages into ranges of values. These ranges must be mutually exclusive (i.e., a patient's age can only be classified into one of the ranges). In addition, the ranges must be exhaustive, meaning that each patient's age will fit into at least one of the categories. For example, we may choose to have ranges of 10, so that the age ranges are 20 to 29, 30 to 39, 40 to 49, 50 to 59, and 60 to 69. We may choose to have ranges of 5, so that the age ranges are 20 to 24, 25 to 29, 30 to 34, etc. The grouping should be devised to provide the greatest possible meaning to the purpose of the study. If the data are to be compared with data in other studies, groupings should be similar to those of other studies in this field of research. Classifying data into groups results in the development of a **grouped frequency distribution**. Table 26-1 presents a grouped frequency distribution of patient ages classified by ranges of 10 years. Note that the range starts at "20" because there are no patient ages lower than 20, nor are there ages higher than 69.

Table 26-1 also includes percentages of patients with an age in each range; the cumulative percentages for the sample should add up to 100%. This table provides an example of a percentage distribution that indicates the percentage of the sample with scores falling into a specific group. Percentage distributions are particularly useful in comparing this study's data with results from other studies.

TABLE 26-1 GROUPED FREQUENCY DISTRIBUTION OF PATIENT AGES WITH PERCENTAGES

Adult Age Range	Frequency (*f*)	Percentage (%)	Cumulative Percentage
20–29	3	15%	15%
30–39	4	20%	35%
40–49	6	30%	65%
50–59	5	25%	90%
60–69	2	10%	100%
Total	20	100%	

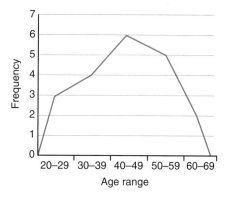

FIGURE 26-1 ■ **FREQUENCY DISTRIBUTION OF PATIENT AGE RANGES.**

As discussed earlier, frequency distributions can be presented in figures. The common figures used to present frequencies include graphs, charts, histograms, and frequency polygons. Figure 26-1 is a line graph of the frequency distribution for age ranges, where the x axis represents the different age ranges and the y axis represents the frequencies (tallies) of patients with ages in each of the ranges.

THE NORMAL CURVE

The theoretical normal curve is an expression of statistical theory. It is a theoretical frequency distribution of all *possible* scores (Figure 26-2). However, no real distribution exactly fits the normal curve. This theoretical normal curve is symmetrical, unimodal, and has continuous values. The mean, median, and mode are equal (see Figure 26-2). The distribution is completely defined by the mean and standard deviation, which are calculated and discussed in Exercises 8 and 27.

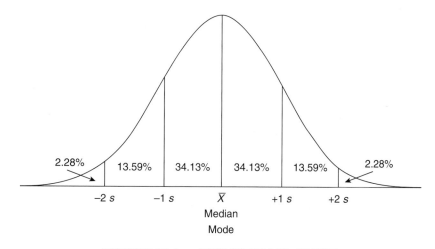

FIGURE 26-2 ■ **THE NORMAL CURVE.**

SKEWNESS

Any frequency distribution that is not symmetrical is referred to as **skewed** or **asymmetrical** (Holmes, 2018). Skewness may be exhibited in the curve in a variety of ways. A distribution may be **positively skewed**, which means that the largest portion of data is below the mean. For example, data on length of enrollment in hospice are positively skewed

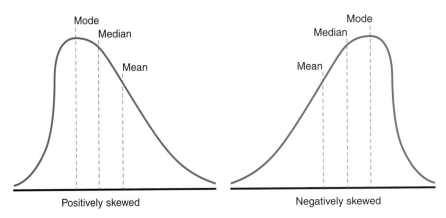

FIGURE 26-3 ■ **EXAMPLES OF POSITIVELY AND NEGATIVELY SKEWED DISTRIBUTIONS.**

because most of the people die within the first 3 weeks of enrollment, whereas increasingly smaller numbers of people survive as time increases. A distribution can also be **negatively skewed**, which means that the largest portion of data is above the mean. For example, data on the occurrence of chronic illness in an older age group are negatively skewed, because more chronic illnesses occur in seniors. Figure 26-3 includes both a positively skewed distribution and a negatively skewed distribution (Gray, Grove & Sutherland, 2017).

In a skewed distribution, the mean, median, and mode are not equal. Skewness interferes with the validity of many statistical analyses; therefore, statistical procedures have been developed to measure the skewness of the distribution of the sample being studied. Few samples will be perfectly symmetrical; however, as the deviation from symmetry increases, the seriousness of the impact on statistical analysis increases. In a positively skewed distribution, the mean is greater than the median, which is greater than the mode. In a negatively skewed distribution, the mean is less than the median, which is less than the mode (see Figure 26-3). The effects of skewness on the types of statistical analyses conducted in a study are discussed later in this exercise.

KURTOSIS

Another term used to describe the shape of the distribution curve is kurtosis. **Kurtosis** explains the degree of peakedness of the frequency distribution, which is related to the spread or variance of scores. An extremely peaked distribution is referred to as **leptokurtic**, an intermediate degree of kurtosis as **mesokurtic**, and a relatively flat distribution as **platykurtic** (see Figure 26-4). Extreme kurtosis can affect the validity of statistical analysis because the scores have little variation. Many computer programs analyze kurtosis before conducting statistical analyses. A kurtosis of zero indicates that the curve is mesokurtic, kurtosis values above zero indicate that the curve is leptokurtic, and values below zero that are negative indicate a platykurtic curve (Gray et al., 2017; Holmes, 2018).

TESTS OF NORMALITY

Skewness and kurtosis should be assessed prior to statistical analysis, and the importance of such non-normality needs to be determined by both the researcher and the statistician. Skewness and kurtosis statistic values of $\geq +1$ or ≥ -1 are fairly severe and could impact the outcomes from parametric analysis techniques. Because the severity of the deviation from symmetry compromises the validity of the parametric tests, nonparametric analysis

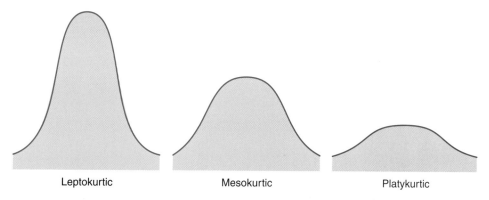

FIGURE 26-4 ▪ EXAMPLES OF KURTOTIC DISTRIBUTIONS.

techniques should be computed instead. Nonparametric statistics have no assumption that the distribution of scores be normally distributed (Daniel, 2000; Pett, 2016).

There are statistics that obtain an indication of *both* the skewness and kurtosis of a given frequency distribution. The Shapiro-Wilk's W test is a formal test of normality that assesses whether a variable's distribution is skewed and/or kurtotic (Kim & Mallory, 2017). Thus this test has the ability to calculate both skewness and kurtosis by comparing the shape of the variable's frequency distribution to that of a perfect normal curve. For large samples ($n > 2000$) the Kolmogorov-Smirnov D test is an alternative test of normality for large samples (Marsaglia, Tsang, & Wang, 2003).

SPSS COMPUTATION

A randomized experimental study examined the impact of a special type of vocational rehabilitation on employment among veterans with felony histories (LePage, Bradshaw, Cipher, Crawford, & Hooshyar, 2014). Age at study enrollment, age at first arrest, years of education, and number of times fired were among the study variables examined. A simulated subset of the study data is presented in Table 26-2.

ID	Age	Age at 1st Arrest	Education	Number Times Fired
TABLE 26-2		AGE, EDUCATION, AND TERMINATION HISTORY AMONG VETERANS WITH FELONIES		
1	46	19	13	2
2	56	23	13	3
3	48	24	12	5
4	50	19	12	6
5	58	21	11	0
6	41	20	12	1
7	56	14	12	1
8	56	12	14	0
9	47	23	12	0
10	52	38	12	3
11	63	16	14	0
12	60	59	12	1
13	62	17	12	3
14	49	19	11	2
15	60	31	13	0
16	56	28	12	3
17	52	43	12	0
18	58	27	14	0
19	43	29	12	0
20	63	42	14	0

This is how our dataset looks in SPSS.

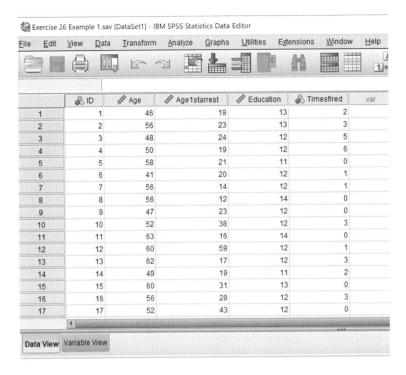

Step 1: From the "Analyze" menu, choose "Descriptive Statistics" and "Frequencies." Move the four study variables over to the right.

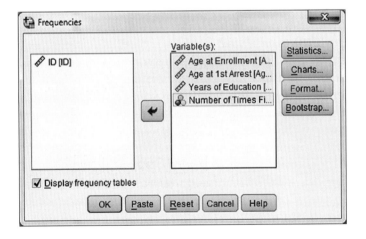

Step 2: Click "Statistics." Check "Skewness" and "Kurtosis." Click "Continue."

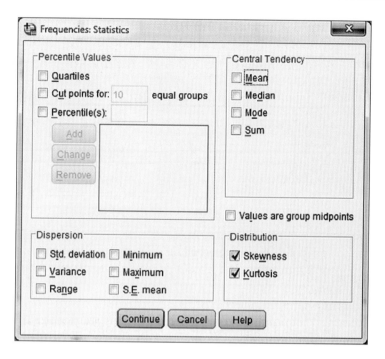

Step 3: Click "Charts." Check "Histograms." Click "Continue" and then "OK."

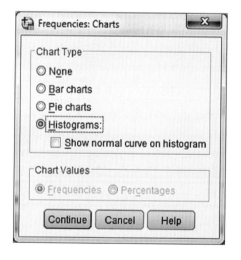

INTERPRETATION OF SPSS OUTPUT

The following tables are generated from SPSS. The first table contains the skewness and kurtosis statistics for the four variables.

Frequencies

Statistics

	Age at Enrollment	Age at 1st Arrest	Years of Education	Number of Times Fired from Job
N Valid	20	20	20	20
Missing	0	0	0	0
Skewness	-.351	1.402	.576	1.133
Std. Error of Skewness	.512	.512	.512	.512
Kurtosis	-.883	2.043	-.575	.576
Std. Error of Kurtosis	.992	.992	.992	.992

The next four tables contain the frequencies, or tallies, of the variable values. The last four tables contain the frequency distributions of the four variables.

Frequency Table

Age at Enrollment

		Frequency	Percent	Valid Percent	Cumulative Percent
Valid	41	1	5.0	5.0	5.0
	43	1	5.0	5.0	10.0
	46	1	5.0	5.0	15.0
	47	1	5.0	5.0	20.0
	48	1	5.0	5.0	25.0
	49	1	5.0	5.0	30.0
	50	1	5.0	5.0	35.0
	52	2	10.0	10.0	45.0
	56	4	20.0	20.0	65.0
	58	2	10.0	10.0	75.0
	60	2	10.0	10.0	85.0
	62	1	5.0	5.0	90.0
	63	2	10.0	10.0	100.0
	Total	20	100.0	100.0	

Age at 1st Arrest

		Frequency	Percent	Valid Percent	Cumulative Percent
Valid	12	1	5.0	5.0	5.0
	14	1	5.0	5.0	10.0
	16	1	5.0	5.0	15.0
	17	1	5.0	5.0	20.0
	19	3	15.0	15.0	35.0
	20	1	5.0	5.0	40.0
	21	1	5.0	5.0	45.0
	23	2	10.0	10.0	55.0
	24	1	5.0	5.0	60.0
	27	1	5.0	5.0	65.0
	28	1	5.0	5.0	70.0
	29	1	5.0	5.0	75.0
	31	1	5.0	5.0	80.0
	38	1	5.0	5.0	85.0
	42	1	5.0	5.0	90.0
	43	1	5.0	5.0	95.0
	59	1	5.0	5.0	100.0
	Total	20	100.0	100.0	

Years of Education

		Frequency	Percent	Valid Percent	Cumulative Percent
Valid	11	2	10.0	10.0	10.0
	12	11	55.0	55.0	65.0
	13	3	15.0	15.0	80.0
	14	4	20.0	20.0	100.0
	Total	20	100.0	100.0	

Number of Times Fired from Job

		Frequency	Percent	Valid Percent	Cumulative Percent
Valid	0	9	45.0	45.0	45.0
	1	3	15.0	15.0	60.0
	2	2	10.0	10.0	70.0
	3	4	20.0	20.0	90.0
	5	1	5.0	5.0	95.0
	6	1	5.0	5.0	100.0
	Total	20	100.0	100.0	

Histogram

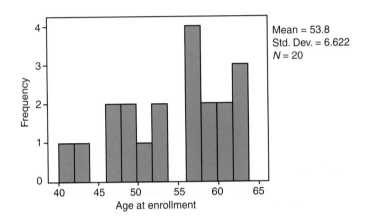

Mean = 53.8
Std. Dev. = 6.622
N = 20

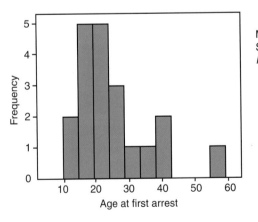

Mean = 26.2
Std. Dev. = 11.624
N = 20

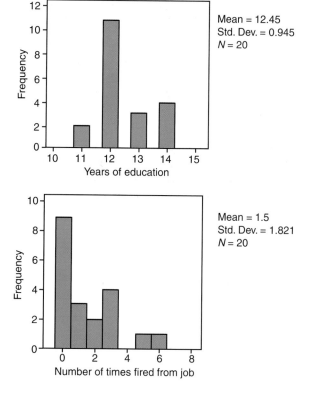

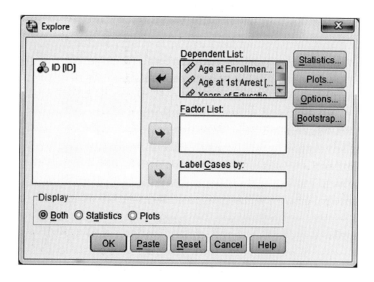

In terms of skewness, the frequency distribution for *Age at enrollment* appears to be negatively skewed, and the other three variables' frequency distributions appear to be positively skewed. The absolute values of the skewness statistics for *Age at first arrest* and *Number of times fired* are greater than 1.0. The kurtosis statistic for *Age at first arrest* is also greater than 1.0. No other skewness or kurtosis statistics were greater than 1.0.

In order to obtain a comparison of the study variables' deviation from normality (and thereby assessing skewness and kurtosis simultaneously), we must compute a Shapiro-Wilk test of normality.

Step 1: From the "Analyze" menu, choose "Descriptive Statistics" and "Explore." Move the four study variables over to the box labeled "Dependent List."

Step 2: Click "Plots." Check "Normality plots with tests." Click "Continue" and "OK."

For this example, SPSS produces many tables and figures. In the interest of saving space, we will focus on the table of interest, titled "Tests of Normality." This table contains the Shapiro-Wilk tests of normality for the four study variables. The last column contains the p values of the Shapiro-Wilk statistics. Of the four p values, three are significant at $p < 0.05$. *Age at enrollment* is the only variable that did not significantly deviate from normality ($p = 0.373$).

Explore

Tests of Normality

	Kolmogorov-Smirnov[a]			Shapiro-Wilk		
	Statistic	df	Sig.	Statistic	df	Sig.
Age at Enrollment	.180	20	.088	.950	20	.373
Age at 1st Arrest	.175	20	.110	.879	20	.017
Years of Education	.333	20	.000	.815	20	.001
Number of Times Fired from Job	.245	20	.003	.808	20	.001

a. Lilliefors Significance Correction

In summary, the skewness statistics as well as the Shapiro-Wilk values for *Age at first arrest* and *Number of times fired from a job* indicated significant deviations from normality. *Age at enrollment*, while appearing to be slightly negatively skewed, did not yield skewness, kurtosis, or Shapiro-Wilk values that indicated deviations from normality. *Years of education* appeared to be positively skewed but did not have an extreme skewness or kurtosis value. However, the Shapiro-Wilk p value was significant at $p = 0.001$. It is common for Shapiro-Wilk values to conflict with skewness and kurtosis statistics, because the Shapiro-Wilk test examines the entire shape of the distribution while skewness and kurtosis statistics examine only skewness and kurtosis, respectively. When a Shapiro-Wilk value is significant *and* visual inspection of the frequency distribution indicates non-normality, the researcher must consider a nonparametric statistical alternative (Pett, 2016). See Exercise 23 for a review of nonparametric statistics that would be appropriate when the normality assumption for a parametric statistic is not met.

STUDY QUESTIONS

1. Define skewness.

2. Define kurtosis.

3. Given this set of numbers, plot the frequency distribution:
   1, 2, 9, 9, 11, 11, 11, 12, 12, 12, 12, 13, 13, 13, 14, 14.

4. How would you characterize the skewness of the distribution in Question 3: positively skewed, negatively skewed, or approximately normal? Provide a rationale for your answer.

5. Given this set of numbers, plot the frequency distribution:
   1, 2, 2, 2, 3, 3, 3, 3, 3, 4, 4, 4, 5, 5, 10, 11.

6. How would you characterize the skewness of the distribution in Question 5: positively skewed, negatively skewed, or approximately normal? Provide a rationale for your answer.

7. Given this set of numbers, plot the frequency distribution:
   4, 4, 4, 5, 5, 5, 5, 5, 5, 5, 5, 5, 6, 6, 6, 6.

8. How would you characterize the kurtosis of the distribution in Question 7: leptokurtic, mesokurtic, or platykurtic? Provide a rationale for your answer.

9. When looking at the frequency distribution for *Age at first arrest* in the example data, where is the mean in relation to the median?

10. What is the mode for *Years of Education*?

Answers to Study Questions

1. Skewness is defined as a frequency distribution that is not symmetrical.

2. Kurtosis is defined as the degree of peakedness of the frequency distribution.

3. The frequency distribution approximates the following plot:

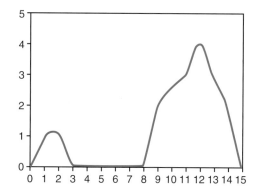

4. The skewness of the distribution in Question 3 is negatively skewed, as evidenced by the "tail" of the distribution appearing below the mean (Gray et al., 2017; Holmes, 2018).

5. The frequency distribution approximates the following plot:

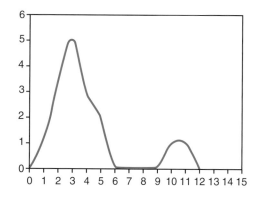

6. The skewness of the distribution in Question 5 is positively skewed, as evidenced by the "tail" of the distribution appearing above the mean.

7. The frequency distribution approximates the following plot:

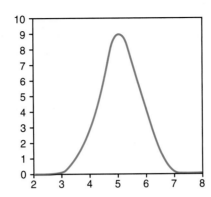

8. The kurtosis of the distribution in Question 7 is leptokurtic, as evidenced by the peakedness of the distribution and the limited variance of the values.

9. The mean, for *Age at First Arrest* is higher than (*above*) the median due to its positively skewed distribution.

10. The mode for *Years of Education* is 12, which is the most frequently occurring value.

DATA FOR ADDITIONAL COMPUTATIONAL PRACTICE FOR QUESTIONS TO BE GRADED

Using the same example from LePage and colleagues (2014), the following data include only the last 15 observations (the first 5 were deleted). The data are presented in Table 26-3.

ID	Age at Enrollment	Age at 1st Arrest	Education	Number Times Fired
TABLE 26-3	AGE, EDUCATION, AND TERMINATION HISTORY AMONG VETERANS WITH FELONIES			
6	41	20	12	1
7	56	14	12	1
8	56	12	14	0
9	47	23	12	0
10	52	38	12	3
11	63	16	14	0
12	60	59	12	1
13	62	17	12	3
14	49	19	11	2
15	60	31	13	0
16	56	28	12	3
17	52	43	12	0
18	58	27	14	0
19	43	29	12	0
20	63	42	14	0

Questions to Be Graded

EXERCISE 26

Name: _____ Class: _____

Date: _____

Answer the following questions with hand calculations using the data presented in Table 26-3 or the SPSS dataset called "Exercise 26 Example 2.sav" available on the Evolve website. Follow your instructor's directions to submit your answers to the following questions for grading. Your instructor may ask you to write your answers below and submit them as a hard copy for grading. Alternatively, your instructor may ask you to submit your answers online.

1. Plot the frequency distribution for *Age at Enrollment* by hand or by using SPSS.

2. How would you characterize the skewness of the distribution in Question 1—positively skewed, negatively skewed, or approximately normal? Provide a rationale for your answer.

3. Compare the original skewness statistic and Shapiro-Wilk statistic with those of the smaller dataset ($n = 15$) for the variable *Age at First Arrest*. How did the statistics change, and how would you explain these differences?

4. Plot the frequency distribution for *Years of Education* by hand or by using SPSS.

5. How would you characterize the kurtosis of the distribution in Question 4—leptokurtic, mesokurtic, or platykurtic? Provide a rationale for your answer.

6. What is the skewness statistic for *Age at Enrollment*? How would you characterize the magnitude of the skewness statistic for *Age at Enrollment*?

7. What is the kurtosis statistic for *Years of Education*? How would you characterize the magnitude of the kurtosis statistic for *Years of Education*?

8. Using SPSS, compute the Shapiro-Wilk statistic for *Number of Times Fired from Job*. What would you conclude from the results?

9. In the SPSS output table titled "Tests of Normality," the Shapiro-Wilk statistic is reported along with the Kolmogorov-Smirnov statistic. Why is the Kolmogorov-Smirnov statistic inappropriate to report for these example data?

10. How would you explain a frequency distribution that yields a low skewness statistic but a statistically significant Shapiro-Wilk statistic ($p < 0.05$)?

Calculating Descriptive Statistics

There are two major classes of statistics: descriptive statistics and inferential statistics. Descriptive statistics are computed to reveal characteristics of the sample data set and to describe study variables. Inferential statistics are computed to gain information about effects and associations in the population being studied. For some types of studies, descriptive statistics will be the only approach to analysis of the data. For other studies, descriptive statistics are the first step in the data analysis process, to be followed by inferential statistics. For all studies that involve numerical data, descriptive statistics are crucial in understanding the fundamental properties of the variables being studied. Exercise 27 focuses only on descriptive statistics and will illustrate the most common descriptive statistics computed in nursing research and provide examples using actual clinical data from empirical publications.

MEASURES OF CENTRAL TENDENCY

A **measure of central tendency** is a statistic that represents the center or middle of a frequency distribution. The three measures of central tendency commonly used in nursing research are the mode, median (MD), and mean ($\overline{X}$). The mean is the arithmetic average of all of a variable's values. The median is the exact middle value (or the average of the middle two values if there is an even number of observations). The mode is the most commonly occurring value or values (see Exercise 8).

The following data have been collected from veterans with rheumatoid arthritis (Tran, Hooker, Cipher, & Reimold, 2009). The values in Table 27-1 were extracted from a larger sample of veterans who had a history of biologic medication use (e.g., infliximab [Remicade], etanercept [Enbrel]). Table 27-1 contains data collected from 10 veterans who had stopped taking biologic medications, and the variable represents the number of years that each veteran had taken the medication before stopping.

Because the number of study subjects represented below is 10, the correct statistical notation to reflect that number is:

$$n = 10$$

Note that the n is lowercase, because we are referring to a sample of veterans. If the data being presented represented the entire population of veterans, the correct notation is the uppercase N. Because most nursing research is conducted using samples, not populations, all formulas in the subsequent exercises will incorporate the sample notation, n.

Mode

The **mode** is the numerical value or score that occurs with the greatest frequency; it does not necessarily indicate the center of the data set. The data in Table 27-1 contain two

TABLE 27-1	DURATION OF BIOLOGIC USE AMONG VETERANS WITH RHEUMATOID ARTHRITIS ($n = 10$)
	Duration of Biologic Use (years)
	0.1
	0.3
	1.3
	1.5
	1.5
	2.0
	2.2
	3.0
	3.0
	4.0

modes: 1.5 and 3.0. Each of these numbers occurred twice in the data set. When two modes exist, the data set is referred to as **bimodal**; a data set that contains more than two modes would be **multimodal** (Gray, Grove, & Sutherland, 2017).

Median

The **median** (*MD*) is the value at the exact center of the ungrouped frequency distribution. It is the 50th percentile. To obtain the *MD*, sort the values from lowest to highest. If the number of values is an uneven number, the *MD* is the exact middle number in the dataset. If the number of values is an even number, the *MD* is the average of the two middle values. Thus the *MD* may not be an actual value in the data set. For example, the data in Table 27-1 consist of 10 observations, and therefore the *MD* is calculated as the average of the two middle values (Grove & Gray, 2019).

$$MD = \frac{(1.5 + 2.0)}{2} = 1.75$$

Mean

The most commonly reported measure of central tendency is the mean. The mean is the sum of the values divided by the number of values being summed. Thus like the *MD*, the mean may not be a member of the data set. The formula for calculating the mean is as follows:

$$\bar{X} = \frac{\sum X}{n}$$

where

$\bar{X}$ = mean
Σ = sigma, the statistical symbol for summation
X = a single value in the sample
n = total number of values in the sample

The mean number of years that the veterans used a biologic medication is calculated as follows:

$$\bar{X} = \frac{(0.1 + 0.3 + 1.3 + 1.5 + 1.5 + 2.0 + 2.2 + 3.0 + 3.0 + 4.0)}{10} = 1.89 \text{ years}$$

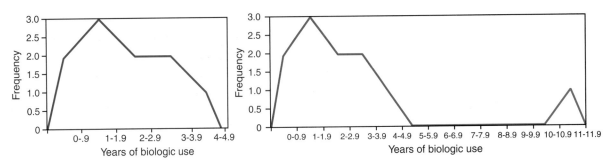

FIGURE 27-1 ■ **FREQUENCY DISTRIBUTION OF YEARS OF BIOLOGIC USE, WITHOUT OUTLIER AND WITH OUTLIER.**

The mean is an appropriate measure of central tendency for approximately normally distributed populations with variables measured at the interval or ratio level. It is also appropriate for ordinal level data such as Likert scale values, where higher numbers represent more of the construct being measured and lower numbers represent less of the construct (such as pain levels, patient satisfaction, depression, and health status (Lenz, Strickland, & Waltz, 2017)).

The mean is sensitive to extreme values such as outliers. An **outlier** is a value in a sample data set that is unusually low or unusually high in the context of the rest of the sample data (Kim & Mallory, 2017). An example of an outlier in the data presented in Table 27-1 might be a value such as 11. The existing values range from 0.1 to 4.0, meaning that no veteran used a biologic beyond 4 years. If an additional veteran were added to the sample and that person used a biologic for 11 years, the mean would be much larger: 2.7 years. Simply adding this outlier to the sample nearly doubled the mean value. The outlier would also change the frequency distribution. Without the outlier, the frequency distribution is approximately normal, as shown in Figure 27-1. Including the outlier changes the shape of the distribution to appear positively skewed.

Although the use of summary statistics has been the traditional approach to describing data or describing the characteristics of the sample before inferential statistical analysis, its ability to clarify the nature of data is limited. For example, using measures of central tendency, particularly the mean, to describe the nature of the data obscures the impact of extreme values or deviations in the data. Thus, significant features in the data may be concealed or misrepresented. Often, anomalous, unexpected, or problematic data and discrepant patterns are evident, but are not regarded as meaningful. Measures of dispersion, such as the range, difference scores, variance, and standard deviation (*SD*), provide important insight into the nature of the data (King & Eckersley, 2019).

MEASURES OF DISPERSION

Measures of dispersion, or variability, are measures of individual differences of the members of the population and sample. They indicate how values in a sample are dispersed around the mean. These measures provide information about the data that is not available from measures of central tendency. They indicate how different the values are—the extent to which individual values deviate from one another. If the individual values are similar, measures of variability are small and the sample is relatively **homogeneous** in terms of those values. **Heterogeneity** (wide variation in values) is important in some statistical procedures, such as correlation. Heterogeneity is determined by measures of variability. The measures most commonly used are range, difference scores, variance, and *SD* (see Exercise 9; Plichta & Kelvin, 2013).

Range

The simplest measure of dispersion is the **range**. In published studies, range is presented in two ways: (1) the range is the set of lowest and highest values, or (2) the range is calculated by subtracting the lowest value from the highest value. The range for the values in Table 27-1 is 0.1 to 4.0, or it can be calculated as follows: $4.0 - 0.1 = 3.9$. In this form, the range is a difference score that uses only the two extreme values for the comparison. Therefore, a very large range can indicate the presence of an outlier.

Difference Scores

Difference scores are obtained by subtracting the mean from each value. Sometimes a difference score is referred to as a **deviation score** because it indicates the extent to which a score (or value) deviates from the mean. Of course, most variables in nursing research are not "scores," yet the term **difference score** is used to represent a value's deviation from the mean. The difference score is positive when the value is above the mean, and it is negative when the value is below the mean (see Table 27-2). Difference scores are the basis for many statistical analyses and can be found within many statistical equations. The formula for difference scores is:

$$X - \bar{X}$$

TABLE 27-2	DIFFERENCE SCORES OF DURATION OF BIOLOGIC USE	
X	**$-\bar{X}$**	**$X - \bar{X}$**
0.1	1.89	−1.79
0.3	1.89	−1.59
1.3	1.89	−0.59
1.5	1.89	−0.39
1.5	1.89	−0.39
2.0	1.89	0.11
2.2	1.89	0.31
3.0	1.89	1.11
3.0	1.89	1.11
4.0	1.89	2.11

Σ of absolute values: 9.5

The **mean deviation** is the average difference score, using the absolute values. The formula for the mean deviation is:

$$\bar{X}_{deviation} = \frac{\sum |X - \bar{X}|}{n}$$

In this example, the mean deviation is 0.95. This value was calculated by taking the sum of the absolute value of each difference score (−1.79, −1.59, −0.59, −0.39, −0.39, 0.11, 0.31, 1.11, 1.11, 2.11) and dividing by 10. The result indicates that, on average, subjects' duration of biologic use deviated from the mean by 0.95 years.

Variance

Variance is another measure commonly used in statistical analysis. The equation for a sample variance (s^2) is below.

$$s^2 = \frac{\sum (X - \bar{X})^2}{n - 1}$$

Note that the lowercase letter s^2 is used to represent a sample variance. The lowercase Greek sigma (σ^2) is used to represent a population variance, in which the denominator is N instead of $n - 1$. Because most nursing research is conducted using samples, not populations, formulas in the subsequent exercises that contain a variance or standard deviation will incorporate the sample notation, using $n - 1$ as the denominator. Moreover, many statistical software packages compute the variance and standard deviation using the sample formulas, not the population formulas, unless otherwise programmed.

The variance is always a positive value and has no upper limit. In general, the larger the variance, the larger the dispersion of sample values. The variance is most often computed to derive the standard deviation because, unlike the variance, the standard deviation reflects important properties about the frequency distribution of the variable it represents. Table 27-3 displays how we would compute a variance by hand, using the biologic duration data.

TABLE 27-3	VARIANCE COMPUTATION OF BIOLOGIC USE		
X	$\bar{X}$	$X - \bar{X}$	$(X - \bar{X})^2$
0.1	1.89	−1.79	3.20
0.3	1.89	−1.59	2.53
1.3	1.89	−0.59	0.35
1.5	1.89	−0.39	0.15
1.5	1.89	−0.39	0.15
2.0	1.89	0.11	0.01
2.2	1.89	0.31	0.10
3.0	1.89	1.11	1.23
3.0	1.89	1.11	1.23
4.0	1.89	2.11	4.45
		Σ	13.41

$$s^2 = \frac{13.41}{9}$$

$$s^2 = 1.49$$

Standard Deviation

Standard deviation is a measure of dispersion that is the square root of the variance. The standard deviation is represented by the notation s or SD. The equation for obtaining a standard deviation is

$$SD = \sqrt{\frac{\sum (X - \bar{X})^2}{n - 1}}$$

Table 27-3 displays the computations for the variance. To compute the SD, simply take the square root of the variance. We know that the variance of biologic duration is $s^2 = 1.49$. Therefore, the s of biologic duration is $SD = 1.22$. The SD is an important statistic, both for understanding dispersion within a distribution and for interpreting the relationship of a particular value to the distribution (Gray et al., 2017).

SAMPLING ERROR

A standard error describes the extent of sampling error. For example, a standard error of the mean is calculated to determine the magnitude of the variability associated with the mean. A small standard error is an indication that the sample mean is close to the population mean, while a large standard error yields less certainty that the sample mean approximates the population mean. The formula for the standard error of the mean $(s_{\bar{X}})$ is:

$$s_{\bar{X}} = \frac{s}{\sqrt{n}}$$

Using the biologic medication duration data, we know that the standard deviation of biologic duration is $s = 1.22$. Therefore, the standard error of the mean for biologic duration is computed as follows:

$$s_{\bar{X}} = \frac{1.22}{\sqrt{10}}$$

$$s_{\bar{X}} = 0.39$$

The standard error of the mean for biologic duration is 0.39.

Confidence Intervals

To determine how closely the sample mean approximates the population mean, the standard error of the mean is used to build a confidence interval. For that matter, a confidence interval can be created for many statistics, such as a mean, proportion, and odds ratio. To build a confidence interval around a statistic, you must have the standard error value and the t value to adjust the standard error. The degrees of freedom (df) to use to compute a confidence interval is $df = n - 1$.

To compute the confidence interval for a mean, the lower and upper limits of that interval are created by multiplying the $s_{\bar{X}}$ by the t statistic, where $df = n - 1$. For a 95% confidence interval, the t value should be selected at $\alpha = 0.05$. For a 99% confidence interval, the t value should be selected at $\alpha = 0.01$.

Using the biologic medication duration data, we know that the standard error of the mean duration of biologic medication use is $s_{\bar{X}} = 0.39$. The mean duration of biologic medication use is 1.89. Therefore, the 95% confidence interval for the mean duration of biologic medication use is computed as follows:

$$\bar{X} \pm s_{\bar{X}} t$$

$$1.89 \pm (0.39)(2.26)$$

$$1.89 \pm 0.88$$

As referenced in Appendix A, the t value required for the 95% confidence interval with $df = 9$ is 2.26 for a two-tailed test. The computation above results in a lower limit of 1.01 and an upper limit of 2.77. This means that our confidence interval of 1.01 to 2.77 estimates the population mean duration of biologic use with 95% confidence (Kline, 2004). Technically and mathematically, it means that if we computed the mean duration of biologic medication use on an infinite number of veterans, exactly 95% of the intervals would contain the true population mean, and 5% would not contain the population mean (Gliner, Morgan, & Leech, 2009). If we were to compute a 99% confidence interval, we would require the t value of 3.25 that is referenced at $\alpha = 0.01$. Therefore, the 99% confidence interval for the mean duration of biologic medication use is computed as follows:

$$1.89 \pm (0.39)(3.25)$$

$$1.89 \pm 1.27$$

As referenced in Appendix A, the *t* value required for the 99% confidence interval with *df* = 9 is 3.25 for a two tailed test. The computation presented previously results in a lower limit of 0.62 and an upper limit of 3.16. This means that our confidence interval of 0.62 to 3.16 estimates the population mean duration of biologic use with 99% confidence.

Degrees of Freedom

The concept of degrees of freedom (*df*) was used in reference to computing a confidence interval. For any statistical computation, **degrees of freedom** are the number of independent pieces of information that are free to vary in order to estimate another piece of information (Zar, 2010). In the case of the confidence interval, the degrees of freedom are $n - 1$. This means that there are $n - 1$ independent observations in the sample that are free to vary (to be any value) to estimate the lower and upper limits of the confidence interval.

SPSS COMPUTATIONS

A retrospective descriptive study examined the duration of biologic use from veterans with rheumatoid arthritis (Tran et al., 2009). The values in Table 27-4 were extracted from a larger sample of veterans who had a history of biologic medication use (e.g., infliximab [Remicade], etanercept [Enbrel]). Table 27-4 contains simulated demographic data collected from 10 veterans who had stopped taking biologic medications. Age at study enrollment, duration of biologic use, race/ethnicity, gender (F = female), tobacco use (F = former use, C = current use, N = never used), primary diagnosis (3 = irritable bowel disease, 4 = psoriatic arthritis, 5 = rheumatoid arthritis, 6 = reactive arthritis), and type of biologic medication used were among the study variables examined.

TABLE 27-4   DEMOGRAPHIC VARIABLES OF VETERANS WITH RHEUMATOID ARTHRITIS

Patient ID	Duration (yrs)	Age	Race/Ethnicity	Gender	Tobacco	Diagnosis	Biologic
1	0.1	42	Caucasian	F	F	5	Infliximab
2	0.3	41	Black, not of Hispanic Origin	F	F	5	Etanercept
3	1.3	56	Caucasian	F	N	5	Infliximab
4	1.5	78	Caucasian	F	F	3	Infliximab
5	1.5	86	Black, not of Hispanic Origin	F	F	4	Etanercept
6	2.0	49	Caucasian	F	F	6	Etanercept
7	2.2	82	Caucasian	F	F	5	Infliximab
8	3.0	35	Caucasian	F	N	3	Infliximab
9	3.0	59	Black, not of Hispanic Origin	F	C	3	Infliximab
10	4.0	37	Caucasian	F	F	5	Etanercept

This is how our dataset looks in SPSS.

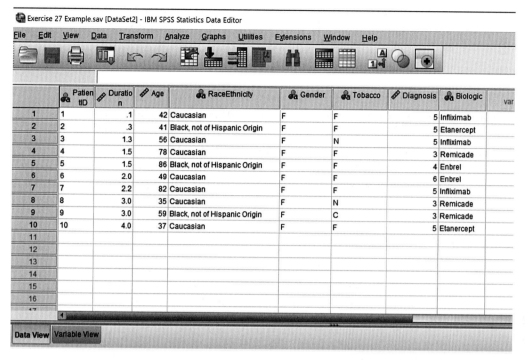

Step 1: For a nominal variable, the appropriate descriptive statistics are frequencies and percentages. From the "Analyze" menu, choose "Descriptive Statistics" and "Frequencies." Move "Race/Ethnicity and Gender" over to the right. Click "OK."

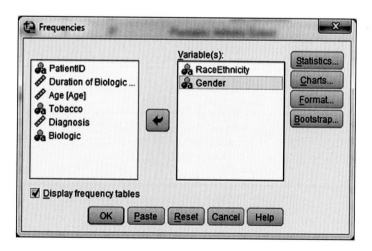

Step 2: For a continuous variable, the appropriate descriptive statistics are means and standard deviations. From the "Analyze" menu, choose "Descriptive Statistics" and "Explore." Move "Duration" over to the right. Click "OK."

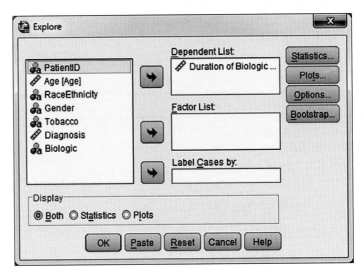

INTERPRETATION OF SPSS OUTPUT

The following tables are generated from SPSS. The first set of tables (from the first set of SPSS commands in Step 1) contains the frequencies of race/ethnicity and gender. Most (70%) were Caucasian, and 100% were female.

Frequencies

Frequency Table

RaceEthnicity

		Frequency	Percent	Valid Percent	Cumulative Percent
	Black, not of Hispanic Origin	3	30.0	30.0	30.0
Valid	Caucasian	7	70.0	70.0	100.0
	Total	10	100.0	100.0	

Gender

	Frequency	Percent	Valid Percent	Cumulative Percent
Valid F	10	100.0	100.0	100.0

The second set of output (from the second set of SPSS commands in Step 2) contains the descriptive statistics for "Duration," including the mean, s (standard deviation), SE, 95% confidence interval for the mean, median, variance, minimum value, maximum value, range, and skewness and kurtosis statistics. As shown in the output, the mean number of years for duration is 1.89, and the SD is 1.22. The 95% CI is 1.02 to 2.76.

Explore

Descriptives

			Statistic	Std. Error
Duration of Biologic Use	Mean		1.890	.3860
	95% Confidence Interval for Mean	Lower Bound	1.017	
		Upper Bound	2.763	
	5% Trimmed Mean		1.872	
	Median		1.750	
	Variance		1.490	
	Std. Deviation		1.2206	
	Minimum		.1	
	Maximum		4.0	
	Range		3.9	
	Interquartile Range		2.0	
	Skewness		.159	.687
	Kurtosis		-.437	1.334

STUDY QUESTIONS

1. Define mean.

2. What does this symbol, s^2, represent?

3. Define outlier.

4. Are there any outliers among the values representing duration of biologic use?

5. List the 95% confidence interval (lower and upper limits) for the mean of duration of biologic use. How would you interpret these values?

6. What percentage of patients were Black, not of Hispanic origin?

7. Can you compute the variance for duration of biologic use by using the information presented in the SPSS output on page 327? If so, calculate the variance.

8. Plot the frequency distribution of duration of biologic use.

9. Where is the median in relation to the mean in the frequency distribution of duration of biologic use? What does this mean about the distribution of values?

10. When would a median be more informative than a mean in describing a variable?

Answers to Study Questions

1. The mean is defined as the arithmetic average of a set of numbers.

2. s^2 represents the sample variance of a given variable.

3. An outlier is a value in a sample data set that is unusually low or unusually high in the context of the rest of the sample data (Gray et al., 2017; Kim & Mallory, 2017).

4. There are no outliers among the values representing duration of biologic use.

5. The 95% CI is 1.02 to 2.76, meaning that our confidence interval of [1.02, 2.76] estimates the population mean duration of biologic use with 95% confidence.

6. 30% of patients were Black, not of Hispanic origin.

7. Yes, the variance for duration of biologic use can be computed by squaring the SD presented in the SPSS table. The SD is listed as 1.22, and, therefore, the variance is 1.22^2 or 1.49.

8. The frequency distribution approximates the following plot:

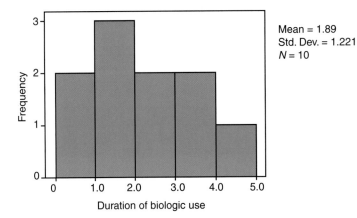

9. The median is 1.75 and the mean is 1.89. Therefore, the median is lower in relation to the mean in the frequency distribution of duration of biologic use, indicating that the distribution is positively skewed.

10. A median can be more informative than a mean in describing a variable when the variable's frequency distribution is positively or negatively skewed. While the mean is sensitive to or increases or decreases based on the values of the outliers, the median is relatively unaffected (Kim & Mallory, 2017).

Questions to Be Graded

Name: _____	Class: _____
Date: _____	

Answer the following questions with hand calculations using the data presented in Table 27-4 or the SPSS dataset called "Exercise 27 Example.sav" available on the Evolve website. Follow your instructor's directions to submit your answers to the following questions for grading. Your instructor may ask you to write your answers below and submit them as a hard copy for grading. Alternatively, your instructor may ask you to submit your answers online.

1. What is the mean age of the sample data?

2. What percentage of patients never used tobacco?

3. What is the standard deviation for age?

4. Are there outliers among the values of age? Provide a rationale for your answer.

5. What is the range of age values?

6. What percentage of patients were taking infliximab?

7. What percentage of patients had rheumatoid arthritis (RA) as their primary diagnosis?

8. Among only those patients who had RA as their primary diagnosis, what percentage were current smokers?

9. List the 95% confidence interval (lower and upper limits) for the mean patient age. How would you interpret these values?

10. Among only those patients who had irritable bowel disease as their primary diagnosis, calculate the mean age.

Calculating Pearson Product-Moment Correlation Coefficient

Correlational analyses identify associations between two variables. There are many different kinds of statistics that yield a measure of correlation. All of these statistics address a research question or hypothesis that involves an association or relationship. Examples of research questions that are answered with correlation statistics are, *Is there an association between weight loss and depression?* and *Is there a relationship between patient satisfaction and health status?* A hypothesis is developed to identify the nature (positive or negative) of the relationship between the variables being studied.

The **Pearson product-moment correlation** was the first of the correlation measures developed and is the most commonly used. As is explained in Exercise 13, this coefficient (statistic) is represented by the letter r, and the value of r is always between -1.00 and $+1.00$. A value of zero indicates no relationship between the two variables. A positive correlation indicates that higher values of x are associated with higher values of y. A negative or inverse correlation indicates that higher values of x are associated with lower values of y. The r value is indicative of the slope of the line (called a regression line) that can be drawn through a standard scatterplot of the two variables (see Exercise 11). The strengths of different relationships are identified in Table 28-1 (Cohen, 1988).

TABLE 28-1 STRENGTH OF ASSOCIATION FOR PEARSON r		
Strength of Association	**Positive Association**	**Negative Association**
Weak association	0.00 to <0.30	0.00 to <−0.30
Moderate association	0.30 to 0.49	−0.49 to −0.30
Strong association	0.50 or greater	−1.00 to −0.50

RESEARCH DESIGNS APPROPRIATE FOR THE PEARSON r

Research designs that may utilize the Pearson r include any associational design (Gliner, Morgan, & Leech, 2009; Kazkin, 2017). The variables involved in the design are often attributional, meaning the variables are characteristics of the participant, such as health status, blood pressure, gender, diagnosis, or race/ethnicity. Regardless of the nature of variables, the variables submitted to a Pearson correlation must be measured as continuous or at the interval or ratio level.

STATISTICAL FORMULA AND ASSUMPTIONS

Use of the Pearson correlation involves the following assumptions:

1. Interval or ratio measurement of both variables (e.g., age, income, blood pressure, cholesterol levels). However, if the variables are measured with a Likert scale, and

the frequency distribution is approximately normally distributed, these data are usually treated as interval-level measurements and are appropriate for the Pearson r (Rasmussen, 1989; de Winter & Dodou, 2010).

2. Normal distribution of at least one variable.
3. Independence of observational pairs.
4. Homoscedasticity.

Data that are **homoscedastic** are evenly dispersed both above and below a line of perfect prediction when variable x predicts variable y (see Exercise 29 for illustrations of homoscedasticity and heteroscedasticity). Homoscedasticity reflects equal variance of both variables. In other words, for every value of x, the distribution of y values should have equal variability. If the data for the two variables being correlated are not homoscedastic, inferences made during significance testing could be invalid (Cohen & Cohen, 1983).

The Pearson product-moment correlation coefficient is computed using one of several formulas—the one below is considered the *computational formula* because it makes computation by hand easier (Zar, 2010):

$$r = \frac{n\sum xy - \sum x \sum y}{\sqrt{\left[n\sum x^2 - \left(\sum x\right)^2\right]\left[n\sum y^2 - \left(\sum y\right)^2\right]}}$$

where

r = Pearson correlation coefficient
n = total number of subjects
x = value of the first variable
y = value of the second variable
xy = x multiplied by y

HAND CALCULATIONS

This example includes data from veterans with a type of inflammatory bowel disease called ulcerative colitis (Flores, Burstein, Cipher, & Feagins, 2015). The two variables are body mass indices (BMI) and the patient's age at the initial diagnosis of ulcerative colitis. The BMI, a measure of body fat based on height and weight that applies to adult men and women, is considered an indicator of obesity when 30 or greater (National Heart, Lung, and Blood Institute, 2019).

The null hypothesis is *There is no correlation between age at diagnosis and BMI among veterans with ulcerative colitis.* A simulated subset of 20 veterans was created for this example so that the computations would be small and manageable. In actuality, studies involving Pearson correlations need to be adequately powered (Cohen, 1988; Taylor & Spurlock, 2018). Observe that the data in Table 28-2 are arranged in columns that correspond to the elements of the formula. The summed values in the last row of Table 28-2 are inserted into the appropriate place in the Pearson r formula.

The computations for the Pearson r are as follows:

Step 1: Plug the values from the bottom row of Table 28-2 into the Pearson r formula below.

$$r = \frac{n\sum xy - \sum x \sum y}{\sqrt{\left[n\sum x^2 - \left(\sum x\right)^2\right]\left[n\sum y^2 - \left(\sum y\right)^2\right]}}$$

TABLE 28-2	BODY MASS INDICES AND AGE AT DIAGNOSIS OF VETERANS WITH ULCERATIVE COLITIS				
Participant Number	x (Age at Diagnosis)	y (BMI)	x^2	y^2	xy
1	33	19.7	1,089	388.09	650.1
2	26	20.1	676	404.01	522.6
3	23	22.9	529	524.41	526.7
4	45	24.4	2,025	595.36	1,098.0
5	33	24.6	1,089	605.16	811.8
6	40	24.8	1,600	615.04	992.0
7	51	25.7	2,601	660.49	1,310.7
8	63	26.2	3,969	686.44	1,650.6
9	34	27.8	1,156	772.84	945.2
10	41	28.1	1,681	789.61	1,152.1
11	36	28.1	1,296	789.61	1,011.6
12	62	28.7	3,844	823.69	1,779.4
13	42	29.5	1,764	870.25	1,239.0
14	46	31.5	2,116	992.25	1,449.0
15	52	31.0	2,704	961.00	1,612.0
16	61	31.7	3,721	1,004.89	1,933.7
17	31	32.2	961	1,036.84	998.2
18	63	35.3	3,969	1,246.09	2,223.9
19	35	36.8	1,225	1,354.24	1,288.0
20	55	36.9	3,025	1,361.61	2,029.5
sum Σ	872	566	41,040	16,481.92	25,224.10

$$r = \frac{20(25,224.1)-(872)(566)}{\sqrt{[(20)(41,040)-872^2][(20)(16,481.92)-566^2]}}$$

Step 2: Solve for r.

$$r = \frac{20(25,224.1)-(872)(566)}{\sqrt{[60,416][9,282.4]}}$$

$$r = \frac{504,482-493,552}{\sqrt{[60,416][9,282.4]}}$$

$$r = \frac{10,930}{23,681.3} = 0.46$$

Step 3: Compute the degrees of freedom.

$$df = n-2$$

$$df = 20-2$$

$$df = 18$$

Step 4: Locate the critical r value in the r distribution table (Appendix B), and compare it to our obtained r value.

The r is 0.46, indicating a moderate positive correlation between BMI and age at diagnosis among veterans with ulcerative colitis. To determine whether this relationship is improbable to have been caused by chance alone, we consult the r probability distribution table in Appendix B. The formula for degrees of freedom (df) for a Pearson r is $n − 2$. With r of 0.46 and $df = 18$, the critical r value at $\alpha = 0.05$, $df = 18$ is 0.444 for a two-tailed test. Our obtained r was 0.46, which exceeds the critical value in the table. Thus the r value of 0.46 is considered statistically significant. It should be noted that if the obtained r was −0.46, it would also be considered statistically significant, because the absolute value of the obtained r is compared to the critical r value. The sign of the r is only used to indicate whether the association is positive or negative.

SPSS COMPUTATIONS

This is how our dataset looks in SPSS.

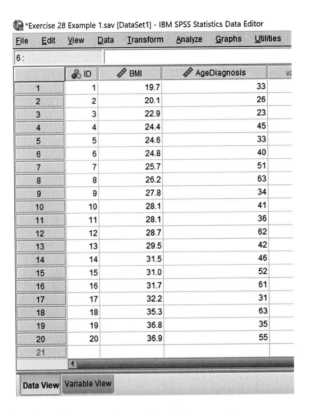

Step 1: From the "Analyze" menu, choose "Correlate" and "Bivariate."

Step 2: Move the two variables, Age at Diagnosis and BMI, over to the right, like the window below. Click "OK."

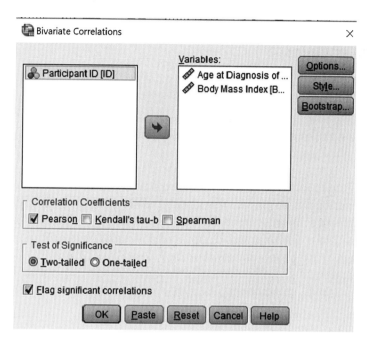

INTERPRETATION OF SPSS OUTPUT

The following table is generated from SPSS. The table contains a correlation matrix that includes the Pearson r between BMI and age at diagnosis, along with the p value and df. The r is listed as 0.46 2 rounded to 0.46, and the p is 0.041.

Correlations

Correlations

		Age at Diagnosis of Ulcerative Colitis	Body Mass Index	
Age at Diagnosis of Ulcerative Colitis	Pearson Correlation	1	.462[*]	**Observe that the upper diagonal is a mirror image of the lower diagonal**
	Sig. (2-tailed)		.041	
	N	20	20	
Body Mass Index	Pearson Correlation	.462[*]	1	
	Sig. (2-tailed)	.041		
	N	20	20	

*. Correlation is significant at the 0.05 level (2-tailed).

The exact p value is .041

FINAL INTERPRETATION IN AMERICAN PSYCHOLOGICAL ASSOCIATION (APA) FORMAT

The following interpretation is written as it might appear in a research article, formatted according to APA guidelines (APA, 2010). A Pearson correlation analysis indicated that there was a significant correlation between BMI and age at diagnosis among veterans with ulcerative colitis, $r(18) = 0.46$, $p = 0.041$. Higher BMI values were associated with older ages at which the diagnosis occurred.

EFFECT SIZE

After establishing the statistical significance of the r, it must subsequently be examined for clinical importance. There are ranges for strength of association suggested by Cohen (1988), as displayed in Table 28-1. One can also assess the magnitude of association by obtaining the **coefficient of determination** for the Pearson correlation. Computing the coefficient of determination simply involves squaring the r value. The r^2 (multiplied by 100%) represents the percentage of variance shared between the two variables (Cohen & Cohen, 1983). In our example, the r was 0.46, and therefore the r^2 was 0.212. This indicates that age at diagnosis and BMI shared 21.2% ($0.212 \times 100\%$) of the same variance. More specifically, 21.2% of the variance in age at diagnosis can be explained by knowing the veteran's BMI, and vice versa—21.2% of the variance in BMI can be explained by knowing the veteran's age at diagnosis.

STUDY QUESTIONS

1. If you have access to SPSS, compute the Shapiro-Wilk test of normality for the variables BMI and age at diagnosis (as demonstrated in Exercise 26). If you do not have access to SPSS, plot the frequency distributions by hand. What do the results indicate with regard to the normality of the distributions?

2. What is the null hypothesis in the example?

3. What was the exact likelihood of obtaining our r value at least as extreme or as close to the one that was actually observed, assuming that the null hypothesis is true?

4. How would you characterize the magnitude of the effect between BMI and age at diagnosis? Provide a rationale for your answer.

5. How much variance in BMI values is explained by knowing the veteran's age at diagnosis? Show your calculations for this value.

6. What kind of design was used in the example?

7. Was the sample size adequate to detect a significant correlation in this example?

8. A researcher computed a Pearson *r* and obtained an *r* of 0.50. How would you characterize the magnitude of the *r* value?

9. A researcher computed a Pearson *r* and obtained an *r* of 0.10. How would you characterize the magnitude of the *r* value? Provide a rationale for your answer.

10. A researcher computed a Pearson *r* on two different samples, one with an *n* of 15, and the other with *n* = 40. In both samples, she obtained an *r* of 0.50. What is the critical tabled *r* for each sample at $\alpha = 0.05$, two-tailed?

Answers to Study Questions

1. As shown in the SPSS output below, the Shapiro-Wilk p values for BMI and age at diagnosis were 0.746 and 0.235, respectively, indicating that the frequency distributions did not significantly deviate from normality. Moreover, visual inspection of the frequency distributions indicates that the variables are approximately normally distributed.

Tests of Normality

	Kolmogorov-Smirnov[a]			Shapiro-Wilk		
	Statistic	df	Sig.	Statistic	df	Sig.
Body Mass Index	.072	20	.200[*]	.970	20	.746
Age at Diagnosis of Ulcerative Colitis	.127	20	.200[*]	.940	20	.235

[*]. This is a lower bound of the true significance.

[a]. Lilliefors Significance Correction

2. The null hypothesis is *There is no correlation between age at diagnosis and BMI among veterans with ulcerative colitis.*

3. The exact likelihood of obtaining our r value at least as extreme or as close to the one that was actually observed, assuming that the null hypothesis is true, was 4.1%. This value was obtained by looking at the SPSS output table titled "Correlations" in the row labeled "Sig. (2-tailed)".

4. The magnitude of the effect between age at diagnosis and BMI would be considered a moderate effect according to the effect size tables in Exercises 24 and 25 and Table 28-1 in this exercise.

5. The r is 0.46, and therefore the r^2 is 0.212. This indicates that age at diagnosis and BMI shared 21.2% (0.212 × 100%) of the same variance. Therefore 21.2% of the variance in BMI values is explained by knowing the veteran's age at diagnosis, and vice versa.

6. The study design was associational or correlational (Gliner, Morgan, & Leech, 2009; Kazdin, 2017).

7. The sample size was indeed adequate to detect a significant correlation, $p = 0.041$.

8. An r of 0.50 is considered a large effect.

9. An r of 0.10 is considered a small effect according to the effect size tables in Exercises 24 and 25 and Table 28-1 in this exercise.

10. For the sample of 15, the df is 13 and the critical tabled r for 13 df at alpha = 0.05 is 0.514 for a two-tailed test. For the sample of 40, the df is 38 and the critical tabled r for 38 df at alpha = 0.05 is 0.312 for a two-tailed test. Therefore, the r in the smaller sample would not have been considered statistically significant, but the r in the larger sample would have been considered

statistically significant. This example demonstrates the importance of having an adequate sample size for a study to prevent a Type II error (Cohen, 1988; Taylor & Spurlock, 2018).

DATA FOR ADDITIONAL COMPUTATIONAL PRACTICE FOR QUESTIONS TO BE GRADED

This example includes survey data from the Centers for Disease Control (CDC) that focused on residential care facilities in the United States in 2010 (CDC, 2010). Residential care facilities primarily consist of persons in assisted living communities who receive housing and supportive services because they cannot live independently but generally do not require the skilled level of care provided by nursing homes. The focus of the first national study of acute care use in residential care facilities by Kahveci and Cipher (2014) was on acute care use (emergency department visits and hospitalizations) among persons in various disease categories, and information regarding the residents' length of stay and visitor frequency was also collected.

Length of stay (LOS) in the facility was coded as 1 = 0 to 3 months; 2 = 3 to 6 months; 3 = 6 months to a year; 4 = 1 to 3 years; 5 = 3 to 5 years; 6 = More than 5 years. Visitor frequency was coded as 1 = Every day; 2 = At least several times a week; 3 = About once a week; 4 = Several times in past month; 5 = At least once in past month; 6 = Not at all in the past 30 days. Therefore higher' values of the length of stay variable represent longer stays in the facility. Higher values of visitor frequency represent fewer visitor frequencies, which are considered inverse scoring.

The null hypothesis is *There is no correlation between length of stay and visitor frequency among residents of residential care facilities.* The data are presented in Table 28-3. A subset of 15 residents was randomly selected for this example so that the computations would be small and manageable. In actuality, studies involving Pearson correlations need to be adequately powered (Aberson, 2019; Cohen, 1988) and in the case of CDC survey data, adjusted for complex sampling. As is reviewed in Exercise 23, analysis of secondary population data requires weighting for complex sampling approaches (Aday & Cornelius, 2006).

TABLE 28-3   LENGTH OF STAY AND FREQUENCY OF VISITORS IN RESIDENTIAL CARE FACILITIES

Resident ID	x (LOS)	y (Visitor Frequency)	x^2	y^2	xy
1	1	2	1	4	2
2	5	5	25	25	25
3	4	3	16	9	12
4	4	5	16	25	20
5	4	2	16	4	8
6	5	4	25	16	20
7	3	3	9	9	9
8	6	4	36	16	24
9	6	5	36	25	30
10	4	2	16	4	8
11	3	4	9	16	12
12	4	3	16	9	12
13	5	5	25	25	25
14	5	6	25	36	30
15	2	3	4	9	6

Questions to Be Graded

Name: _____ Class: _____

Date: _____

Answer the following questions with hand calculations using the data presented in Table 28-3 or the SPSS dataset called "Exercise 28 Example 2.sav" available on the Evolve website. Follow your instructor's directions to submit your answers to the following questions for grading. Your instructor may ask you to write your answers below and submit them as a hard copy for grading. Alternatively, your instructor may ask you to submit your answers online.

1. If you have access to SPSS, compute the Shapiro-Wilk test of normality for the variables visitor frequency and length of stay (as demonstrated in Exercise 26). If you do not have access to SPSS, plot the frequency distributions by hand. What do the results indicate?

2. What is the null hypothesis in the example?

3. What is the Pearson r between visitor frequency and length of stay?

4. Is the r significant at $\alpha = 0.05$? Provide a rationale for your answer.

5. If using SPSS, what is the exact likelihood of obtaining an *r* value at least as extreme or as close to the one that was actually observed, assuming that the null hypothesis is true?

6. How would you characterize the magnitude of the effect between length of stay and visitor frequency? Provide a rationale for your answer.

7. What was the research design of this example?

8. Write your interpretation of the results, as you would in an APA-formatted journal.

9. How much variance in visitor frequency is explained by knowing the resident's length of stay and vice versa? Discuss the clinical importance of this value.

10. Can the researchers make a statement regarding the extent to which length of stay caused the frequency of visitors in residential care? Provide a rationale for your answer.

Calculating Simple Linear Regression

Simple linear regression is a procedure that provides an estimate of the value of a dependent variable (outcome) based on the value of an independent variable (predictor). Knowing that estimate with some degree of accuracy, we can use regression analysis to predict the value of one variable if we know the value of the other variable (Cohen & Cohen, 1983). The regression equation is a mathematical expression of the influence that a predictor has on a dependent variable, based on some theoretical framework. For example, in Exercise 14, Figure 14-1 illustrates the linear relationship between gestational age and birth weight. As shown in the scatterplot, there is a strong positive relationship between the two variables. Advanced gestational ages predict higher birth weights.

A regression equation can be generated with a data set containing subjects' x and y values. Once this equation is generated, it can be used to predict future subjects' y values, given only their x values. In simple or bivariate regression, predictions are made in cases with two variables. The score on variable y (dependent variable, or outcome) is predicted from the same subject's known score on variable x (independent variable, or predictor; Gray, Grove, & Sutherland, 2017).

RESEARCH DESIGNS APPROPRIATE FOR SIMPLE LINEAR REGRESSION

Research designs that may utilize simple linear regression include any associational design (Gliner, Morgan, & Leach, 2009; Plichta & Kelvin, 2013). The variables involved in the design are attributional, meaning the variables are characteristics of the participant, such as health status, blood pressure, gender, diagnosis, or ethnicity. Regardless of the nature of variables, the dependent variable submitted to simple linear regression must be measured as continuous, at the interval or ratio level.

STATISTICAL FORMULA AND ASSUMPTIONS

Use of simple linear regression involves the following assumptions (Zar, 2010; Plichta & Kelvin, 2013):

1. Normal distribution of the dependent (y) variable
2. Linear relationship between x and y
3. Independent observations
4. No (or little) multicollinearity
5. Homoscedasticity

349

Data that are **homoscedastic** are evenly dispersed both above and below a plotted line of perfect prediction when variable x predicts variable y. If the data for the predictor and dependent variable are not homoscedastic, inferences made during significance testing could be invalid (Cohen & Cohen, 1983; Zar, 2010). Visual examples of homoscedasticity and heteroscedasticity are presented in Exercise 30.

In simple linear regression, the dependent variable is continuous, and the predictor can be any scale of measurement; however, if the predictor is nominal, it must be correctly coded. Once the data are ready, the parameters a and b are computed to obtain a regression equation. To understand the mathematical process, recall the algebraic equation for a straight line:

$$y = bx + a$$

where

$$y = \text{the dependent variable (outcome)}$$

$$x = \text{the independent variable (predictor)}$$

$$b = \text{the slope of the line}$$

$$a = y\text{-intercept (the point where the regression line intersects the } y\text{-axis)}$$

No single regression line can be used to predict with complete accuracy every y value from every x value. In fact, you could draw an infinite number of lines through the scattered paired values (Zar, 2010). However, the purpose of the regression equation is to develop the line to allow the highest degree of prediction possible—the line of best fit. The procedure for developing the line of best fit is the **method of least squares** (Tabachnick & Fidell, 2013). The formulas for the beta (b) and slope (a) of the regression equation are computed as follows. Note that once the b is calculated, that value is inserted into the formula for a.

$$b = \frac{n\sum xy - \sum x \sum y}{n\sum x^2 - \left(\sum x\right)^2}$$

$$a = \frac{\sum y - b\sum x}{n}$$

HAND CALCULATIONS

This example uses data collected from a study of students enrolled in a registered nurse to bachelor of science in nursing (RN to BSN) program (Mancini, Ashwill, & Cipher, 2015). The predictor in this example is number of academic degrees (beyond their Associate Degree in Nursing [ADN]) obtained by the student prior to enrollment, and the dependent variable was number of months it took for the student to complete the RN to BSN program. The null hypothesis is *Number of degrees does not predict the number of months until completion of an RN to BSN program.*

The data are presented in Table 29-1. A simulated subset of 20 students was selected for this example so that the computations would be small and manageable. In actuality, studies involving linear regression need to be adequately powered (Aberson, 2019; Cohen, 1988). Observe that the data in Table 29-1 are arranged in columns that correspond to

Student ID	x (Number of Degrees)	y (Months to Completion)	x^2	xy
1	1	17	1	17
2	2	9	4	18
3	0	17	0	0
4	1	9	1	9
5	0	16	0	0
6	1	11	1	11
7	0	15	0	0
8	0	12	0	0
9	1	15	1	15
10	1	12	1	12
11	1	14	1	14
12	1	10	1	10
13	1	17	1	17
14	0	20	0	0
15	2	9	4	18
16	2	12	4	24
17	1	14	1	14
18	2	10	4	20
19	1	17	1	17
20	2	11	4	22
sum Σ	20	267	30	238

TABLE 29-1 ENROLLMENT GPA AND MONTHS TO COMPLETION IN AN RN TO BSN PROGRAM

the elements of the formula. The summed values in the last row of Table 29-1 are inserted into the appropriate place in the formula for b.

The computations for the b and a are as follows:

Step 1: Calculate b.

From the values in Table 29-1, we know that $n = 20$, $\Sigma x = 20$, $\Sigma y = 267$, $\Sigma x^2 = 30$, and $\Sigma xy = 238$. These values are inserted into the formula for b, as follows:

$$b = \frac{20(238)-(20)(267)}{20(30)-20^2}$$

$$b = -2.90$$

Step 2: Calculate a.

From Step 1, we now know that $b = -2.90$, and we plug this value into the formula for a.

$$a = \frac{267-(-2.9)(20)}{20}$$

$$a = 16.25$$

Step 3: Write the new regression equation:

$$y = -2.90x + 16.25$$

Step 4: Calculate R.

The multiple R is defined as the correlation between the actual y values and the predicted y values using the new regression equation. The predicted y value using the new equation is represented by the symbol $\hat{y}$ to differentiate from y, which represents the actual y values in the data set. We can use our new regression equation from Step 3 to compute predicted program completion time in months for each student, using their number of academic degrees prior to enrollment in the RN to BSN Program. For example, Student #1 had earned 1 academic degree prior to enrollment, and the predicted months to completion for Student 1 is calculated as:

$$\hat{y} = -2.90(1) + 16.25$$

$$\hat{y} = 13.35$$

Thus, the predicted $\hat{y}$ is 13.35 months. This procedure would be continued for the rest of the students, and the Pearson correlation between the actual months to completion (y) and the predicted months to completion ($\hat{y}$) would yield the multiple R value. In this example, the $R = 0.638$. The higher the R, the more likely that the new regression equation accurately predicts y, because the higher the correlation, the closer the actual y values are to the predicted $\hat{y}$ values. Figure 29-1 displays the regression line where the x axis represents possible numbers of degrees, and the y axis represents the predicted months to program completion ($\hat{y}$ values).

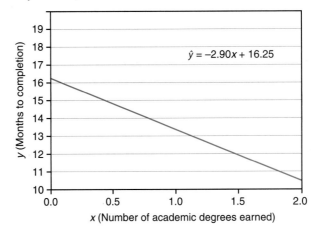

FIGURE 29-1 ▪ **REGRESSION LINE REPRESENTED BY NEW REGRESSION EQUATION.**

Step 5: Determine whether the predictor significantly predicts y.

$$t = R\sqrt{\frac{n-2}{1-R^2}}$$

To know whether the predictor significantly predicts y, the beta must be tested against zero. In simple regression, this is most easily accomplished by using the R value from Step 4:

$$t = .638\sqrt{\frac{20-2}{1-.407}}$$

$$t = 3.52$$

The t value is then compared to the t probability distribution table (see Appendix A). The df for this t statistic is $n - 2$. The critical t value at alpha (α) = 0.05, $df = 18$ is 2.10 for a two-tailed test. Our obtained t was 3.52, which exceeds the critical value in the table, thereby indicating a significant association between the predictor (x) and outcome (y).

Step 6: Calculate R^2.

After establishing the statistical significance of the R value, it must subsequently be examined for clinical importance. This is accomplished by obtaining the **coefficient of determination** for regression—which simply involves squaring the R value. The R^2 represents the percentage of variance explained in y by the predictor. Cohen describes R^2 values of 0.02 as small, 0.13 as moderate, and 0.26 or higher as large effect sizes (Cohen, 1988). In our example, the R was 0.638, and, therefore, the R^2 was 0.407. Multiplying 0.407 × 100% indicates that 40.7% of the variance in months to program completion can be explained by knowing the student's number of earned academic degrees at admission (Cohen & Cohen, 1983).

The R^2 can be very helpful in testing more than one predictor in a regression model. Unlike R, the R^2 for one regression model can be compared with another regression model that contains additional predictors (Cohen & Cohen, 1983). The R^2 is discussed further in Exercise 30.

The standardized beta (β) is another statistic that represents the magnitude of the association between x and y. β has limits just like a Pearson r, meaning that the standardized β cannot be lower than −1.00 or higher than 1.00. This value can be calculated by hand but is best computed with statistical software. The standardized beta (β) is calculated by converting the x and y values to z scores and then correlating the x and y value using the Pearson r formula. The standardized beta (β) is often reported in the literature instead of the unstandardized b, because b does not have lower or upper limits and therefore the magnitude of b cannot be judged. β, on the other hand, is interpreted as a Pearson r and the descriptions of the magnitude of β can be applied, as recommended by Cohen (1988). In this example, the standardized beta (β) is −0.638. Thus, the magnitude of the association between x and y in this example is considered a large predictive association (Cohen, 1988; Tabachnick & Fidell, 2013).

SPSS COMPUTATIONS

This is how our dataset looks in SPSS.

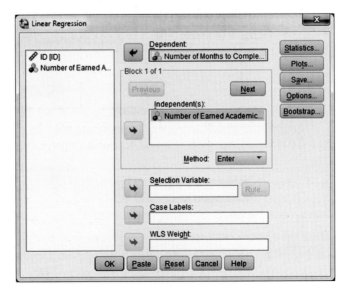

Step 1: From the "Analyze" menu, choose "Regression" and "Linear."

Step 2: Move the predictor, Number of Degrees, to the space labeled "Independent(s)." Move the dependent variable, Number of Months to Completion, to the space labeled "Dependent." Click "OK."

INTERPRETATION OF SPSS OUTPUT

The following tables are generated from SPSS. The first table contains the multiple R and the R^2 values. The multiple R is 0.638, indicating that the correlation between the actual y values and the predicted y values using the new regression equation is 0.638. The R^2 is 0.407, indicating that 40.7% of the variance in months to program completion can be explained by knowing the student's number of earned academic degrees at enrollment.

Regression

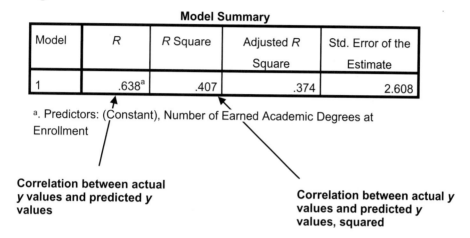

Model Summary

Model	R	R Square	Adjusted R Square	Std. Error of the Estimate
1	.638[a]	.407	.374	2.608

[a]. Predictors: (Constant), Number of Earned Academic Degrees at Enrollment

Correlation between actual y values and predicted y values

Correlation between actual y values and predicted y values, squared

The second table contains the analysis of variance (ANOVA) table. As presented in Exercises 18 and 33, the ANOVA is usually performed to test for differences between group means. However, ANOVA can also be performed for regression, where the null hypothesis is that *knowing the value of x explains no information about y*. This table indicates that knowing the value of x explains a significant amount of variance in y. The contents of the ANOVA table are rarely reported in published manuscripts, because the significance of each predictor is presented in the last SPSS table titled "Coefficients" (see below).

ANOVA[a]

Model		Sum of Squares	df	Mean Square	F	Sig.
1	Regression	84.100	1	84.100	12.363	.002[b]
	Residual	122.450	18	6.803		
	Total	206.550	19			

a. Dependent Variable: Number of Months to Complete Program

b. Predictors: (Constant), Number of Earned Academic Degrees at Enrollment

The third table contains the b and a values, standardized beta (β), t, and exact p value. The a is listed in the first row, next to the label "Constant." The β is listed in the second row, next to the name of the predictor. The remaining information that is important to extract when interpreting regression results can be found in the second row. The standardized beta (β) is −0.638. This value has limits just like a Pearson r, meaning that the standardized β cannot be lower than −1.00 or higher than 1.00. The t value is −3.516, and the exact p value is 0.002.

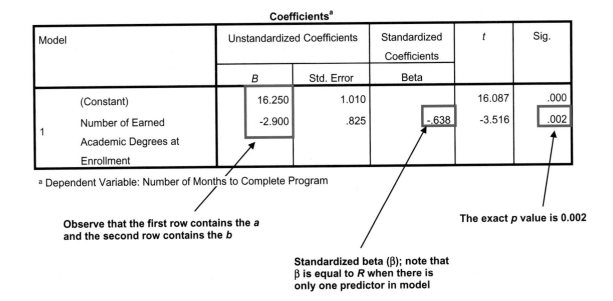

Coefficients[a]

Model		Unstandardized Coefficients		Standardized Coefficients	t	Sig.
		B	Std. Error	Beta		
1	(Constant)	16.250	1.010		16.087	.000
	Number of Earned Academic Degrees at Enrollment	-2.900	.825	-.638	-3.516	.002

[a] Dependent Variable: Number of Months to Complete Program

**Observe that the first row contains the *a*
and the second row contains the *b***

**Standardized beta (β); note that
β is equal to *R* when there is
only one predictor in model**

The exact *p* value is 0.002

FINAL INTERPRETATION IN AMERICAN PSYCHOLOGICAL ASSOCIATION (APA) FORMAT

The following interpretation is written as it might appear in a research article, formatted according to APA guidelines (APA, 2010). Simple linear regression was performed with number of earned academic degrees as the predictor and months to program completion as the dependent variable. The student's number of degrees significantly predicted months to completion among students in an RN to BSN program, $\beta = -0.638$, $p = 0.002$, and R^2 = 40.7%. Higher numbers of earned academic degrees significantly predicted shorter program completion time.

STUDY QUESTIONS

1. If you have access to SPSS, compute the Shapiro-Wilk test of normality for months to completion (as demonstrated in Exercise 26). If you do not have access to SPSS, plot the frequency distributions by hand. What do the results indicate?

2. State the null hypothesis for the example where number of degrees was used to predict time to BSN program completion.

3. In the formula $y = bx + a$, what does "b" represent?

4. In the formula $y = bx + a$, what does "a" represent?

5. Using the new regression equation, $\hat{y} = -2.90x + 16.25$, compute the predicted months to program completion if a student's number of earned degrees is 0. Show your calculations.

6. Using the new regression equation, $\hat{y} = -2.90x + 16.25$, compute the predicted months to program completion if a student's number of earned degrees is 2. Show your calculations.

7. What was the correlation between the actual y values and the predicted y values using the new regression equation in the example?

8. What was the exact likelihood of obtaining a t value at least as extreme as or as close to the one that was actually observed, assuming that the null hypothesis is true?

9. How much variance in months to completion is explained by knowing the student's number of earned degrees?

10. How would you characterize the magnitude of the R^2 in the example? Provide a rationale for your answer.

Answers to Study Questions

1. The Shapiro-Wilk *p* value for months to RN to BSN program completion was 0.16, indicating that the frequency distribution did not significantly deviate from normality. Moreover, visual inspection of the frequency distribution indicates that months to completion is approximately normally distributed. See SPSS output below for the histogram of the distribution and the test of normality table.

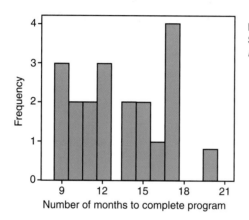

Mean = 13.35
Std. Dev. = 3.297
n = 20

Tests of Normality						
	Kolmogorov-Smirnova[a]			Shapiro-Wilk		
	Statistic	df	Sig.	Statistic	df	Sig.
Number of Months to Complete Program	.159	20	.200*	.931	20	.160
*. This is a lower bound of the true significance.						
a. Lilliefors Significance Correction						

2. The null hypothesis is: *The number of earned academic degrees does not predict the number of months until completion of an RN to BSN program.*

3. In the formula $y = bx + a$, "*b*" represents the slope of the regression line.

4. In the formula $y = bx + a$, "*a*" represents the *y*-intercept, or the point at which the regression line intersects the *y*-axis.

5. The predicted months to program completion if a student's number of academic degrees is 0 is calculated as: $\hat{y} = -2.90(0) + 16.25 = 16.25$ months.

6. The predicted months to program completion if a student's number of academic degrees is 2 is calculated as: $\hat{y} = -2.90(2) + 16.25 = 10.45$ months.

7. The correlation between the actual *y* values and the predicted *y* values using the new regression equation in the example, also known as the multiple *R*, is 0.638.

8. The exact likelihood of obtaining a *t* value at least as extreme as or as close to the one that was actually observed, assuming that the null hypothesis is true, was 0.2%. This value was obtained by looking at the SPSS output table titled "Coefficients" in the last value of the column labeled "Sig."

9. 40.7% of the variance in months to completion is explained by knowing the student's number of earned academic degrees at enrollment. This value is seen in the Model Summary Table under the column labeled R^2. The value is multiplied by 100% to report as a percentage.

10. The magnitude of the R^2 in this example, 0.407, would be considered a large effect according to the effect size tables in Exercises 24 and 25 of this text.

DATA FOR ADDITIONAL COMPUTATIONAL PRACTICE FOR THE QUESTIONS TO BE GRADED

Using the example from Mancini and colleagues (2015), students enrolled in an RN to BSN program were assessed for demographics at enrollment. The predictor in this example is age at program enrollment, and the dependent variable was number of months it took for the student to complete the RN to BSN program. The null hypothesis is: *Student age at enrollment does not predict the number of months until completion of an RN to BSN program.* The data are presented in Table 29-2. A simulated subset of 20 students was randomly selected for this example so that the computations would be small and manageable.

TABLE 29-2 AGE AT ENROLLMENT AND MONTHS TO COMPLETION IN AN RN TO BSN PROGRAM

Student ID	x (Student Age)	y (Months to Completion)	x^2	xy
1	23	17	529	391
2	24	9	576	216
3	24	17	576	408
4	26	9	676	234
5	31	16	961	496
6	31	11	961	341
7	32	15	1,024	480
8	33	12	1,089	396
9	33	15	1,089	495
10	34	12	1,156	408
11	34	14	1,156	476
12	35	10	1,225	350
13	35	17	1,225	595
14	39	20	1,521	780
15	40	9	1,600	360
16	42	12	1,764	504
17	42	14	1,764	588
18	44	10	1,936	440
19	51	17	2,601	867
20	24	11	576	264
sum	**677**	**267**	**24,005**	**9,089**

Questions to Be Graded

Name: _____ Class: _____

Date: _____

Answer the following questions with hand calculations using the data presented in Table 29-2 or the SPSS dataset called "Exercise 29 Example 2.sav" available on the Evolve website. Follow your instructor's directions to submit your answers to the following questions for grading. Your instructor may ask you to write your answers below and submit them as a hard copy for grading. Alternatively, your instructor may ask you to submit your answers online.

1. If you have access to SPSS, compute the Shapiro-Wilk test of normality for the variable age (as demonstrated in Exercise 26). If you do not have access to SPSS, plot the frequency distributions by hand. What do the results indicate?

2. State the null hypothesis where age at enrollment is used to predict the time for completion of an RN to BSN program.

3. What is *b* as computed by hand (or using SPSS)?

4. What is *a* as computed by hand (or using SPSS)?

5. Write the new regression equation.

6. How would you characterize the magnitude of the obtained R^2 value? Provide a rationale for your answer.

7. How much variance in months to RN to BSN program completion is explained by knowing the student's enrollment age?

8. What was the correlation between the actual y values and the predicted y values using the new regression equation in the example?

9. Write your interpretation of the results as you would in an APA-formatted journal.

10. Given the results of your analyses, would you use the calculated regression equation to predict future students' program completion time by using enrollment age as x? Provide a rationale for your answer.

Calculating Multiple Linear Regression

Multiple linear regression analysis is an extension of simple linear regression in which more than one independent variable is entered into the analysis. Interpretations of multiple regression findings are much the same as with simple linear regression, which is reviewed in Exercise 29. The beta (β) values of each predictor are tested for significance, and a multiple R and R^2 are computed. In multiple linear regression, however, when all predictors are tested simultaneously, each β has been adjusted for every other predictor in the regression model. The β represents the independent relationship between that predictor and y, even after controlling for (or accounting for) the presence of every other predictor in the model (Cohen & Cohen, 1983; Stevens, 2009)).

In multiple linear regression, relationships between multiple predictors and y are tested simultaneously with a series of matrix algebra calculations. Therefore, multiple linear regression is best conducted using a statistical software package; however, full explanations and examples of the matrix algebraic computations of multiple linear regression are presented in Stevens (2009) and Tabachnick and Fidell (2013).

RESEARCH DESIGNS APPROPRIATE FOR MULTIPLE LINEAR REGRESSION

Research designs that may utilize multiple linear regression include any associational design (Gliner, Morgan, & Leech, 2009; Kazdin, 2017). The variables involved in the design are usually attributional, meaning the variables are characteristics of the participant, such as health status, blood pressure, gender, diagnosis, or ethnicity. Regardless of the nature of variables, the dependent variable submitted to multiple linear regression must be measured as continuous or measured at the interval or ratio level (see Exercise 1; Gray, Grove, & Sutherland, 2017). Although the predictor can be any scale of measurement, if it is nominal, it must be correctly coded which is described later in this exercise.

STATISTICAL FORMULA AND ASSUMPTIONS

Use of multiple linear regression involves the following assumptions (Zar, 2010; Tabachnick & Fidell, 2013):

1. Normal distribution of the dependent (y) variable
2. Linear relationship between x and y
3. Independent observations
4. Homoscedasticity (discussed later in this exercise)

5. Interval or ratio measurement of the dependent variable; however, if the variables are measured with a Likert scale, and the frequency distribution is approximately normally distributed, these data are usually considered interval level measurement and are appropriate to serve as the outcome in a linear regression model (Rasmussen, 1989; Waltz, Strickland, & Lenz, 2017).

Multiple Linear Regression Equation

The parameters a and β (a beta is computed for each predictor) are computed to obtain a regression equation. The equation looks similar to that of the simple linear regression equation presented in Exercise 29, but has been expanded to reflect the presence of multiple predictors:

$$y = \beta_1 x_1 + \beta_2 x_2 + \beta_3 x_3 \ldots + a$$

where

y = the dependent variable
x_1, x_2, x_3, etc. = the independent variables (predictors)
$\beta_1, \beta_2, \beta_3$, etc. = the slopes of the line for each predictor
a = y-intercept (the point where the regression line intersects the y-axis)

Multiple linear regression can be computed by hand, but requires knowledge of matrix algebra. Therefore, we will use SPSS to compute the regression equation and other important parameters such as the R and R^2.

Homoscedasticity and Heteroscedasticity

Data that are **homoscedastic** are evenly dispersed both above and below a plotted line of perfect prediction when variable x predicts variable y. Homoscedasticity reflects equal variance of both variables. In other words, for every value of x, the distribution of y values should have equal variability. If the data for the predictor and dependent variable are not homoscedastic, inferences made during significance testing could be invalid (Cohen & Cohen, 1983; Zar, 2010).

This assumption can be checked by visual examination of a plot of the standardized residuals (the errors) by the regression standardized predicted value. Ideally, residuals are randomly scattered around 0 (the horizontal line representing perfectly accurate prediction) providing a relatively even distribution. **Heteroscedasticity** is indicated when the residuals are not evenly scattered around the line. Heteroscedasticity manifested itself in all kinds of uneven shapes. When the plot of residuals appears to deviate substantially from normal, more formal tests for heteroscedasticity should be performed. Formal tests for heteroscedasticity include the Breusch-Pagan Test (Breusch & Pagan, 1979) and White's Test (White, 1980).

Take for example the plots in Figures 30-1 and 30-2 that follow. Two multiple linear regression analyses were performed, and the predicted y values were plotted against the residuals (actual y − predicted y). Homoscedasticity occurs when the observations (seen as dots) are equally distributed above the line and below the line. It should look like a "bird's nest," such as the shape exhibited in Figure 30-1, and not a cone or triangle, such as the shape in Figure 30-2.

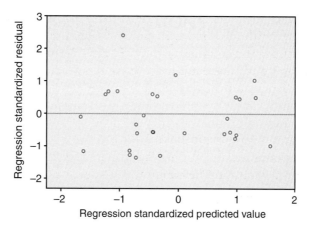

FIGURE 30-1 ■ **EXAMPLE OF HOMOSCEDASTICITY.**

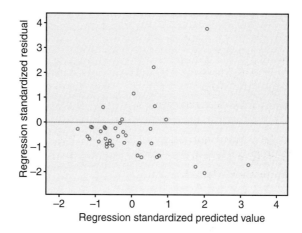

FIGURE 30-2 ■ **EXAMPLE OF HETEROSCEDASTICITY.**

Multicollinearity

Multicollinearity occurs when the predictors in a multiple regression equation are strongly correlated (Cohen & Cohen, 1983). Multicollinearity is minimized by carefully selecting the predictors and thoroughly determining the interrelationships among predictors prior to the regression analysis. Multicollinearity does not affect predictive power (the capacity of the predictors to predict values of the dependent variable in that specific sample); rather it causes problems related to generalizability (Zar, 2010). If multicollinearity is present, the equation will not have predictive validity. The amount of variance explained by each variable in the equation will be inflated. The β values will not remain consistent across samples when cross-validation (the process of testing a new regression equation's ability to predict new data) is performed (Cohen & Cohen, 1983; Zar, 2010).

The first step in identifying multicollinearity is to examine the correlations among the predictor variables. Therefore, you would perform multiple correlation analyses before conducting the regression analyses. The correlation matrix is carefully examined for evidence of multicollinearity. SPSS provides two statistics (tolerance and VIF [variance inflation factor]) that describe the extent to which your model has a multicollinearity problem. A tolerance of less than 0.20 or 0.10 and/or a VIF of 5 or 10 and above indicates a multicollinearity problem (Allison, 1999).

Dummy Coding of Nominal Predictors

In multiple linear regression, the dependent variable is continuous, and the predictor can be any scale of measurement; however, if the predictor is nominal, it must be correctly coded. To use categorical predictors in regression analysis, a coding system is developed to represent group membership. Categorical variables of interest in nursing that might be used in regression analysis include gender, income, ethnicity, social status, level of education, and diagnosis. If the variable is dichotomous, such as gender, members of one category are assigned the number 1, and all others are assigned the number 0. In this case, for gender the coding could be:

$$1 = \text{female}, 0 = \text{male}$$

The process of creating dichotomous variables from categorical variables is called dummy coding. If the categorical variable has three values, two dummy variables are used; for example, social class could be classified as lower class, middle class, or upper class. The first dummy variable ($x1$) would be classified as:

$$1 = \text{lower class}$$

$$0 = \text{not lower class}$$

The second dummy variable ($x2$) would be classified as

$$1 = \text{middle class}$$

$$0 = \text{not middle class}$$

The three social classes would then be specified in the equation in the following manner:

$$\text{Lower class } x1 = 1, x2 = 0$$

$$\text{Middle class } x1 = 0, x2 = 1$$

$$\text{Upper class } x1 = 0, x2 = 0$$

When more than three categories define the values of the variable, increased numbers of dummy variables are used. The number of dummy variables is always one less than the number of categories (Aiken & West, 1991)—otherwise multicollinearity will be very high.

SPSS COMPUTATIONS

This example uses data collected from a study of students enrolled in an RN to BSN program (Mancini, Ashwill, & Cipher, 2015). The predictors in this example are student age at enrollment, number of prior academic degrees earned at the time of enrollment, and type of program (1 = in-seat; 0 = online). The dependent variable is number of months it took for the student to complete the RN to BSN program. The null hypothesis is *Age, number of degrees earned, and type of program do not predict the number of months until completion of an RN to BSN program.*

The data are presented in Table 30-1. A simulated subset of 20 students was randomly selected for this example so that the computations would be small and manageable. In actuality, studies involving linear regression need to be adequately powered (Aberson,

TABLE 30-1	PREDICTORS OF MONTHS TO COMPLETION IN AN RN TO BSN PROGRAM			
Student ID	Student Age	In-Seat Program	Number of Degrees	Months to Completion
1	23	0	1	17
2	24	1	2	9
3	24	0	0	17
4	26	1	1	9
5	31	1	0	16
6	31	1	1	11
7	32	0	0	15
8	33	1	0	12
9	33	0	1	15
10	34	1	1	12
11	34	0	1	14
12	35	1	1	10
13	35	0	1	17
14	39	0	0	20
15	40	1	2	9
16	42	1	2	12
17	42	0	1	14
18	44	1	2	10
19	51	0	1	17
20	24	1	2	11

2019; Cohen, 1988; Gaskin & Happell, 2014). See Exercises 24 and 25 for more information regarding statistical power. Observe that the dichotomous predictor, program type, has been properly coded as 1 or 0.

This is how our data set looks in SPSS.

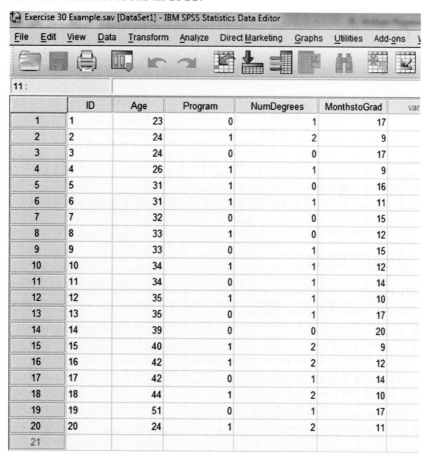

Step 1: From the "Analyze" menu, choose "Regression" and "Linear."

Step 2: Move the predictors Age, Program, and Number Degrees, to the space labeled "Independent(s)." Move the dependent variable, Number of Months to Completion, to the space labeled "Dependent."

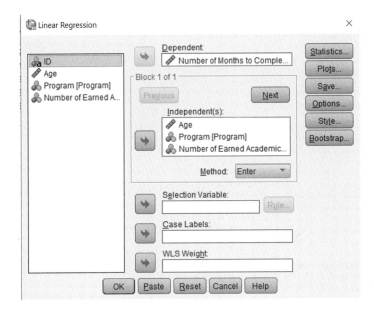

Step 3: Click "Statistics." Check the box labeled "Collinearity diagnostics." Click "Continue."

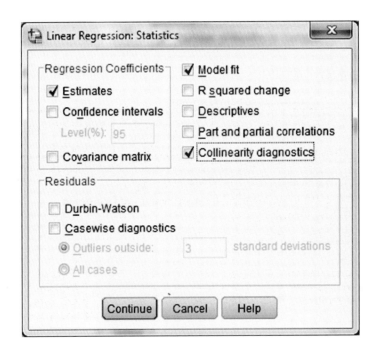

Step 4: Click "Plots." Move the variable "ZPRED" (standardized predictor values) to the box labeled "X." Move the variable "ZRESID" (standardized residual values) to the box labeled "Y." Click "Continue" and "OK."

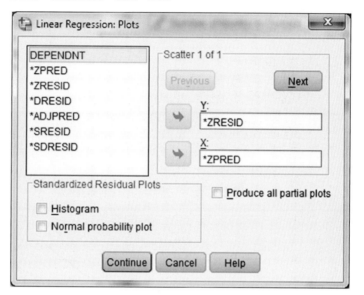

INTERPRETATION OF SPSS OUTPUT

The following tables and figure are generated from SPSS. The first table contains the multiple R and the R^2 values. The multiple R is 0.855, indicating that the correlation between the actual y values and the predicted y values using the new regression equation is 0.875. The R^2 is 0.766, indicating that 76.6% of the variance in months to program completion can be explained by knowing the student's age, number of prior degrees, and program type. The adjusted R^2 is 0.723, which is slightly lower because it reflects an elimination of increases in R^2 that occurred due to chance by simply adding predictors to the model (Allison, 1999).

Regression

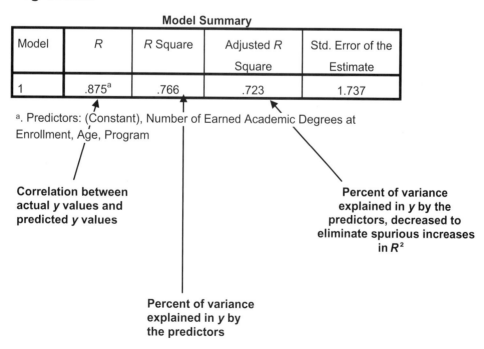

Model Summary

Model	R	R Square	Adjusted R Square	Std. Error of the Estimate
1	.875[a]	.766	.723	1.737

a. Predictors: (Constant), Number of Earned Academic Degrees at Enrollment, Age, Program

Correlation between actual y values and predicted y values

Percent of variance explained in y by the predictors

Percent of variance explained in y by the predictors, decreased to eliminate spurious increases in R^2

The second table contains the analysis of variance (ANOVA) table. As presented in Exercise 33, the ANOVA is usually performed to test for differences between group means; however, ANOVA can also be performed for regression, where the null hypothesis is that *knowing the value of x explains no information about y.* This table indicates that knowing the value of x explains a significant amount of variance in y. The contents of the ANOVA table are rarely reported in published manuscripts, because the significance of each predictor is presented in the last SPSS table titled "Coefficients" (see below).

ANOVA[a]

Model		Sum of Squares	df	Mean Square	F	Sig.
1	Regression	158.294	3	52.765	17.495	.000[b]
	Residual	48.256	16	3.016		
	Total	206.550	19			

[a]. Dependent Variable: Number of Months to Complete Program

[b]. Predictors: (Constant), Number of Earned Academic Degrees at Enrollment, Age, Program type

The third table contains the b and a values, standardized beta (β), t, exact p values, and collinearity diagnostics. The a is listed in the first row, next to the label "Constant." The b is listed in the following rows, next to the name of each predictor. The remaining information that is important to extract when interpreting regression results can be found in the second through fourth rows, which list the standardized β and the p values. It should be noted that although that the p value in the "ANOVA" table and the p value listed in the "Coefficients" table for the predictor Program are ".000". However, p is never zero and should more accurately be written as less than 0.001 or < 0.001. Finally, the collinearity diagnostics, tolerance, and VIF (variance inflation factor) are listed for each predictor. A tolerance of less than 0.20 or 0.10 and/or a VIF of 5 or 10 and above indicates a multicollinearity problem (Allison, 1999). Here, there does not appear to be a multicollinearity problem, as the tolerance values are greater than 0.70, and the VIF values are less than 2.0.

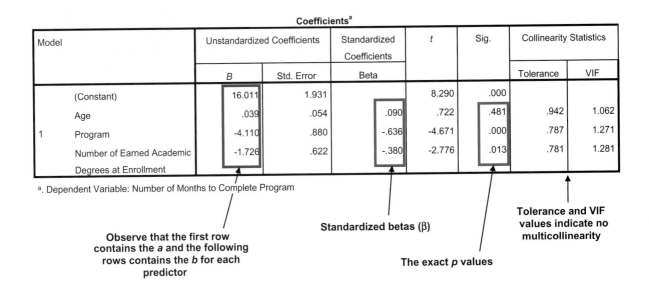

Coefficients[a]

Model		Unstandardized Coefficients		Standardized Coefficients	t	Sig.	Collinearity Statistics	
		B	Std. Error	Beta			Tolerance	VIF
1	(Constant)	16.011	1.931		8.290	.000		
	Age	.039	.054	.090	.722	.481	.942	1.062
	Program	-4.110	.880	-.636	-4.671	.000	.787	1.271
	Number of Earned Academic Degrees at Enrollment	-1.726	.622	-.380	-2.776	.013	.781	1.281

[a]. Dependent Variable: Number of Months to Complete Program

Observe that the first row contains the *a* and the following rows contains the *b* for each predictor

Standardized betas (β)

The exact *p* values

Tolerance and VIF values indicate no multicollinearity

The last figure in the output is the scatterplot that assists us in identifying heteroscedasticity. Recall that homoscedasticity occurs when the observations (seen as dots in the figure) are equally distributed above a horizontal line representing perfectly accurate prediction drawn at $y = 0$ and below the line at $y = 0$. In this example, our data appear to have met the homoscedasticity assumption, because the values appear to be evenly dispersed above and below the line.

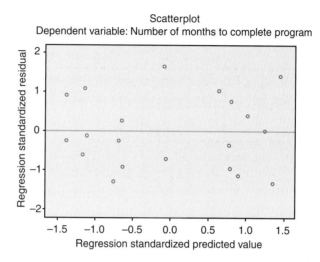

Scatterplot
Dependent variable: Number of months to complete program

FINAL INTERPRETATION IN AMERICAN PSYCHOLOGICAL ASSOCIATION (APA) FORMAT

The following interpretation is written as it might appear in a research article, formatted according to APA guidelines (APA, 2010). Multiple linear regression was performed with enrollment age, number of prior academic degrees earned, and program type as the predictors and months to RN to BSN program completion as the dependent variable. Collinearity diagnostics indicated no multicollinearity, and visual inspection of the scatterplot of the residuals revealed no heteroscedasticity. Number of prior degrees earned and program type significantly predicted months to completion among students in an RN to BSN program, $R^2 = 76.6\%$, adjusted $R^2 = 72.3\%$. Higher numbers of earned academic degrees significantly predicted shorter program completion time ($\beta = -0.38$, $p = 0.013$). Enrollment in the in-seat program also significantly predicted shorter program completion time ($\beta = -0.636$, $p < 0.001$). Age did not significantly predict program completion time.

STUDY QUESTIONS

1. If you have access to SPSS, compute Pearson correlations between the predictors (age, number of degrees, and program type). Is there any indication of multicollinearity? Provide a rationale for your answer.

2. State the null hypothesis for this study where age, number of degrees, and program type are used to predict the time for RN to BSN program completion.

3. Write the newly computed regression equation, predicting months to completion.

4. Using the new regression equation, compute the predicted months to program completion if a student's enrollment age = 40, number of degrees = 1, and enrolled in the in-seat program. Show your calculations.

5. Using the new regression equation, compute the predicted months to program completion if a student's enrollment age = 23, number of degrees = 0, and enrolled in the online program. Show your calculations.

6. What was the correlation between the actual y values and the predicted y values using the new regression equation in the example?

7. What was the exact likelihood of obtaining our t value for program type that is at least as extreme or as close to the one that was actually observed, assuming that the null hypothesis is true?

8. Which predictor has the strongest association with y? Provide a rationale for your answer.

9. How much variance in months to completion is explained by the three model predictors?

10. How would you characterize the magnitude of the R^2 in the example? Provide a rationale for your answer.

Answers to Study Questions

1. There is no evidence of a multicollinearity problem, as the largest correlation between the three predictors is $r = 0.426$. This means that the most variance shared between any two variables is 18.1% (calculated by squaring 0.426).

2. The null hypothesis is: *Age, number of earned academic degrees, and type of program do not predict the number of months until completion of an RN to BSN program.*

3. The newly computed regression equation is: $\hat{y} = 0.039x_1 + -4.11x_2 + -1.73x_3 + 16.01$ where x_1 = age, x_2 = program type, x_3 = number degrees, and a = 16.01.

4. The predicted months to program completion if a student's enrollment age = 40, number of degrees = 1, and enrolled in the in-seat program is:

$$\hat{y} = 0.039(40) + -4.11(1) + -1.73(1) + 16.01 = 1.56 - 4.11 - 1.73 + 16.01 = 11.73$$

$$\hat{y} = 11.73 \text{ months}$$

5. The predicted months to program completion if a student's enrollment age = 23, number of degrees = 0, and enrolled in the online program is:

$$\hat{y} = 0.039(23) + -4.11(0) + -1.73(0) + 16.01 = 0.897 + 0 + 0 + 16.01 = 16.91$$

$$\hat{y} = 16.91 \text{ months}$$

6. The multiple R is 0.875. This value can be observed in the "Model Summary" table of the SPSS output.

7. The exact likelihood of obtaining our t value for program type that is at least as extreme or as close to the one that was actually observed, assuming that the null hypothesis is true, is less than 0.1%. The p value for program type is listed in the SPSS output as ".000". However, p is never zero and should more accurately be written as less than 0.001 or < 0.001. When converted to a percentage, this would mean that $0.001 \times 100\%$ = less than 0.1%. value can be observed in the "Coefficients" table of the SPSS output, in the row labeled "Program Type".

8. The predictor type of program has the strongest association with y, with a standardized β of −0.636. The other two predictors had lower standardized beta values as presented in the "Coefficients" Table.

9. 76.6% of the variance in months to completion is explained by the three model predictors.

10. The magnitude of the R^2, 0.766, or 76.6%, is considered a large effect according to the effect size tables in Exercises 24 and 25 (Tables 24-1 and 25-1).

DATA FOR ADDITIONAL COMPUTATIONAL PRACTICE FOR QUESTIONS TO BE GRADED

Using the same example from Mancini and colleagues (2015), the following data include only the two significant predictors from the previous analysis. The significant predictors were number of earned academic degrees at program enrollment and program type (in-seat/online) and the dependent variable was number of months it took for the student to complete the RN to BSN program. The data are presented in Table 30-2.

TABLE 30-2	PREDICTORS OF MONTHS TO COMPLETION IN AN RN TO BSN PROGRAM		
Student ID	**In-Seat Program**	**Number of Degrees**	**Months to Completion**
1	0	1	17
2	1	2	9
3	0	0	17
4	1	1	9
5	1	0	16
6	1	1	11
7	0	0	15
8	1	0	12
9	0	1	15
10	1	1	12
11	0	1	14
12	1	1	10
13	0	1	17
14	0	0	20
15	1	2	9
16	1	2	12
17	0	1	14
18	1	2	10
19	0	1	17
20	1	2	11

Questions to Be Graded

Name: _____	Class: _____
Date: _____	

Answer the following questions with hand calculations using the data presented in Table 30-2 or the SPSS dataset called "Exercise 30 Example 2.sav" available on the Evolve website. Follow your instructor's directions to submit your answers to the following questions for grading. Your instructor may ask you to write your answers below and submit them as a hard copy for grading. Alternatively, your instructor may ask you to submit your answers online.

1. Write the newly computed regression equation, predicting months to RN to BSN program completion.

2. Why have the values in the equation changed slightly from the first analysis?

3. Using SPSS, create the scatterplot of predicted values and residuals that assists us in identifying heteroscedasticity. Do the data meet the homescedasticity assumption? Provide a rationale for your answer.

379

4. Using the new regression equation, compute the predicted months to RN to BSN program completion if a student's number of degrees is 1 and is enrolled in the online program. Show your calculations.

5. Using the new regression equation, compute the predicted months to RN to BSN program completion if a student's number of degrees is 2 and is enrolled in the in-seat program. Show your calculations.

6. What was the correlation between the actual y values and the predicted y values using the new regression equation in the example?

7. Which predictor has the strongest association with y? Provide a rationale for your answer.

8. How much variance in months to completion is explained by the two model predictors?

9. Write your interpretation of the results as you would in an APA-formatted journal.

10. Given the results of your analyses, would you use the calculated regression equation to predict future students' RN to BSN program completion time by using program type and number of degrees as the predictors?

Calculating *t*-tests for Independent Samples

One of the most common statistical tests chosen to investigate significant differences between two independent samples is the independent samples *t*-test. The samples are independent if the study participants in one group are unrelated or different participants than those in the second group. The dependent variable in an independent samples *t*-test must be scaled as interval or ratio. If the dependent variable is measured with a Likert scale, and the frequency distribution is approximately normally distributed, these data are usually considered interval level measurement and are appropriate for an independent samples *t*-test (see Exercise 1; Rasmussen, 1989; Waltz, Strickland, & Lenz, 2017; de Winter & Dodou, 2010).

RESEARCH DESIGNS APPROPRIATE FOR THE INDEPENDENT SAMPLES *t*-TEST

Research designs that may utilize the independent samples *t*-test include the randomized experimental, quasi-experimental, and comparative designs (Gliner, Morgan, & Leech, 2009). The independent variable (the *grouping* variable for the *t*-test) may be active or attributional. An **active independent variable** refers to an intervention, treatment, or program. An **attributional independent variable** refers to a characteristic of the participant, such as gender, diagnosis, or ethnicity. Regardless of the nature of the independent variable, the independent samples *t*-test only compares two groups at a time.

Example 1: Researchers conduct a randomized experimental study where the participants are randomized to either a novel weight loss intervention or a placebo. The number of pounds lost from baseline to post-treatment for both groups is measured. The research question is: *Is there a difference between the two groups in weight lost?* The active independent variable is the weight loss intervention, and the dependent variable is number of pounds lost over the treatment span.

Null hypothesis: *There is no difference between the intervention and the control (placebo) groups in weight lost.*

Example 2: Researchers conduct a retrospective comparative descriptive study where a chart review of patients is done to identify patients who recently underwent a colonoscopy. The patients were divided into two groups: those who used statins continuously in the past year, and those who did not. The dependent variable is the number of polyps found during the colonoscopy, and the independent variable is statin use. Her research question is: *Is there a significant difference between the statin users and nonusers in number of colon polyps found?*

Null hypothesis: *There is no difference between the group taking statins versus the group not taking statins (control) in number of colon polyps found.*

STATISTICAL FORMULA AND ASSUMPTIONS

Use of the independent samples *t*-test involves the following assumptions (Zar, 2010):

1. Sample means from the population are normally distributed.
2. The dependent variable is measured at the interval/ratio level.
3. The two samples have equal variance.
4. All observations within each sample are independent.

The formula and calculation of the independent samples *t*-test are presented in this exercise.

The formula for the independent samples *t*-test is:

$$t = \frac{\bar{X}_1 - \bar{X}_2}{s_{X1-X2}}$$

where

$\bar{X}_1$ = mean of group 1
$\bar{X}_2$ = mean of group 2
"s_{X1-X2}" = to the standard error of the difference between the two groups

To compute the *t*-test, one must compute the denominator in the formula, which is the standard error of the difference between the means. If the two groups have different sample sizes, then one must use this formula:

$$s_{\bar{X}_1 - \bar{X}_2} \sqrt{\frac{(n_1 - 1)s_1^2 + (n_2 - 1)s_2^2}{n_1 + n_2 - 2}\left(\frac{1}{n_1} + \frac{1}{n_2}\right)}$$

where

n_1 = group 1 sample size
n_2 = group 2 sample size
s_1 = group 1 variance
s_2 = group 2 variance

If the two groups have the same number of subjects in each group, then one can use this simplified formula:

$$s_{\bar{X}_1 - \bar{X}_2} = \sqrt{\frac{s_1^2 + s_2^2}{n}}$$

where

n = the sample size in each group and not the total sample of both groups

HAND CALCULATIONS

A randomized experimental study examined the impact of a special type of vocational rehabilitation on employment variables among spinal cord injured veterans, in which post-treatment wages and hours worked were examined (Ottomanelli et al., 2012). Participants were randomized to receive supported employment or treatment as usual (subsequently referred to as "Control"). Supported employment refers to a type of specialized interdisciplinary vocational rehabilitation designed to help people with disabilities obtain and maintain community-based competitive employment in their chosen occupation (Bond, 2004).

The data from this study are presented in Table 31-1. A simulated subset was selected for this example so that the computations would be small and manageable. In actuality, studies involving independent samples *t*-tests need to be adequately powered (Aberson, 2019; Cohen, 1988). See Exercises 24 and 25 for more information regarding statistical power.

TABLE 31-1   POST-TREATMENT WEEKLY HOURS WORKED BY TREATMENT AND CONTROL GROUPS

Participant # Treatment Group	Weekly Hours Worked Treatment Group	Participant # Control Group	Weekly Hours Worked Control Group
1	25	11	8
2	27	12	9
3	19	13	15
4	20	14	17
5	40	15	24
6	25	16	15
7	40	17	18
8	35	18	9
9	30	19	18
10	15	20	16

The independent variable in this example is the treatment (or intervention) Supported Employment Vocational Rehabilitation, and the treatment group is compared with the control group that received usual or standard care. The dependent variable was number of weekly hours worked post-treatment. The null hypothesis is: *There is no difference between the treatment and control groups in post-treatment weekly hours worked among veterans with spinal cord injuries.*

The computations for the independent samples *t*-test are as follows:

Step 1: Compute means for both groups, which involves the sum of scores for each group divided by the number in the group.

$$\text{The mean for Group 1, Treatment Group: } \bar{X}_1 = 27.6$$

$$\text{The mean for Group 2, Control Group: } \bar{X}_2 = 14.9$$

Step 2: Compute the numerator of the *t*-test:

$$27.6 - 14.9 = \mathbf{12.7}$$

It does not matter which group is designated as "Group 1" or "Group 2."

Another possible correct method for Step 2 is to subtract Group 1's mean from Group 2's mean, such as: $\bar{X}_2 - \bar{X}_1$: $14.9 - 27.6 = \mathbf{-12.7}$

This will result in the exact same *t*-test results and interpretation, only the *t*-test value will be negative instead of positive. The sign of the *t*-test does not matter in the interpretation of the results—only the *magnitude* of the *t*-test.

Step 3: Compute the standard error of the difference.
  a. Compute the variances for each group:

$$s^2 \text{ for Group 1} = 74.71$$

$$s^2 \text{ for Group 2} = 24.99$$

  b. Plug into the standard error of the difference formula:

$$s_{\bar{X}_1 - \bar{X}_2} = \sqrt{\frac{s_1^2 + s_2^2}{n}}$$

$$s_{\bar{X}_1 - \bar{X}_2} = \sqrt{\frac{74.71 + 24.99}{10}}$$

$$s_{\bar{X}_1 - \bar{X}_2} = \mathbf{3.16}$$

Step 4: Compute *t* value:

$$t = \frac{\bar{X}_1 - \bar{X}_2}{s_{\bar{X}_1 - \bar{X}_2}}$$

$$t = \frac{12.7}{3.16}$$

$$t = \mathbf{4.02}$$

Step 5: Compute the degrees of freedom:

$$df = n_1 + n_2 - 2$$
$$df = 10 + 10 - 2$$
$$df = 18$$

Step 6: Locate the critical *t* value in the *t* distribution table (Appendix A) and compare it to the obtained *t* value.

The critical *t* value for a two-tailed test with 18 degrees of freedom at alpha (α) = 0.05 is 2.101. This means that if we viewed the *t* distribution for $df = 18$, the middle 95% of the distribution would be marked by -2.10 and 2.10. The obtained *t* is 4.02, exceeding the critical value, which means our *t*-test is statistically significant and represents a real difference between the two groups. Therefore, we can reject our null hypothesis. It should be noted that if the obtained *t* was -4.02, it would also be considered statistically significant, because the absolute value of the obtained *t* is compared to the critical *t* tabled value (Zar, 2010).

SPSS COMPUTATIONS

This is how our dataset looks in SPSS.

	ID	Group	Hours	var	va
1	1	1	25		
2	2	1	27		
3	3	1	19		
4	4	1	20		
5	5	1	40		
6	6	1	25		
7	7	1	40		
8	8	1	35		
9	9	1	30		
10	10	1	15		
11	11	2	8		
12	12	2	9		
13	13	2	15		
14	14	2	17		
15	15	2	24		
16	16	2	15		
17	17	2	18		
18	18	2	9		
19	19	2	18		
20	20	2	16		
21					

Data View Variable View

Step 1: From the "Analyze" menu, choose "Compare Means" and "Independent Samples T Test". Move the dependent variable, Hours Worked, over to the right, like the window below.

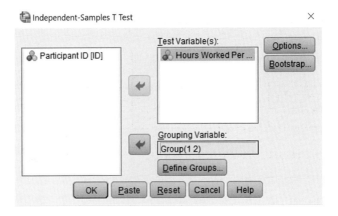

Step 2: Move the independent variable, Group, into the space titled "Grouping Variable." Click "Define Groups" and enter 1 and 2 to represent the coding chosen to differentiate between the two groups. Click Continue and OK.

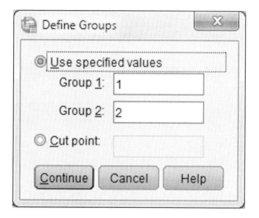

INTERPRETATION OF SPSS OUTPUT

The following tables are generated from SPSS. The first table contains descriptive statistics for hours worked, separated by the two groups. The second table contains the *t*-test results.

T-Test

Group Statistics

	Treatment Group	N	Mean	Std. Deviation	Std. Error Mean
Hours Worked Per Week	Supported Employment	10	27.60	8.644	2.733
	Control	10	14.90	4.999	1.581

Observe the means for the two groups

The first table displays descriptive statistics that allow us to observe the means for both groups. This table is important because it indicates that the participants in the treatment group (Supported Employment) worked 27.60 weekly hours on average, and the participants in the Control group worked 14.90 weekly hours on average.

Independent Samples Test

		Levene's Test for Equality of Variances		t-test for Equality of Means						
									95% Confidence Interval of the Difference	
		F	Sig.	t	df	Sig. (2-tailed)	Mean Difference	Std. Error Difference	Lower	Upper
Hours Worked Per Week	Equal variances assumed	3.267	.087	4.022	18	.001	12.700	3.158	6.066	19.334
	Equal variances not assumed			4.022	14.415	.001	12.700	3.158	5.946	19.454

Observe that the *t* value is 4.022   **The exact *p* value is .001**

The last table contains the actual *t*-test value, the *p* value, along with the values that compose the *t*-test formula. The first value in the table is the Levene's test for equality of variances. The Levene's test is a statistical test of the equal variances assumption. The *p* value is 0.087, indicating the there was no significant difference between the two groups' variances. If there had been a significant difference, the second row of the table, titled "Equal variances not assumed," would be reported in the results (Zar, 2010).

Following the Levene's test results are the *t*-test value of 4.022 and the *p* value of .001, otherwise known as the probability of obtaining a statistical value at least as extreme or as close to the one that was actually observed, assuming that the null hypothesis is true. Following the *t*-test value, the next value in the table is 12.70, which is the mean difference that we computed in Step 2 of our hand calculations. The next value in the table is 3.16, the value we computed in Steps 3a and 3b of our hand calculations.

FINAL INTERPRETATION IN AMERICAN PSYCHOLOGICAL ASSOCIATION (APA) FORMAT

The following interpretation is written as it might appear in a research article, formatted according to APA guidelines (APA, 2010). An independent samples *t*-test computed on hours worked revealed that veterans who received supported employment worked significantly more hours post-treatment than veterans in the control group, $t(18) = 4.02$, $p = 0.001$; $\bar{X} = 27.6$ versus 14.9, respectively. Thus, the particular type of vocational rehabilitation approach implemented to increase the work activity of spinal cord injured veterans appeared to have been more effective than standard practice.

STUDY QUESTIONS

1. Is the dependent variable in the Ottomanelli et al. (2012) example normally distributed? Provide a rationale for your answer.

2. If you have access to SPSS, compute the Shapiro-Wilk test of normality for the dependent variable, hours worked (as demonstrated in Exercise 26). What do the results indicate?

3. Do the data meet criteria for "independent samples"? Provide a rationale for your answer.

4. What is the null hypothesis in the example?

5. What was the exact likelihood of obtaining a *t*-test value at least as extreme or as close to the one that was actually observed, assuming that the null hypothesis is true?

6. If the Levene's test for equality of variances was significant at $p \leq 0.05$, what SPSS output would the researcher need to report?

7. What does the numerator of the independent samples *t*-test represent?

8. What does the denominator of the independent samples *t*-test represent?

9. What kind of design was implemented in the example?

10. Was the sample size adequate to detect differences between the two groups in this example? Provide a rationale for your answer.

Answers to Study Questions

1. The data appear slightly positively skewed as noted by a hand-drawn frequency distribution and using SPSS. See below for the SPSS frequency distribution.

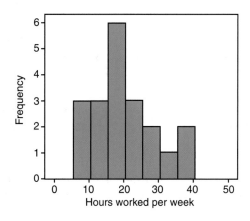

Mean = 21.25
Std. Dev. = 9.469
N = 20

2. As shown below, the Shapiro-Wilk p value for hours worked was 0.142, indicating that the frequency distribution did not significantly deviate from normality.

	Tests of Normality					
	Kolmogorov-Smirnov[a]			Shapiro-Wilk		
	Statistic	df	Sig.	Statistic	df	Sig.
Hours Worked Per Week	.153	20	.200*	.928	20	.142

*. This is a lower bound of the true significance.

a. Lilliefors Significance Correction

3. Yes, the data meet criteria for "independent samples" because the dependent variable data were collected from two mutually exclusive groups of study participants. In addition, the study participants were randomly assigned to either the intervention or control group, which makes the groups independent.

4. The null hypothesis is: *There is no difference between the treatment and control groups in post-treatment weekly hours worked among veterans with spinal cord injuries.*

5. The exact likelihood of obtaining a t-test value at least as extreme or as close to the one that was actually observed, assuming that the null hypothesis is true, was 0.1%. This value can be found in the "Independent Samples t-test" table in the SPSS output, where the exact p value is reported as 0.001. The value is calculated as follows: $0.001 \times 100\% = 0.1\%$.

6. If the Levene's test for equality of variances was significant at $p \leq 0.05$, the researcher would need to report the second row of SPSS output, containing the t-test value that has been adjusted for unequal variances.

7. The numerator represents the mean difference between the two groups (see formula for the independent samples *t*-test).

8. The denominator represents the extent to which there is dispersion among the values of the dependent variable.

9. The study design in the example was a randomized experimental design as evidenced by the fact that the participants were randomly assigned to receiving the treatment or the control conditions (Gray et al., 2017; Kazdin, 2017; Shadish, Cook, & Campbell, 2002).

10. The sample size was adequate to detect differences between the two groups, because a significant difference was found, $p = 0.001$. However, this sample is considered small, and as emphasized in Exercises 24 and 25, it is strongly recommended that a power analysis be conducted prior to the study beginning, in order to avoid the risk of Type II error (Taylor & Spurlock, 2018).

DATA FOR ADDITIONAL COMPUTATIONAL PRACTICE FOR QUESTIONS TO BE GRADED

Using the same example from Ottomanelli and colleagues (2012), participants were randomized to receive the Supported Employment treatment or usual care ("Control"). A simulated subset was selected for this example so that the computations would be small and manageable. The independent variable in this example is the type of treatment received (Supported Employment) or the Control group and the dependent variable was the amount of weekly wages earned post-treatment. The null hypothesis is: *There is no difference between the treatment and control groups in post-treatment weekly wages earned among veterans with spinal cord injuries.*

Compute the independent samples *t*-test on the data in Table 31-2 below.

TABLE 31-2	POST-TREATMENT WEEKLY WAGES EARNED BY TREATMENT GROUP		
Participant # Treatment Group	Weekly Wages Earned Treatment Group	Participant # Control Group	Weekly Wages Earned Control Group
1	$200	11	$75
2	$225	12	$70
3	$157	13	$125
4	$165	14	$140
5	$330	15	$200
6	$210	16	$165
7	$330	17	$149
8	$290	18	$75
9	$250	19	$150
10	$170	20	$135

Questions to Be Graded

Name: _____ Class: _____

Date: _____

Answer the following questions with hand calculations using the data presented in Table 31-2 or the SPSS dataset called "Exercise 31 Example 2.sav" available on the Evolve website. Follow your instructor's directions to submit your answers to the following questions for grading. Your instructor may ask you to write your answers below and submit them as a hard copy for grading. Alternatively, your instructor may ask you to submit your answers online.

1. Do the example data meet the assumptions for the independent samples *t*-test? Provide a rationale for your answer.

2. If calculating by hand, draw the frequency distributions of the dependent variable, wages earned. What is the shape of the distribution? If using SPSS, what is the result of the Shapiro-Wilk test of normality for the dependent variable?

3. What are the means for two group's wages earned?

4. What is the independent samples *t*-test value?

395

5. Is the *t*-test significant at $a = 0.05$? Specify how you arrived at your answer.

6. If using SPSS, what is the exact likelihood of obtaining a *t*-test value at least as extreme or as close to the one that was actually observed, assuming that the null hypothesis is true?

7. Which group earned the most money post-treatment?

8. Write your interpretation of the results as you would in an APA-formatted journal.

9. What do the results indicate regarding the impact of the supported employment vocational rehabilitation on wages earned?

10. Was the sample size adequate to detect significant differences between the two groups in this example? Provide a rationale for your answer.

Calculating *t*-tests for Paired (Dependent) Samples

A paired samples *t*-test (also referred to as a dependent samples *t*-test) is a statistical procedure that compares two sets of data from one group of people. The paired samples *t*-test was introduced in Exercise 17, which is focused on understanding these results in research reports. This exercise focuses on calculating and interpreting the results from paired samples *t*-tests. When samples are related, the formula used to calculate the *t* statistic is different from the formula for the independent samples *t*-test (see Exercise 31).

RESEARCH DESIGNS APPROPRIATE FOR THE PAIRED SAMPLES *t*-TEST

The term *paired samples* refers to a research design that repeatedly assesses the same group of people, an approach commonly referred to as **repeated measures**. Paired samples can also refer to naturally occurring pairs, such as siblings or spouses. The most common research design that may utilize a paired samples *t*-test is the one-group pretest–posttest design, wherein a single group of subjects is assessed at baseline and once again after receiving an intervention (Gliner, Morgan, & Leech, 2009; Gray, Grove, & Sutherland, 2017). Another design that may utilize a paired samples *t*-test is where one group of participants is exposed to one level of an intervention and then those scores are compared with the same participants' responses to another level of the intervention, resulting in paired scores. This is called a **one-sample crossover design** (Gliner et al., 2009).

Example 1: A researcher conducts a one-sample pretest–posttest study wherein she assesses her sample for health status at baseline, and again post-treatment. Her research question is: *Is there a difference in health status from baseline to post-treatment?* The dependent variable is health status.

Null hypothesis: *There is no difference between the baseline and post-treatment health status scores.*

Example 2: A researcher conducts a crossover study wherein subjects receive a randomly generated order of two medications. One is a standard FDA-approved medication to reduce blood pressure, and the other is an experimental medication. The dependent variable is reduction in blood pressure (systolic and diastolic), and the independent variable is medication type. Her research question is: *Is there a difference between the experimental medication and the control medication in blood pressure reduction?*

Null hypothesis: *There is no difference between the two medication trials in blood pressure reduction.*

STATISTICAL FORMULA AND ASSUMPTIONS

Use of the paired samples *t*-test involves the following assumptions (Zar, 2010):

1. The distribution of values is normal or approximately normal.
2. The dependent variable(s) is (are) measured at interval or ratio levels.
3. Repeated measures data are collected from one group of subjects, resulting in paired scores.
4. The differences between the paired scores are independent.

The formula for the paired samples *t*-test is:

$$t = \frac{\bar{D}}{s_{\bar{D}}}$$

where:

$\bar{D}$ = the mean difference of the paired data
$s_{\bar{D}}$ = the standard error of the difference

To compute the *t*-test, one must compute the denominator in the formula, the standard error of the difference:

$$s_{\bar{D}} = \frac{s_D}{\sqrt{n}}$$

where:

s_D = the standard deviation of the differences between the paired data
n = the number of subjects in the sample (or number of paired scores in the case of sibling or spousal data)

HAND CALCULATIONS

Using an example from a study of adults with gastroesophageal reflux disease (GERD), symptoms of gastroesophageal reflux were examined over time (Dunbar et al., 2016). Twelve adults with GERD were followed over a period of 2 weeks while being required to be free of all proton-pump inhibitor medications (the "intervention"). A subset of these data ($n = 10$) are presented in Table 32-1. One of the dependent variables was esophageal

TABLE 32-1	ESOPHAGEAL IMPENDANCE VALUES AT BASELINE AND 2-WEEK FOLLOW-UP		
Participant #	Esophageal Impedance, Baseline	Esophageal Impedance, 2-Week Follow-up	Difference Scores
1	2249	773	1476
2	3993	1329	2664
3	1422	1113	309
4	3676	1670	2006
5	2004	1231	773
6	3271	2660	611
7	2130	1784	346
8	2947	2000	947
9	2000	850	1150
10	3021	1674	1347

impedance, which is an index of mucosal integrity, where higher numbers are more desirable and indicative of healthy esophageal functioning. Impedance was measured with a pH electrode positioned 5 cm above the lower esophageal sphincter. For this example, the null hypothesis is: *There is no change in esophageal impedance from baseline to follow-up for patients with GERD who had stopped taking proton-pump inhibitor medications.*

The computations for the *t*-test are as follows:

Step 1: Compute the difference between each subject's pair of data (see last column of Table 32-1).

Step 2: Compute the mean of the difference scores, which becomes the numerator of the *t*-test:

$$\bar{D} = 11629.00 \div 10$$

$$\bar{D} = 1162.90$$

Step 3: Compute the standard error of the difference.
   a. Compute the standard deviation of the difference scores

$$s = \sqrt{\frac{\sum(X - \bar{X})^2}{n-1}}$$

$$s = \sqrt{\frac{4995908.90}{10-1}}$$

$$s = 745.05$$

   b. Plug into the standard error of the difference formula

$$s_{\bar{D}} = \frac{s_D}{\sqrt{n}}$$

$$s_{\bar{D}} = \frac{745.05}{\sqrt{10}}$$

$$s_{\bar{D}} = \frac{745.05}{3.16}$$

$$s_{\bar{D}} = 235.78$$

Step 4: Compute *t* value:

$$t = \frac{\bar{D}}{s_{\bar{D}}}$$

$$t = \frac{1162.90}{235.78}$$

$$t = 4.93$$

Step 5: Compute the degrees of freedom:

$$df = n - 1$$

$$df = 10 - 1$$

$$df = 9$$

Step 6: Locate the critical *t* value on the *t* distribution table and compare it to the obtained *t*.

The critical *t* value for 9 degrees of freedom at alpha (α) = 0.05 is 2.262 (rounded to 2.26) for a two-tailed test. Our obtained *t* is 4.93, exceeding the critical value (Appendix A), which means our *t*-test is statistically significant and represents a real difference between the two pairs. Therefore we can reject our null hypothesis. This means that if we viewed the *t* distribution for *df* = 9, the middle 95% of the distribution would be marked by -2.26 and 2.26. It should be noted that if the obtained *t* was -4.93, it would also be considered statistically significant, because the absolute value of the obtained *t* is compared to the critical *t* value (Gray et al., 2017).

SPSS COMPUTATIONS

This is how our dataset looks in SPSS.

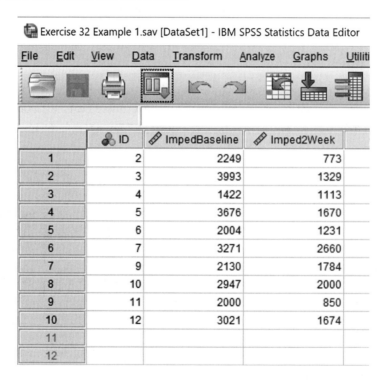

Step 1: From the Analyze menu, choose "Compare Means" and "Paired-Samples T Test."

Step 2: Move both variables over to the right, as in the window below. Click "OK."

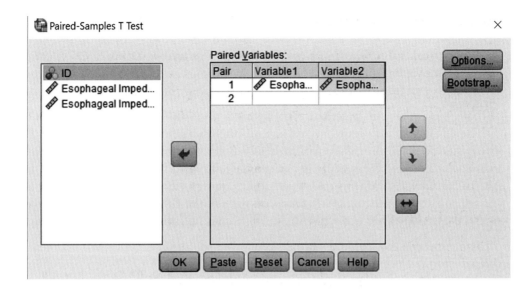

INTERPRETATION OF SPSS OUTPUT

The following tables are generated from SPSS. The first table contains descriptive statistics for the two variables. The second table contains the Pearson product-moment correlation between the two variables. The last table contains the *t*-test results.

T-Test

Paired Samples Statistics		Mean	N	Std. Deviation	Std. Error Mean
Pair 1	Esophageal Impedance, Baseline	2671.30	10	832.819	263.360
	Esophageal Impedance, 2-Week Follow-up	1508.40	10	571.268	180.651

Paired Samples Correlations		N	Correlation	Sig.
Pair 1	Esophageal Impedance, Baseline & Esophageal Impedance, 2-Week Follow-up	10	.489	.152

Paired Samples Test		Paired Differences							
					95% Confidence Interval of the Difference				Sig.
		Mean	Std. Deviation	Std. Error Mean	Lower	Upper	t	df	(2-tailed)
Pair 1	Esophageal Impedance, Baseline – Esophageal Impedance, 2-Week Follow-up	1162.900	745.051	235.606	629.923	1695.877	4.936	9	.001

The first table displays descriptive statistics that allow us to note the means at baseline and follow-up. This table is important because we can observe that the mean impedance at baseline was 2671.30, and the mean impedance at follow-up was 1508.40, indicating a decrease in esophageal impedance. Recall that higher numbers are indicative of healthy esophageal functioning, and therefore a decrease over time is undesirable for persons with GERD.

The second table displays the Pearson product-moment correlation coefficient that was computed between the two variables. It is common that the two variables are significantly correlated, because the sample is being assessed twice, and therefore it is logical that a person's follow-up value is affected by his or her baseline value in a repeated measures design. Although this table is a standard part of the SPSS output for a paired samples *t*-test, the contents are not reported in the results of published studies.

The last table contains the actual *t*-test value, along with the values that compose the *t*-test formula. Note that the first value in the table, 1162.90, was the mean difference that we computed in Step 2 of our hand calculations. The next two values in the table, 745.05 and 235.61, were the values we computed in Steps 3a and 3b of our hand calculations. The *t*-test value of 4.936 is slightly higher than what we obtained in our hand calculations. This is because we rounded to the hundredth decimal place in our hand calculations, when the standard error value is actually 235.606, which yields a *t*-test value of 1162.90 ÷ 235.606 = 4.936. Therefore, 4.936 (rounded to 4.94) is more accurate and will be reported as 4.94 in the interpretation below. The last value in the table is the *p* value, otherwise known as the probability of obtaining a statistical value at least as extreme or as close to the one that was actually observed, assuming that the null hypothesis is true. SPSS has printed a value of ".001," indicating a 0.1% probability of obtaining a *t*-test value at least as extreme or as close to the one that was actually observed, assuming that the null hypothesis is true (Gray et al., 2017).

FINAL INTERPRETATION IN AMERICAN PSYCHOLOGICAL ASSOCIATION (APA) FORMAT

The following interpretation is written as it might appear in a research article, formatted according to APA (2010) guidelines. A paired samples *t*-test computed on esophageal impedance revealed that the patients with GERD undergoing the withdrawal of proton-pump inhibitors had significantly lower impedance from baseline to post-treatment, $t(9) = 4.94$, $p = 0.001$; $\overline{X} = 2671.30$ versus 1508.40, respectively. Thus, the removal of proton-pump inhibiting medications appeared to play a role in the deterioration of the esophageal mucosal integrity.

STUDY QUESTIONS

1. Are the example data normally distributed? Provide a rationale for your answer.

2. If you have access to SPSS, compute the Shapiro-Wilk tests of normality for the two variables (as demonstrated in Exercise 26). If you do not have access to SPSS, plot the frequency distributions by hand. What do the results indicate?

3. Do the data meet criteria for "paired samples"? Provide a rationale for your answer.

4. On average, did esophageal impedance improve or deteriorate over time? Provide a rationale for your answer.

5. What was the exact likelihood of obtaining a *t*-test value at least as extreme or as close to the one that was actually observed, assuming that the null hypothesis is true?

6. Why do you think the baseline and follow-up variables were correlated?

7. What is the numerator for the paired samples *t*-test in this example? What does the numerator of the paired samples *t*-test represent?

8. What is the denominator for the paired samples *t*-test in this example? What does the denominator of the paired samples *t*-test represent?

9. Why would a one-sample crossover design also be suitable for a paired samples *t*-test?

10. The researchers concluded that the removal of proton-pump inhibiting medications appeared to deteriorate the mucosal integrity of the esophagus. What are some alternative explanations for these changes? (These alternative scientific explanations would apply to any one-sample repeated measures design.) Document your response.

Answers to Study Questions

1. Yes, the data are approximately normally distributed as noted by the two SPSS frequency distributions below.

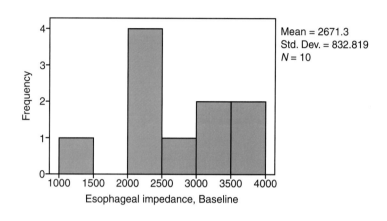

Mean = 2671.3
Std. Dev. = 832.819
N = 10

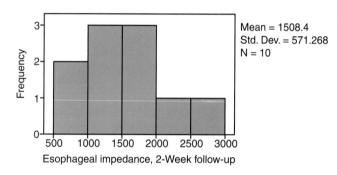

Mean = 1508.4
Std. Dev. = 571.268
N = 10

2. The Shapiro-Wilk p values for baseline and follow-up esophageal impedance were 0.67 and 0.70, respectively, indicating that the two frequency distributions did not significantly deviate from normality. Moreover, visual inspection of the frequency distributions in the answer to Question 1 indicates that the variables are approximately normally distributed.

Tests of Normality						
	Kolmogorov-Smirnov[a]			Shapiro-Wilk		
	Statistic	df	Sig.	Statistic	df	Sig.
Esophageal Impedance, Baseline	.194	10	.200[*]	.950	10	.670
Esophageal Impedance, 2-Week Follow-up	.123	10	.200[*]	.953	10	.701

[*]. This is a lower bound of the true significance.
a. Lilliefors Significance Correction

3. Yes, the data meet criteria for "paired samples" because the two esophageal impedance values were collected from the same single group of study participants over time.

4. The mean impedance at baseline was 2671.30, and the mean impedance at follow-up was 1508.40, indicating a decrease in esophageal impedance, and therefore an undesirable trend for persons with GERD. As noted earlier, higher numbers are more desirable and indicative of healthy esophageal functioning.

5. The exact likelihood of obtaining a *t*-test value at least as extreme as or as close to the one that was actually observed, assuming that the null hypothesis is true, was 0.1%.

6. The baseline and follow-up variables were correlated because the sample of patients was assessed twice, and therefore it is logical that a person's follow-up value is affected by his or her baseline value in a repeated measures design (Gray et al., 2017; Kim & Mallory, 2017).

7. As shown in the SPSS output, the numerator of the *t*-test in this example is 1162.90. The numerator represents the mean difference between the two variables (see formula for the paired samples *t*-test).

8. As shown in the SPSS output, the denominator of the *t*-test in this example is 235.606 (rounded to 235.61). The denominator represents the extent to which there is dispersion among the entire dataset's values.

9. A one-sample crossover design also would be suitable for a paired samples *t*-test because one group of participants is exposed to one level of an intervention and then those scores are compared with the same participants' responses to another level of the intervention. This meets criteria for "paired samples" because the two variables were collected from the same single group of people (Gliner et al., 2009).

10. When changes occur in a one-sample pretest–posttest design, we cannot be certain that the intervention caused the changes. Other explanations may include the passing of time, the inadvertent use of other treatments during the time elapsed from baseline to post-treatment, or statistical regression (a phenomenon that refers to artificially high baseline levels that naturally decrease to the actual population mean at post-treatment, or vice versa; Gliner et al., 2009; Gray et al., 2017; Shadish, Cook, & Campbell, 2002).

DATA FOR ADDITIONAL COMPUTATIONAL PRACTICE FOR QUESTIONS TO BE GRADED

Using an example from a study examining the gastroesophageal reflux among 12 adults with gastroesophageal reflux disease (GERD), changes over time were investigated (Dunbar et al., 2016). These data are presented in Table 32-2. The independent variable in this example is intervention over time, meaning that all of the participants were followed over time while being required to be free of all proton-pump inhibitor medications for two weeks (the "intervention"). The dependent variable was esophageal reflux symptoms, measured by the GERD Health-Related Quality of Life (HRQL) questionnaire, a validated instrument for GERD symptom severity with higher scores representing more GERD symptoms (Velanovich, 2007). The data in Table 32-2 were transformed to approximate normality. The null hypothesis is: *There is no change in esophageal reflux symptoms from baseline to follow-up for patients with GERD.*

Compute the paired samples *t*-test on the data in Table 32-2 below.

TABLE 32-2	ESOPHAGEAL SYMPTOM SCORES AT BASELINE AND 2-WEEK FOLLOW-UP		
Participant #	Esophageal Symptom Scores, Baseline	Esophageal Symptom Scores, 2-Week Follow-up	Difference Scores
1	.00	3.00	3.00
2	5.00	4.69	−.31
3	4.12	5.39	1.26
4	1.00	1.73	.73
5	4.36	4.47	.11
6	3.32	4.00	.68
7	.00	3.74	3.74
8	1.41	2.00	.59
9	.00	2.24	2.24
10	1.41	2.00	.59
11	2.00	4.24	2.24
12	.00	2.00	2.00

Name: _____ Class: _____

Date: _____

Answer the following questions with hand calculations using the data presented in Table 32-2 or the SPSS dataset called "Exercise 32 Example 2.sav" available on the Evolve website. Follow your instructor's directions to submit your answers to the following questions for grading. Your instructor may ask you to write your answers below and submit them as a hard copy for grading. Alternatively, your instructor may ask you to submit your answers online.

1. Do the example data meet the assumptions for the paired samples *t*-test? Provide a rationale for your answer.

2. If calculating by hand, draw the frequency distributions of the GERD-HRQL scores at baseline and follow-up. What are the shapes of the distributions? If using SPSS, what are the results of the Shapiro-Wilk tests of normality for these scores?

3. What are the means for the baseline and follow-up GERD Health-Related Quality of Life (HRQL) questionnaire scores, respectively?

4. What is the paired samples *t*-test value?

5. Is the *t*-test significant at α = 0.05? Use the table in Appendix A to specify how you arrived at your answer.

6. If using SPSS, what is the exact likelihood of obtaining a *t*-test value at least as extreme as or as close to the one that was actually observed, assuming that the null hypothesis is true?

7. On average, did the GERD HRQL scores improve or deteriorate over time? Provide a rationale for your answer.

8. Write your interpretation of the results as you would in an American Psychological Association (APA, 2010) formatted journal.

9. What do the results indicate regarding the impact of the removal of proton-pump inhibitors among persons with GERD?

10. What are the weaknesses of the design in this example?

Calculating Analysis of Variance (ANOVA) and Post Hoc Analyses Following ANOVA

Analysis of variance (ANOVA) is a statistical procedure that compares data between two or more groups or conditions to investigate the presence of differences between those groups on some continuous dependent variable (see Exercise 18). In this exercise, we will focus on the **one-way ANOVA**, which involves testing one independent variable and one dependent variable (as opposed to other types of ANOVAs, such as factorial ANOVAs that incorporate multiple independent variables).

Why ANOVA and not a *t*-test? Remember that a *t*-test is formulated to compare two sets of data or two groups at one time (see Exercise 23 for guidance on selecting appropriate statistics). Thus, data generated from a clinical trial that involves four experimental groups, Treatment 1, Treatment 2, Treatments 1 and 2 combined, and a Control, would require 6 *t*-tests. Consequently, the chance of making a Type I error (alpha error) increases substantially (or is inflated) because so many computations are being performed. Specifically, the chance of making a Type I error is the number of comparisons multiplied by the alpha level. Thus, ANOVA is the recommended statistical technique for examining differences between more than two groups (Kim & Mallory, 2017; Zar, 2010).

ANOVA is a procedure that culminates in a statistic called the *F* statistic. It is this value that is compared against an *F* distribution (see Appendix C) in order to determine whether the groups significantly differ from one another on the dependent variable. The formulas for ANOVA actually compute two estimates of variance: One estimate represents differences between the groups/conditions, and the other estimate represents differences among (within) the data.

RESEARCH DESIGNS APPROPRIATE FOR THE ONE-WAY ANOVA

Research designs that may utilize the one-way ANOVA include the randomized experimental, quasi-experimental, and comparative designs (Gliner, Morgan, & Leech, 2009). The independent variable (the "grouping" variable for the ANOVA) may be active or attributional. An active independent variable refers to an intervention, treatment, or program. An attributional independent variable refers to a characteristic of the participant, such as gender, diagnosis, or ethnicity. The ANOVA can compare two groups or more. In the case of a two-group design, the researcher can either select an independent samples *t*-test or a one-way ANOVA to answer the research question. The results will always yield the same conclusion, regardless of which test is computed; however, when examining differences between more than two groups, the one-way ANOVA is the preferred statistical test (Gray, Grove, & Sutherland, 2017).

Example 1: A researcher conducts a randomized experimental study wherein she randomizes participants to receive a high-dosage weight loss pill, a low-dosage weight loss pill, or a placebo. She assesses the number of pounds lost from baseline to post-treatment for the three groups. Her research question is: *Is there a difference between the three groups in weight lost?* The independent variables are the treatment conditions (high-dose weight loss pill, low-dose weight loss pill, and placebo) and the dependent variable is number of pounds lost over the treatment span.

Null hypothesis: *There is no difference in weight lost among the high-dose weight loss pill, low-dose weight loss pill, and placebo groups in a population of overweight adults.*

Example 2: A nurse researcher working in dermatology conducts a retrospective comparative study wherein she conducts a chart review of patients and divides them into three groups: psoriasis, psoriatric symptoms, or control. The dependent variable is health status and the independent variable is disease group (psoriasis, psoriatic symptoms, and control). Her research question is: *Is there a difference between the three groups in levels of health status?*

Null hypothesis: *There is no difference in health status among the psoriasis, psoriatric symptoms, and control groups of selected patients.*

STATISTICAL FORMULA AND ASSUMPTIONS

Use of the ANOVA involves the following assumptions (Zar, 2010):

1. Sample means from the population are normally distributed.
2. The groups are mutually exclusive.
3. The dependent variable is measured at the interval/ratio level.
4. The groups should have equal variance, termed "homogeneity of variance."
5. All observations within each sample are independent.

The dependent variable in an ANOVA must be scaled as interval or ratio. If the dependent variable is measured with a Likert scale and the frequency distribution is approximately normally distributed, these data are usually considered interval-level measurements and are appropriate for an ANOVA (see Exercise 1; de Winter & Dodou, 2010; Rasmussen, 1989; Waltz, Strickland, & Lenz, 2017).

The basic formula for the *F* without numerical symbols is:

$$F = \frac{\text{Mean Square Between Groups}}{\text{Mean Square Within Groups}}$$

The term *mean square (MS)* is used interchangeably with the word *variance*. The formulas for ANOVA compute two estimates of variance: the between groups variance and the within groups variance. The **between groups variance** represents differences between the groups/conditions being compared, and the **within groups variance** represents differences among (within) each group's data. Therefore, the formula is $F = MS$ between/MS within.

HAND CALCULATIONS

Using an example from a study of students enrolled in an RN to BSN program, a subset of graduates from the program were examined (Mancini, Ashwill, & Cipher, 2015). The data are presented in Table 33-1. A simulated subset was selected for this example so that

TABLE 33-1	**MONTHS FOR COMPLETION OF RN TO BSN PROGRAM BY HIGHEST DEGREE STATUS**				
Participant #	Associate's Degree	Participant #	Bachelor's Degree	Participant #	Master's Degree
1	17	10	16	19	17
2	19	11	15	20	21
3	24	12	16	21	20
4	18	13	12	22	21
5	24	14	16	23	12
6	24	15	12	24	16
7	16	16	16	25	20
8	16	17	12	26	18
9	20	18	10	27	12

the computations would be small and manageable. In actuality, studies involving one-way ANOVAs need to be adequately powered (Aberson, 2019; Cohen, 1988). See Exercises 24 and 25 for more information regarding statistical power.

The independent variable in this example is highest degree obtained prior to enrollment (Associate's, Bachelor's, or Master's degree), and the dependent variable was number of months it took for the student to complete the RN to BSN program. The null hypothesis is *There is no difference among the groups (highest degree of Associate's, Bachelor's, or Master's) in the months these nursing students require to complete an RN to BSN program.*

The computations for the ANOVA are as follows:

Step 1: Compute correction term, C.
Square the grand sum (G), and divide by total N:

$$C = \frac{460^2}{27} = 7,837.04$$

Step 2: Compute Total Sum of Squares.
Square every value in dataset, sum, and subtract C:

$$(17^2 + 19^2 + 24^2 + 18^2 + 24^2 + 16^2 + 16^2 + \ldots + 12^2) - 7,837.04$$
$$= 8,234 - 7,837.04 = 396.96$$

Step 3: Compute Between Groups Sum of Squares.
Square the sum of each column and divide by N. Add each, and then subtract C:

$$\frac{178^2}{9} + \frac{125^2}{9} + \frac{157^2}{9} - 7,837.04$$
$$(3,520.44 + 1,736.11 + 2,738.78) - 7,837.04 = 158.29$$

Step 4: Compute Within Groups Sum of Squares.
Subtract the Between Groups Sum of Squares (Step 3) from Total Sum of Squares (Step 2):

$$396.96 - 158.29 = 238.67$$

TABLE 33-2 ANOVA SUMMARY TABLE				
Source of Variation	SS	df	MS	F
Between Groups	158.29	2	79.15	7.96
Within Groups	238.67	24	9.94	
Total	396.96	26		

Step 5: Create ANOVA Summary Table (see Table 33-2).

   a. Insert the sum of squares values in the first column.
   b. The degrees of freedom are in the second column. Because the *F* is a ratio of two separate statistics (mean square between groups and mean square within groups) both have different *df* formulas—one for the *numerator* and one for the *denominator*:

$$\text{Mean square between groups } df = \text{number of groups} - 1$$

$$\text{Mean square within groups } df = N - \text{number of groups}$$

For this example, the *df* for the numerator is $3 - 1 = 2$.

The *df* for the denominator is $27 - 3 = 24$.

   c. The mean square between groups and mean square within groups are in the third column. These values are computed by dividing the *SS* by the *df*. Therefore, the *MS* between = 158.29 ÷ 2 = 79.15. The *MS* within = 238.67 ÷ 24 = 9.94.
   d. The *F* is the final column and is computed by dividing the *MS* between by the *MS* within. Therefore, F = 79.15 ÷ 9.94 = 7.96.

Step 6: Locate the critical *F* value on the *F* distribution table (see Appendix C) and compare it to our obtained F = 7.96 value. The critical *F* value for 2 and 24 *df* at α = 0.05 is 3.40, which indicates the *F* value in this example is statistically significant. Researchers report ANOVA results in a study report using the following format: $F(2,24) = 7.96$, $p < 0.05$. Researchers report the exact *p* value instead of "$p < 0.05$," but this usually requires the use of computer software due to the tedious nature of *p* value computations.

Our obtained F = 7.96 exceeds the critical value in the table, which indicates that the *F* is statistically significant and that the population means are not equal. Therefore, we can reject our null hypothesis that *the three groups spent the same amount of time completing the RN to BSN program.* However, the *F* does not indicate which groups differ from one another, and this *F* value does not identify which groups are significantly different from one another. Further testing, termed multiple comparison tests or post hoc tests, is required to complete the ANOVA process and determine all the significant differences among the study groups (Kim & Mallory, 2017; Plichta & Kelvin, 2013).

Post Hoc Tests

Post hoc tests have been developed specifically to determine the location of group differences after ANOVA is performed on data from more than two groups. These tests were developed to reduce the incidence of a Type I error. Frequently used post hoc tests are the Newman-Keuls test, the Tukey Honestly Significant Difference (HSD) test, the Scheffé test, and the Dunnett test (Zar, 2010; see Exercise 18 for examples). When these tests are calculated, the alpha level is reduced in proportion to the number of additional tests required to locate statistically significant differences. For example, for several of the afore-mentioned post hoc tests, if many groups' mean values are being compared, the magnitude of the difference is set higher than if only two groups are being compared. Thus, post hoc tests are tedious to perform by hand and are best handled with statistical computer software programs. Accordingly, the rest of this example will be presented with the assistance of SPSS.

SPSS COMPUTATIONS

The following screenshot is a replica of what your SPSS window will look like. The data for ID numbers 18 through 27 are viewable by scrolling down in the SPSS screen.

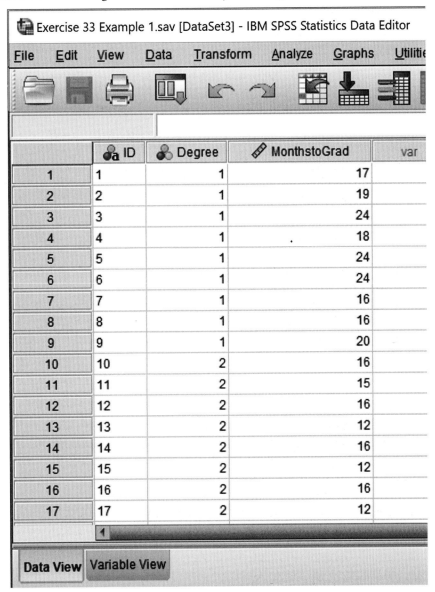

Step 1: From the "Analyze" menu, choose "Compare Means" and "One-Way ANOVA." Move the dependent variable, Number of Months to Complete Program, over to the right, as in the window below.

Step 2: Move the independent variable, Highest Degree at Enrollment, to the right in the space labeled "Factor."

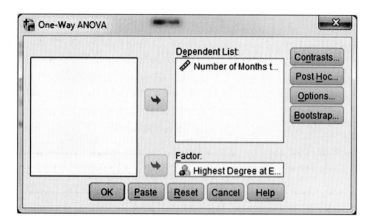

Step 3: Click "Options." Check the boxes next to "Descriptive" and "Homogeneity of variance test." Click "Continue" and "OK."

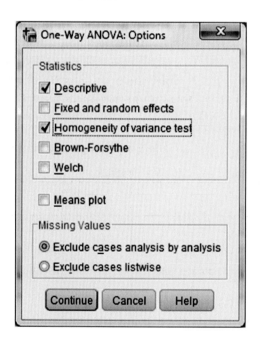

INTERPRETATION OF SPSS OUTPUT

The following tables are generated from SPSS. The first table contains descriptive statistics for months to completion, separated by the three groups. The second table contains the Levene's test of homogeneity of variances. The third table contains the ANOVA summary table, along with the F and p values.

The first table displays descriptive statistics that allow us to observe the means for the three groups. This table is important because it indicates that the students with an Associate's degree took an average of 19.78 months to complete the program, compared to 13.89 months for students with a Bachelor's and 17.44 months for students with a Master's degree.

One Way

Descriptives

Number of Months to Complete Program

	N	Mean	Std. Deviation	Std. Error	95% Confidence Interval for Mean		Minimum	Maximum
					Lower Bound	Upper Bound		
Associate's	9	19.78	3.420	1.140	17.15	22.41	16	24
Bachelor's	9	13.89	2.369	.790	12.07	15.71	10	16
Master's	9	17.44	3.539	1.180	14.72	20.17	12	21
Total	27	17.04	3.907	.752	15.49	18.58	10	24

Observe the means for the three groups

The second table contains the Levene's test for equality of variances. The Levene's test is a statistical test of the equal variances assumption (Kim & Mallory, 2017). As is shown on the first row of the table, the p value is 0.488, indicating there was no significant difference among the three groups' variances; thus, the data have met the equal variances assumption for ANOVA.

Test of Homogeneity of Variances

Number of Months to Complete Program

	Levene Statistic	df1	df2	Sig.
Based on Mean	.740	2	24	.488
Based on Median	.524	2	24	.599
Based on Median and with adjusted df	.524	2	23.030	.599
Based on trimmed mean	.729	2	24	.493

The last table contains the contents of the ANOVA summary table, which looks much like Table 33-2. This table contains an additional value that we did not compute by hand—the exact p value, which is 0.002. Because the SPSS output indicates that we have a significant ANOVA, post hoc testing must be performed.

ANOVA

Number of Months to Complete Program

	Sum of Squares	df	Mean Square	F	Sig.
Between Groups	158.296	2	79.148	7.959	.002
Within Groups	238.667	24	9.944		
Total	396.963	26			

Observe that the *F* is 7.96   **The exact *p* value is .002**

Return to the ANOVA window and click "Post Hoc." You will see a window similar to the one below. Select the "LSD" and "Tukey" options. Click "Continue" and "OK."

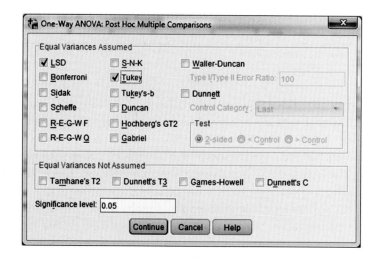

The following output is added to the original output. This table contains post hoc test results for two different tests: the LSD (Least Significant Difference) test and the Tukey HSD (Honestly Significant Difference) test. The LSD test, the original post hoc test, explores all possible pairwise comparisons of means using the equivalent of multiple *t*-tests. However, the LSD test, in performing a set of multiple *t*-tests, may report inaccurate *p* values, because they have not been adjusted for multiple computations (Zar, 2010). Consequently, researchers should exercise caution when choosing the LSD post hoc test following an ANOVA.

The Tukey HSD comparison test, on the other hand, is a more *conservative* test, meaning that it requires a larger difference between two groups to indicate a significant difference than some of the other post hoc tests available. By requiring a larger difference between the groups, the Tukey HSD procedure might yield more accurate *p* values of 0.062 to reflect the multiple comparisons (Kim & Mallory, 2017; Zar, 2010).

Post Hoc Tests

Multiple Comparisons

Dependent Variable: Number of Months to Complete Program

	(I) Highest Degree at Enrollment	(J) Highest Degree at Enrollment	Mean Difference (I-J)	Std. Error	Sig.	95% Confidence Interval	
						Lower Bound	Upper Bound
Tukey HSD	Associate's	Bachelor's	5.889*	1.487	.002	2.18	9.60
		Master's	2.333	1.487	.278	-1.38	6.05
	Bachelor's	Associate's	-5.889*	1.487	.002	-9.60	-2.18
		Master's	-3.556	1.487	.062	-7.27	.16
	Master's	Associate's	-2.333	1.487	.278	-6.05	1.38
		Bachelor's	3.556	1.487	.062	-.16	7.27
LSD	Associate's	Bachelor's	5.889*	1.487	.001	2.82	8.96
		Master's	2.333	1.487	.130	-.73	5.40
	Bachelor's	Associate's	-5.889*	1.487	.001	-8.96	-2.82
		Master's	-3.556*	1.487	.025	-6.62	-.49
	Master's	Associate's	-2.333	1.487	.130	-5.40	.73
		Bachelor's	3.556*	1.487	.025	.49	6.62

* The mean difference is significant at the 0.05 level.

Observe the "Mean Difference" column. Any difference noted with an asterisk (*) is significant at $p < 0.05$. The p values of each comparison are listed in the "Sig." column, and values below 0.05 indicate a significant difference between the pair of groups. Observe the p values for the comparison of the Bachelor's degree group versus the Master's degree group. The Tukey HSD test indicates no significant difference between the groups, with a p of 0.062; however, the LSD test indicates that the groups significantly differed, with a p of 0.025. This example enables you see the difference in results obtained when calculating a conservative versus a lenient post hoc test. However, it should be noted that because an *a priori* power analysis was not conducted, there is a possibility that these analyses are underpowered. See Exercises 24 and 25 for more information regarding the consequences of low statistical power.

FINAL INTERPRETATION IN AMERICAN PSYCHOLOGICAL ASSOCIATION (APA) FORMAT

The following interpretation is written as it might appear in a research article, formatted according to APA guidelines (APA, 2010). A one-way ANOVA performed on months to program completion revealed significant differences among the three groups, $F(2,24) = 7.96$, $p = 0.002$. Post hoc comparisons using the Tukey HSD comparison test indicated that the students in the Associate's degree group took significantly longer to complete the program than the students in the Bachelor's degree group (19.8 versus 13.9 months, respectively). However, there were no significant differences in program completion time between the Associate's degree group and the Master's degree group or between the Bachelor's degree group and the Master's degree group.

STUDY QUESTIONS

1. Is the dependent variable in the Mancini et al. (2015) example normally distributed? Provide a rationale for your answer.

2. What are the two instances that must occur to warrant post hoc testing following an ANOVA?

3. Do the data in this example meet criteria for homogeneity of variance? Provide a rationale for your answer.

4. What is the null hypothesis in the example?

5. What was the exact likelihood of obtaining an F value at least as extreme as or as close to the one that was actually observed, assuming that the null hypothesis is true?

6. Do the data meet criteria for "mutual exclusivity"? Provide a rationale for your answer.

7. What does the numerator of the F ratio represent?

8. What does the denominator of the F ratio represent?

9. How would our final interpretation of the results have changed if we had chosen to report the LSD post hoc test instead of the Tukey HSD test?

10. Was the sample size adequate to detect differences among the three groups in this example? Provide a rationale for your answer.

Answers to Study Questions

1. Yes, the data are approximately normally distributed as noted by the frequency distribution generated from SPSS, below. The Shapiro-Wilk (covered in Exercise 26) p value for months to completion was 0.151, indicating that the frequency distribution did not significantly deviate from normality.

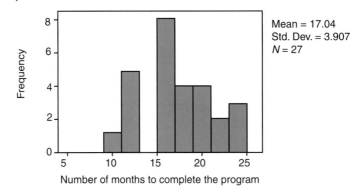

2. The two instances that must occur to warrant post hoc testing following an ANOVA are (1) the ANOVA was performed on data comparing more than two groups, and (2) the F value is statistically significant (Gray et al., 2017; Zar, 2010).

3. Yes, the data met criteria for homogeneity of variance because the Levene's test for equality of variances yielded a p of 0.488 (see the Test of Homogeneity of Variances Table in this exercise), indicating no significant differences in variance between the groups.

4. The null hypothesis is: *There is no difference between groups (Associate's, Bachelor's, and Master's degree groups) in months until completion of an RN to BSN program.*

5. The exact likelihood of obtaining an F value at least as extreme as or as close to the one that was actually observed, assuming that the null hypothesis is true, was 0.2%. The calculations include the following: $0.002 \times 100\% = 0.2\%$.

6. Yes, the data met criteria for mutual exclusivity because a student could only belong to one of the three groups of the highest degree obtained prior to enrollment (Associate, Bachelor's, and Master's degree).

7. The numerator represents the between groups variance or the differences between the groups/conditions being compared.

8. The denominator represents within groups variance or the extent to which there is dispersion among the dependent variables.

9. The final interpretation of the results would have changed if we had chosen to report the LSD post hoc test instead of the Tukey HSD test. The results of the LSD test indicated that the students in the Master's degree group took significantly longer to complete the program than the students in the Bachelor's degree group ($p = 0.025$). Review the results of the Post Hoc Tests Table in this exercise to identify the answer.

10. The sample size was most likely adequate to detect differences among the three groups overall because a significant difference was found, $p = 0.002$. However, there was a discrepancy between the results of the LSD post hoc test and the Tukey HSD test. The difference between the Master's degree group and the Bachelor's degree group was significant according to the results of the LSD test but not the Tukey HSD test. Therefore, it is possible that with only 27 total students in this example, the data were underpowered for the multiple comparisons following the ANOVA (Aberson, 2019; Cohen, 1988).

DATA FOR ADDITIONAL COMPUTATIONAL PRACTICE FOR QUESTIONS TO BE GRADED

Using the example from Ottomanelli and colleagues (2012) study, participants were randomized to receive Supported Employment or treatment as usual. A third group, also a treatment as usual group, consisted of a nonrandomized observational group of participants. A simulated subset was selected for this example so that the computations would be small and manageable. The independent variable in this example is treatment group (Supported Employment, Treatment as Usual–Randomized, and Treatment as Usual–Observational/Not Randomized), and the dependent variable was the number of hours worked post-treatment. Supported employment refers to a type of specialized interdisciplinary vocational rehabilitation designed to help people with disabilities obtain and maintain community-based competitive employment in their chosen occupation (Bond, 2004).

The null hypothesis is: *There is no difference between among the Supported Employment, Treatment as Usual–Randomized, and Treatment as Usual–Observational groups in post-treatment number of hours worked among veterans with spinal cord injuries.*

Compute the ANOVA on the data in Table 33-3 below.

TABLE 33-3	POST-TREATMENT HOURS WORKED BY TREATMENT GROUP				
Participant #	Supported Employment	Participant #	TAU Observational	Participant #	TAU Randomized
1	8	6	15	11	25
2	9	7	18	12	28
3	15	8	9	13	35
4	17	9	18	14	30
5	24	10	16	15	15

"TAU" = Treatment as Usual.

Questions to Be Graded

Name: _____ Class: _____

Date: _____

Answer the following questions with hand calculations using the data presented in Table 33-3 or the SPSS dataset called "Exercise 33 Example 2.sav" available on the Evolve website. Follow your instructor's directions to submit your answers to the following questions for grading. Your instructor may ask you to write your answers below and submit them as a hard copy for grading. Alternatively, your instructor may ask you to submit your answers online.

1. Do the data meet criteria for homogeneity of variance? Provide a rationale for your answer.

2. If calculating by hand, draw the frequency distribution of the dependent variable, hours worked at a job. What is the shape of the distribution? If using SPSS, what is the result of the Shapiro-Wilk test of normality for the dependent variable?

3. What are the means for three groups' hours worked on a job?

4. What are the F value and the group and error df for this set of data?

5. Is the *F* significant at $\alpha = 0.05$? Specify how you arrived at your answer.

6. If using SPSS, what is the exact likelihood of obtaining an *F* value at least as extreme as or as close to the one that was actually observed, assuming that the null hypothesis is true?

7. Which group worked the most weekly job hours post-treatment? Provide a rationale for your answer.

8. Write your interpretation of the results as you would in an APA-formatted journal.

9. Is there a difference in your final interpretation when comparing the results of the LSD post hoc test versus Tukey HSD test? Provide a rationale for your answer.

10. If the researcher decided to combine the two Treatment as Usual groups to represent an overall "Control" group, then there would be two groups to compare: Supported Employment versus Control. What would be the appropriate statistic to address the difference in hours worked between the two groups? Provide a rationale for your answer.

Calculating Sensitivity and Specificity

An important part of building evidence-based practice is the ability to differentiate between people who have a disease and those who do not. This is accomplished by using the most accurate and precise measure or test to promote quality outcomes. Regardless of whether the test is used by clinicians or researchers, the same issue is raised—how good is the screening test in separating patients with and without a disease? This question is best answered by current, quality research to determine the sensitivity and specificity of the test (Gordis, 2014).

The accuracy of a screening test or a test used to confirm a diagnosis is evaluated in terms of its ability to correctly assess the presence or absence of a disease or condition as compared with a gold standard. The gold standard is the most accurate means of currently diagnosing a particular disease and serves as a basis for comparison with newly developed diagnostic or screening tests (Campo, Shiyko, & Lichtman, 2010). As shown in Table 34-1, there are four possible outcomes of a screening test for a disease: (1) **sensitivity**, or true positive, which accurately identifies the presence of a disease; (2) **false positive**, which indicates a disease is present when it is not; (3) **specificity**, or true negative, which indicates accurately that a disease is not present; or (4) **false negative**, which indicates that a disease is not present when it is (Gordis, 2014).

TABLE 34-1 RESULTS OF SENSITIVITY AND SPECIFICITY OF SCREENING TESTS		
	Disease Present	**Disease Not Present**
Positive test	a (true positive)	b (false positive)
Negative test	c (false negative)	d (true negative)

where:

a = The number of people who have the disease and the test is positive (true positive)
b = The number of people who do not have the disease and the test is positive (false positive)
c = The number of people who have the disease and the test is negative (false negative)
d = The number of people who do not have the disease and the test is negative (true negative)

STATISTICAL FORMULA AND ASSUMPTIONS

Sensitivity and Specificity

Sensitivity and specificity can be calculated based on research findings and clinical practice outcomes to determine the most accurate diagnostic or screening tool to use in identifying the presence or absence of a disease for a population of patients. The

TABLE 34-2 STRUCTURE OF DATA FOR SENSITIVITY AND SPECIFICITY CALCULATIONS		
	Disease Present	**Disease Not Present**
Positive test	a	b
Negative test	c	d

calculations for sensitivity and specificity are provided as follows. Table 34-2 displays the following notation to assist the researcher in calculating the sensitivity and specificity of a screening test.

The disease variable (present/absent) is often called the state variable. It is always dichotomous. The screening test variable can be either dichotomous or continuous (such as a lab value). If the screening test is continuous, sensitivity and specificity are repeatedly calculated for each individual test value (Melnyk & Fineout-Overholt, 2019).

$$\text{Sensitivity calculation} = \text{probability of having the disease}$$
$$= a/(a+c)$$
$$= \text{true positive rate}$$

$$\text{Specificity calculation} = \text{probability of the absence of disease}$$
$$= d/(b+d)$$
$$= \text{true negative rate}$$

$$\text{False positive calculation} = \text{probability of no disease but having a positive test}$$
$$= b/(b+d)$$
$$= \text{false positive rate}$$

$$\text{False negative calculation} = \text{probability of having disease but having negative test}$$
$$= c/(c+a)$$
$$= \text{false negative rate}$$

Sensitivity is the proportion of patients with the disease who have a positive test result, or true positive. The ways the researcher or clinician might refer to the test sensitivity include the following:

- A highly sensitive test is very good at identifying the patient with a disease.
- If a test is highly sensitive, it has a low percentage of false negatives.
- Low sensitivity test is limited in identifying the patient with a disease.
- If a test has low sensitivity, it has a high percentage of false negatives.
- If a sensitive test has negative results, the patient is less likely to have the disease.

Specificity of a screening or diagnostic test is the proportion of patients without the disease who have a negative test result, or true negative. The ways the researcher or clinician might refer to the test specificity include the following:

- A highly specific test is very good at identifying patients without a disease.
- If a test is very specific, it has a low percentage of false positives.
- Low specificity test is limited in identifying patients without a disease.
- If a test has low specificity, it has a high percentage of false positives.
- If a specific test has positive results, the patient is more likely to have the disease.

Likelihood Ratios

Likelihood ratios (LRs) are additional calculations that can help researchers to determine the accuracy of diagnostic or screening tests, which are based on the sensitivity and specificity results. LRs are calculated to determine the likelihood that a positive test result is a true positive and a negative test result is a true negative.

The ratio of the true positive results to false positive results is known as the **positive LR** (Boyko, 1994; Melnyk & Fineout-Overholt, 2019). The positive LR is calculated as follows:

$$\text{Positive LR} = \text{Sensitivity} \div (1 - \text{Specificity})$$

The ratio of true negative results to false negative results is known as the **negative LR**, and it is calculated as follows:

$$\text{Negative LR} = (1 - \text{Sensitivity}) \div \text{Specificity}$$

An LR greater than 1.0 represents an increase in the likelihood of the disease, while an LR of less than 1.0 represents a decrease in the likelihood of the disease. The very high LRs (or LRs that are >10) rule in the disease or indicate that the patient has the disease. The very low LRs (or LRs that are <0.1) virtually rule out the chance that the patient has the disease (Boyko, 1994; Campo et al., 2010). Understanding sensitivity, specificity, and LR increases the researcher's ability to read clinical studies and to determine the most accurate diagnostic test to use in research and clinical practice (Straus, Glasziou, Richardson, & Haynes, 2011).

Receiver Operating Characteristic Curves

In studies that compute sensitivity and specificity, a receiver operating characteristic (ROC), or ROC curve, is often created. An **ROC curve** is a descriptive graph that plots the true positive rate against the false positive rate. The x-axis represents the false positive rate (1 − specificity), and the y-axis represents the true positive rate (sensitivity). The actual rates are plotted and a line is drawn between the numbers. The larger the area under that line, the more accurate the test. The actual area under the line can be calculated by a value called the C statistic. The **C statistic**, or area under the curve, is the probability that the test result from a randomly selected person with the disease will be positive (Austin & Steyerberg, 2012).

HAND CALCULATIONS

A retrospective comparative study examined whether longer antibiotic treatment courses were associated with candiduria (the presence of *Candida* species in the urine) among 97 veterans with a spinal cord injury (Goetz, Howard, Cipher, & Revankar, 2010). Using urine cultures from a sample of spinal cord–injured veterans, two groups were created: those with evidence of candiduria and those with no evidence of candiduria. Each veteran was also divided into two groups based on having had a history of recent antibiotic use for more than 2 weeks or no history of recent antibiotic use. As shown in Table 34-3, to analyze the sensitivity and specificity of these data, the presence of candiduria will be

TABLE 34-3   CANDIDURIA AND ANTIBIOTIC USE IN VETERANS WITH SPINAL CORD INJURIES

	Candiduria	No Candiduria
Antibiotic use	15	43
No antibiotic use	0	39

considered the disease, also called the state variable. The screening test variable is the presence of antibiotic use.

The computations for sensitivity, specificity, positive LR, and negative LR are as follows:

Sensitivity Calculation

$$\text{Sensitivity} = a/(a + c)$$
$$15/(15 + 0) = 1 \times 100\% = 100\%$$

Specificity Calculation

$$\text{Specificity} = d/(b + d)$$
$$39/(43 + 39) = 0.476 \times 100\% = 47.6\%$$

Positive LR Calculation

$$\text{Positive LR} = \text{Sensitivity} \div (1 - \text{Specificity})$$
$$1.0 \div (1 - 0.476) = 1.91$$

Negative LR Calculation

$$\text{Negative LR} = (1 - \text{Sensitivity}) \div \text{Specificity}$$
$$(1 - 1) \div 0.476 = 0$$

The sensitivity of the test was 100%, indicating that the proportion of patients with candiduria who were correctly identified as "positive" by their antibiotic use was 100%. The specificity of the test was 47.6%, indicating that the proportion of patients without candiduria who were correctly identified as "negative" by their antibiotic use was 47.6%. The positive LR was 1.91, indicating an increase in the likelihood of candiduria among those with antibiotic use. The negative LR was 0, indicating a very low likelihood of candiduria among those who did not take antibiotics.

SPSS COMPUTATIONS

The following screenshot is a replica of what your SPSS window will look like. The data for subjects 18 through 97 are viewable by scrolling down in the SPSS screen. The values in the data set must be coded as "1" or "0."

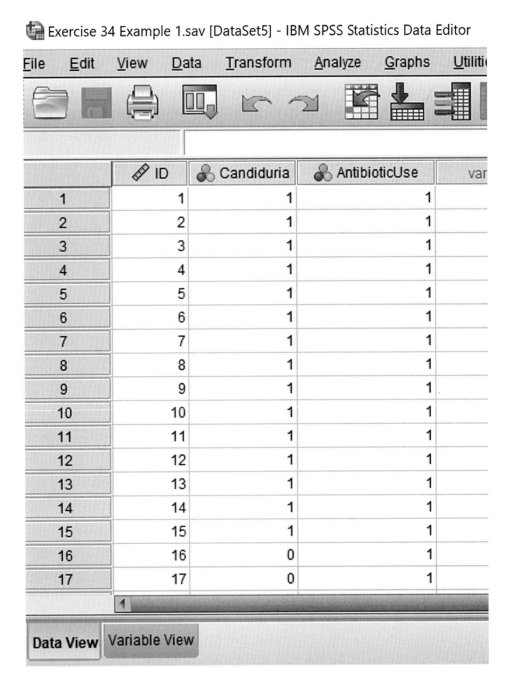

Step 1: From the "Analyze" menu, choose "Descriptive Statistics" and "Crosstabs." Move the two variables to the right, where either variable can be in the "Row" or "Column" space. Click "OK."

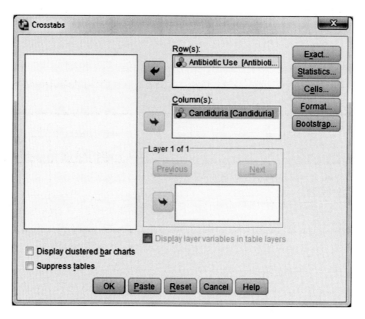

Step 2: From the "Analyze" menu, choose "ROC Curve." Move "Antibiotic Use" to the box labeled "Test Variable," and move "Candiduria" to the box labeled "State Variable." Enter the number "1" next to the box labeled "Value of State Variable." Check all of the boxes underneath ("ROC Curve," "With diagonal reference line," "Standard error and confidence interval," and "Coordinate points of the ROC Curve"). Click "OK."

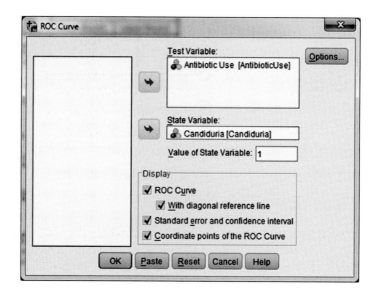

INTERPRETATION OF SPSS OUTPUT

The following tables are generated from SPSS. The first table contains the contingency table, similar to Table 34-3 presented previously. The following tables and figure are generated from the ROC Curve menu.

Crosstabs

Antibiotic Use * Candiduria Crosstabulation

Count

		Candiduria		Total
		No Candiduria	Candiduria	
Antibiotic Use	No Antibiotic Use	39	0	39
	History of Antibiotic Use	43	15	58
Total		82	15	97

The first table is the cross-tabulation table of the two variables. The values are the same as in Table 34-3. The next set of output is generated from the ROC menu selections. The first table contains the number of veterans who tested positive and negative for candiduria.

ROC Curve

Case Processing Summary

Candiduria	Valid N (listwise)
Positive[a]	15
Negative	82

Larger values of the test result variable(s) indicate stronger evidence for a positive actual state.

a. The positive actual state is Candiduria.

The second table contains the ROC curve, where the x-axis represents the false positive rate ($1 -$ specificity), and the y-axis represents the true positive rate (sensitivity). The blue line represents our actual data, and the black line is the reference line that represents a 50/50 chance of accurately predicting candiduria. The greater the distance the blue line is from the black line, the more accurate the test.

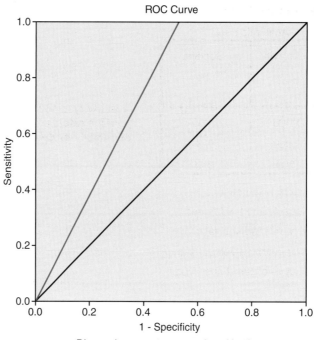

Diagonal segments are produced by ties.

In the table titled "Area Under the Curve," the first value labeled "Area" is also considered the *C* statistic. The area under the curve is the probability that the antibiotic use from a randomly selected veteran with candiduria will be positive. For the example data, the probability that the antibiotic use from a randomly selected veteran with candiduria will be positive is 73.8%. The *p* value is 0.004, indicating that knowing the test value (antibiotic use) is significantly better than guessing. The 95% confidence interval for the *C* statistic was 0.633–0.843, which can be interpreted as the interval of 63.3% to 84.3% estimates the population *C* statistic with 95% confidence (Kline, 2004).

Area Under the Curve

Test Result Variable(s):   Antibiotic Use

Area	Std. Error[a]	Asymptotic Sig.[b]	Asymptotic 95% Confidence Interval	
			Lower Bound	Upper Bound
.738	.054	.004	.633	.843

The *C* statistic is .738, or 73.8%

[a]. Under the nonparametric assumption

[b]. Null hypothesis: true area = 0.5

Coordinates of the Curve

Test Result Variable(s): Antibiotic Use

Positive if Greater Than or Equal To[a]	Sensitivity	1 - Specificity
-1.00	1.000	1.000
.50	1.000	.524
2.00	.000	.000

[a]. The smallest cutoff value is the minimum observed test value minus 1, and the largest cutoff value is the maximum observed test value plus 1. All the other cutoff values are the averages of two consecutive ordered observed test values.

Sensitivity is 100%, and 1 – Specificity (false positive rate) is 52.4%, making the value of Specificity 47.6%.

The last table contains the sensitivity and 1 – specificity of antibiotic use, which is listed as 1.00 and 0.524, respectively. Because 1 – specificity is 0.524, the specificity equals 0.476, or 47.6%.

STUDY QUESTIONS

1. Discuss the sensitivity of a screening test and its importance in diagnosing a disease.

2. Discuss the specificity of a screening test and its importance in diagnosing a disease.

3. Define false positive rate.

4. What is the difference between a "test" variable and a "state" variable when calculating sensitivity and specificity?

5. Define the C statistic and how it relates to sensitivity and specificity.

6. The specificity of the screening test for candiduria was 47.6%. What are the implications for the ability of the test to identify patients without candiduria?

7. What was the false positive rate of the screening test for candiduria?

8. What was the false negative rate of the screening test for candiduria?

9. In the ROC curve for the candiduria example, what were the coordinates used to represent the blue line?

10. List the 95% confidence interval of the C statistic, and state your interpretation of that interval.

Answers to Study Questions

1. Sensitivity indicates the portion of patients with the disease and who have positive test results. The higher the sensitivity of a screening test, the more likely the test is to be positive when a person has a disease, true positive (Straus et al., 2011).

2. Specificity of a test indicates the proportion of the patients who do not have a disease and have negative test results. The higher the specificity of a screening test, the more likely the test is to be negative when a person does not have a disease, true negative. A test that is both sensitive and specific identifies the patients with disease and rules out those that do not have disease (Straus et al., 2011).

3. The false positive rate is defined as the number of people who do not have the disease and the test is positive for the disease.

4. The "test" variable is the screening variable, and the "state" variable is the disease state or the gold standard. It is important to define these two variables so that the calculations for sensitivity and specificity are correct.

5. The C statistic is the actual area under a ROC curve. The value is interpreted as the probability that the test result from a randomly selected person with the disease will be positive (Austin & Steyerberg, 2012).

6. The specificity of the screening test for candiduria, or true negative rate, was 47.6%. Thus, the antibiotic screening test is limited in identifying patients without a disease.

7. The false positive rate of the screening test for candiduria is calculated as: $1 - 0.476 = 0.524 \times 100\% = 52.4\%$.

8. The false negative rate of the screening test for candiduria is calculated as: $1 - 1 = 0$ or $0 \times 100\% = 0\%$.

9. The coordinates of the ROC curve that were used to represent the blue line are 0,0 and 1,0.524. The line was subsequently drawn to connect these two coordinates.

10. The 95% confidence interval of the C statistic was 0.633–0.843, or 63.3%–84.3%. Thus, the interval of 63.3% to 84.3% estimates the population C statistic with 95% confidence. These values are identified in the SPSS Table Area Under the Curve.

DATA FOR ADDITIONAL COMPUTATIONAL PRACTICE FOR QUESTIONS TO BE GRADED

This additional example uses data presented by Spurlock and Hunt (2008) in a retrospective study to examine the ability of nursing students' performance on the HESI Exam (Health Education Systems, Inc.) to predict their performance on the NCLEX-RN (National Council Licensure Examination for Registered Nurses). Most nursing programs use comprehensive examinations such as the HESI Exit Exam to assess students' preparedness for the NCLXES-RN. The two variables in this example are HESI Exam pass/fail and NCLEX-RN pass/fail at first attempt. The "state" variable, or gold standard, in this example is NCLEX-RN pass or fail. The screening test variable is HESI pass or fail. These data are presented in Table 34-4 as a contingency table.

TABLE 34-4 HESI AND NCLEX-RN PERFORMANCE		
	NCLEX Pass	**NCLEX Fail**
HESI Pass	129	13
HESI Fail	26	11

Questions to Be Graded

Name: _____ Class: _____

Date: _____

Answer the following questions with hand calculations using the data presented in Table 34-4 or the SPSS dataset called "Exercise 34 Example 2.sav" available on the Evolve website. Follow your instructor's directions to submit your answers to the following questions for grading. Your instructor may ask you to write your answers below and submit them as a hard copy for grading. Alternatively, your instructor may ask you to submit your answers online.

1. Compute the sensitivity value using the data from Table 34-4. Show your calculations.

2. Compute the specificity value. Show your calculations.

3. Compute the false positive rate. Show your calculations.

4. Compute the false negative rate. Show your calculations.

5. Using SPSS, create a ROC curve and list the C statistic. How would you interpret the value?

6. What does the p value for the C statistic indicate?

7. What was the 95% confidence interval of the C statistic? State your interpretation of that interval.

8. In the ROC curve for the NCLEX example, what were the coordinates used to represent the blue line?

9. What was the positive LR, and how would you interpret that value?

10. What was the negative LR, and how would you interpret that value?

Calculating Pearson Chi-Square

The **Pearson chi-square test** (χ^2) compares differences between groups on variables measured at the nominal level. The χ^2 compares the frequencies that are observed with the frequencies that are expected. When a study requires that researchers compare proportions (percentages) in one category versus another category, the χ^2 is a statistic that will reveal if the difference in proportion is statistically improbable.

A **one-way** χ^2 is a statistic that compares different levels of one variable only. For example, a researcher may collect information on gender and compare the proportions of males to females. If the one-way χ^2 is statistically significant, it would indicate that proportions of one gender are significantly higher than proportions of the other gender than what would be expected by chance (Daniel, 2000; Pett, 2015). If more than two groups are being examined, the χ^2 does not determine where the differences lie; it only determines that a significant difference exists. Further testing on pairs of groups with the χ^2 would then be warranted to identify the significant differences.

A **two-way** χ^2 is a statistic that tests whether proportions in levels of one nominal variable are significantly different from proportions of the second nominal variable. For example, the presence of advanced colon polyps was studied in three groups of patients: those having a normal body mass index (BMI), those who were overweight, and those who were obese (Siddiqui, Sahdala, Nazario, Mahgoub, Patel, Cipher, & Spechler, 2009). The research question tested was: *Is there a difference between the three groups (normal weight, overweight, and obese) on the presence of advanced colon polyps?* The results of the χ^2 test indicated that a larger proportion of obese patients fell into the category of having advanced colon polyps compared to normal weight and overweight patients, suggesting that obesity may be a risk factor for developing advanced colon polyps. Further examples of two-way χ^2 tests are reviewed in Exercise 19.

RESEARCH DESIGNS APPROPRIATE FOR THE PEARSON χ^2

Research designs that may utilize the Pearson χ^2 include the randomized experimental, quasi-experimental, and comparative designs (Gliner, Morgan, & Leech, 2009). The variables may be active, attributional, or a combination of both. An active variable refers to an intervention, treatment, or program. An attributional variable refers to a characteristic of the participant, such as gender, diagnosis, or race/ethnicity. Regardless of the whether the variables are active or attributional, all variables submitted to χ^2 calculations must be measured at the nominal level.

443

STATISTICAL FORMULA AND ASSUMPTIONS

Use of the Pearson χ^2 involves the following assumptions (Daniel, 2000):

1. Only one datum entry is made for each subject in the sample. Therefore, if repeated measures from the same subject are being used for analysis, such as pretests and post-tests, χ^2 is not an appropriate test.
2. The variables must be categorical (nominal), either inherently or transformed to categorical from quantitative values.
3. For each variable, the categories are mutually exclusive and exhaustive. No cells may have an *expected* frequency of zero. In the actual data, the *observed* cell frequency may be zero. However, the Pearson χ^2 test is not sensitive to small sample sizes, and other tests, such as the Fisher's exact test, are more appropriate when testing very small samples (Daniel, 2000; Yates, 1934).

The test is distribution-free, or nonparametric, which means that no assumption has been made for a normal distribution of values in the population from which the sample was taken (Daniel, 2000).

The formula for a two-way χ^2 is:

$$\chi^2 = \frac{n[(A)(D)-(B)(C)]^2}{(A+B)(C+D)(A+C)(B+D)}$$

A **contingency table** is a table that displays the relationship between two or more categorical variables (Daniel, 2000). The contingency table is labeled as follows.

	Columns	
	A	B
Rows	---	---
	C	D

With any χ^2 analysis, the degrees of freedom (*df*) must be calculated to determine the significance of the value of the statistic. The following formula is used for this calculation:

$$df = (R-1)(C-1)$$

where

R = Number of rows
C = Number of columns

HAND CALCULATIONS

A retrospective comparative study examined whether longer antibiotic treatment courses were associated with increased antimicrobial resistance in patients with spinal cord injury (Lee et al., 2014). Using urine cultures from a sample of spinal cord—injured veterans, two groups were created: those with evidence of antibiotic resistance and those with no evidence of antibiotic resistance. Each veteran was also divided into two groups based on having had a history of recent (in the past 6 months) antibiotic use for more than 2 weeks or no history of recent antibiotic use.

TABLE 35-1	ANTIBIOTIC RESISTANCE BY ANTIBIOTIC USE	
	Antibiotic Use	**No Recent Use**
Resistant	8	7
Not resistant	6	21

The data are presented in Table 35-1. The null hypothesis is: *There is no difference between antibiotic users and non-users on the presence of antibiotic resistance.*

The computations for the Pearson χ^2 test are as follows:

Step 1: Create a contingency table of the two nominal variables:

	Used Antibiotics	**No Recent Use**	**Totals**	
Resistant	8	7	15	
Not resistant	6	21	27	
Totals	14	28	42	←Total n

Step 2: Fit the cells into the formula:

$$\chi^2 = \frac{n[(A)(D)-(B)(C)]^2}{(A+B)(C+D)(A+C)(B+D)}$$

$$\chi^2 = \frac{42[(8)(21)-(7)(6)]^2}{(8+7)(6+21)(8+6)(7+28)}$$

$$\chi^2 = \frac{666,792}{158,760}$$

$$\chi^2 = 4.20$$

Step 3: Compute the degrees of freedom:

$$df = (2-1)(2-1) = 1$$

Step 4: Locate the critical χ^2 value in the χ^2 distribution table (Appendix D) and compare it to the obtained χ^2 value.

The obtained χ^2 value is compared with the tabled χ^2 values in Appendix D. The table includes the critical values of χ^2 for specific degrees of freedom at selected levels of significance. If the value of the statistic is equal to or greater than the value identified in the χ^2 table, the difference between the two variables is statistically significant. The critical χ^2 for $df = 1$ is 3.8415 that was rounded to 3.84, and our obtained χ^2 is 4.20, thereby exceeding the critical value and indicating a significant difference between antibiotic users and non-users on the presence of antibiotic resistance.

Furthermore, we can compute the rates of antibiotic resistance among antibiotic users and non-users by using the numbers in the contingency table from Step 1. The antibiotic resistance rate among the antibiotic users can be calculated as 8 ÷ 14 = 0.571 × 100% = 57.1%. The antibiotic resistance rate among the non-antibiotic users can be calculated as 7 ÷ 28 = 0.25 × 100% = 25%.

SPSS COMPUTATIONS

The following screenshot is a replica of what your SPSS window will look like. The data for subjects 18 through 42 are viewable by scrolling down in the SPSS screen.

 Exercise 35 Example 1.sav [DataSet4] - IBM SPSS Statistics Data Editor

File   Edit   View   Data   Transform   Analyze   Graphs   Utilities

	ID	Resistant	AntibioticUse	var
1	1	1	0	
2	2	1	0	
3	3	1	0	
4	4	1	0	
5	5	1	0	
6	6	1	0	
7	7	1	0	
8	8	1	1	
9	9	1	1	
10	10	1	1	
11	11	1	1	
12	12	1	1	
13	13	1	1	
14	14	1	1	
15	15	1	1	
16	16	0	0	
17	17	0	0	

Data View   Variable View

Step 1: From the "Analyze" menu, choose "Descriptive Statistics" and "Crosstabs." Move the two variables to the right, where either variable can be in the "Row" or "Column" space.

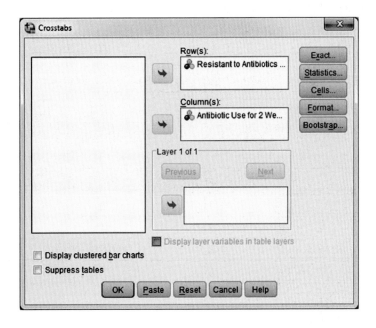

Step 2: Click "Statistics" and check the box next to "Chi-square." Click "Continue" and "OK."

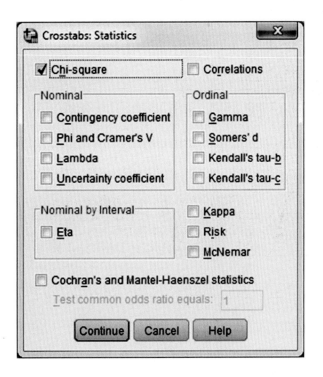

INTERPRETATION OF SPSS OUTPUT

The following tables are generated from SPSS. The first table contains the contingency table, similar to Table 35-1 above. The second table contains the χ^2 results.

Crosstabs

Resistant to Antibiotics * Antibiotic Use for 2 Weeks or More Crosstabulation

Count

		Antibiotic Use for 2 Weeks or More		Total
		No Antibiotic Use	History of >2 Weeks of Antibiotic Use	
Resistant to Antibiotics	Not Resistant	21	6	27
	Resistant	7	8	15
Total		28	14	42

Chi-Square Tests

	Value	df	Asymp. Sig. (2-sided)	Exact Sig. (2-sided)	Exact Sig. (1-sided)
Pearson Chi-Square	4.200[a]	1	.040		
Continuity Correction[b]	2.917	1	.088		
Likelihood Ratio	4.135	1	.042		
Fisher's Exact Test				.085	.045
Linear-by-Linear Association	4.100	1	.043		
N of Valid Cases	42				

[a]. 0 cells (0.0%) have expected count less than 5. The minimum expected count is 5.00.

[b]. Computed only for a 2x2 table

Observe that the χ^2 value is 4.20   **The exact p value is .04**

The last table contains the χ^2 value in addition to other statistics that test associations between nominal variables. The Pearson χ^2 test is located in the first row of the table, which contains the χ^2 value, *df*, and *p* value.

FINAL INTERPRETATION IN AMERICAN PSYCHOLOGICAL ASSOCIATION (APA) FORMAT

The following interpretation is written as it might appear in a research article, formatted according to APA guidelines (APA, 2010). A Pearson χ^2 analysis indicated that antibiotic users had significantly higher rates of antibiotic resistance than those who did not use antibiotics, $\chi^2(1, N = 42) = 4.20$, $p = 0.04$ (57.1% versus 25%, respectively). This finding suggests that extended antibiotic use may be a risk factor for developing resistance, and further research is needed to investigate resistance as a direct effect of antibiotics.

STUDY QUESTIONS

1. Do the example data meet the assumptions for the Pearson χ^2 test? Provide a rationale for your answer.

2. Was the null hypothesis accepted or rejected? Provide a rationale for your answer.

3. What was the exact likelihood of obtaining a χ^2 value at least as extreme or as close to the one that was actually observed, assuming that the null hypothesis is true?

4. Using the numbers in the contingency table, calculate the percentage of antibiotic users who were resistant.

5. Using the numbers in the contingency table, calculate the percentage of non-antibiotic users who were resistant.

6. Using the numbers in the contingency table, calculate the percentage of resistant veterans who used antibiotics for more than 2 weeks.

7. Using the numbers in the contingency table, calculate the percentage of resistant veterans who had no recent history of antibiotic use.

8. Was this an appropriate research design for a chi-square analysis? Provide a rationale for your answer.

9. What result would have been obtained if the variables in the SPSS Crosstabs window had been switched, with Antibiotic Use being placed in the "Row" and Resistance being placed in the "Column"?

10. Was the sample size adequate to detect differences between the two groups in this example? Provide a rationale for your answer.

Answers to Study Questions

1. Yes, the data meet the assumptions of the Pearson χ^2:

   a. Only one datum per participant was entered into the contingency table, and no participant was counted twice.
   b. Both antibiotic use and resistance are categorical (nominal-level data).
   c. For each variable, the categories are mutually exclusive and exhaustive. It was not possible for a participant to belong to both groups, and the two categories (recent antibiotic user and non-user) included all study participants.

2. The null hypothesis is rejected. The critical χ^2 value for 1 degree of freedom at alpha = 0.05 is 3.84 (see Appendix D that includes the critical values for the chi-square distribution). Our obtained χ^2 is 4.20, exceeding the critical value in the table. If using SPSS, note that the p value is listed as 0.04, which is less than $\alpha = 0.05$, indicating a significant result.

3. The exact likelihood of obtaining a χ^2 value at least as extreme as or as close to the one that was actually observed, assuming that the null hypothesis is true, was $0.04 \times 100\% = 4.0\%$.

4. The percentage of antibiotic users who were resistant is calculated as $8 \div 14 = 0.5714 \times 100\% = 57.14\% = 57.1\%$.

5. The percentage of non-antibiotic users who were resistant is calculated as $7 \div 28 = 0.25 \times 100\% = 25\%$.

6. The percentage of antibiotic-resistant veterans who used antibiotics for more than 2 weeks is calculated as $8 \div 15 = 0.533 \times 100\% = 53.3\%$.

7. The percentage of resistant veterans who had no recent history of antibiotic use is calculated as $7 \div 15 = 0.4666 \times 100\% = 46.7\%$.

8. The study design in the example was a retrospective comparative design (Gliner et al., 2009; Gray, Grove, & Sutherland, 2017). Both of the variables (antibiotic resistance and history of antibiotic use) were nominal (yes/no). Therefore the design was appropriate for a chi-square analysis.

9. Switching the variables in the SPSS Crosstabs window would have resulted in the exact same χ^2 result.

10. The sample size was adequate to detect differences between the two groups, because a significant difference was found, $p = 0.04$, which is smaller than alpha = 0.05.

DATA FOR ADDITIONAL COMPUTATIONAL PRACTICE FOR QUESTIONS TO BE GRADED

A retrospective comparative study examining the presence of candiduria (presence of *Candida* species in the urine) among 97 adults with a spinal cord injury is presented as an additional example. The differences in the use of antibiotics were investigated with the Pearson χ^2 test (Goetz, Howard, Cipher, & Revankar, 2010). These data are presented in Table 35-2 as a contingency table.

TABLE 35-2	CANDIDURIA AND ANTIBIOTIC USE IN ADULTS WITH SPINAL CORD INJURIES		
	Candiduria	**No Candiduria**	**Totals**
Antibiotic use	15	43	58
No antibiotic use	0	39	39
Totals	15	82	97

Questions to Be Graded

Name: _____ Class: _____

Date: _____

Answer the following questions with hand calculations using the data presented in Table 35-2 or the SPSS dataset called "Exercise 35 Example 2.sav" available on the Evolve website. Follow your instructor's directions to submit your answers to the following questions for grading. Your instructor may ask you to write your answers below and submit them as a hard copy for grading. Alternatively, your instructor may ask you to submit your answers online.

1. Do the example data in Table 35-2 meet the assumptions for the Pearson χ^2 test? Provide a rationale for your answer.

2. Compute the χ^2 test. What is the χ^2 value?

3. Is the χ^2 significant at $\alpha = 0.05$? Specify how you arrived at your answer.

4. If using SPSS, what is the exact likelihood of obtaining the χ^2 value at least as extreme as or as close to the one that was actually observed, assuming that the null hypothesis is true?

5. Using the numbers in the contingency table, calculate the percentage of antibiotic users who tested positive for candiduria.

6. Using the numbers in the contingency table, calculate the percentage of non-antibiotic users who tested positive for candiduria.

7. Using the numbers in the contingency table, calculate the percentage of veterans with candiduria who had a history of antibiotic use.

8. Using the numbers in the contingency table, calculate the percentage of veterans with candiduria who had no recent history of antibiotic use.

9. Write your interpretation of the results as you would in an APA-formatted journal.

10. Was the sample size adequate to detect differences between the two groups in this example? Provide a rationale for your answer.

Calculating Odds Ratio and 95% Confidence Intervals

When both the predictor and the dependent variable are dichotomous (having only two values), the odds ratio is a commonly used statistic to obtain an indication of association. The **odds ratio** (*OR*) is defined as the ratio of the odds of an event occurring in one group to the odds of it occurring in another group (Gordis, 2014). Put simply, the *OR* is a way of comparing whether the odds of a certain event is the same for two groups. For example, the use of angiotensin converting enzyme inhibitors (ACE inhibitors) in a sample of veterans was examined in relation to having advanced adenomatous colon polyps (Kedika et al., 2011). The *OR* was 0.63, indicating that ACE inhibitor use was associated with a lower likelihood of developing adenomatous colon polyps in veterans.

The *OR* can also be computed when the dependent variable is dichotomous and the predictor is continuous and would be computed by performing logistic regression analysis. **Logistic regression** analysis tests a predictor (or set of predictors) with a dichotomous dependent variable. The output yields an adjusted *OR,* meaning that each predictor's *OR* represents the relationship between that predictor and *y*, after adjusting for the presence of the other predictors in the model (Tabachnick & Fidell, 2013). As is the case with multiple linear regression, each predictor serves as a covariate to every other predictor in the model. Logistic regression is best conducted using a statistical software package. Full explanations and examples of the mathematical computations of logistic regression are presented in Tabachnick and Fidell (2013). Exercise 36 focuses on the odds ratio that involves two dichotomous variables.

RESEARCH DESIGNS APPROPRIATE FOR THE ODDS RATIO

Research designs that may utilize the odds ratio include the randomized experimental, quasi-experimental, comparative, and associational designs (Gliner, Morgan, & Leech, 2009). The variables may be active, attributional, or a combination of both. An active variable refers to an intervention, treatment, or program. An attributional variable refers to a characteristic of the participant, such as gender, diagnosis, or race/ethnicity. Regardless of whether the variables are active or attributional, the dependent variable submitted to *OR* calculations must be dichotomous.

STATISTICAL FORMULA AND ASSUMPTIONS

Use of the odds ratio involves the following assumptions (Gordis, 2014):

1. Only one datum entry is made for each subject in the sample. Therefore, if repeated measures from the same subject are being used for analysis, such as pretests and posttests, the odds ratio is not an appropriate test.

2. The variables must be dichotomous, either inherently or transformed to categorical from quantitative values.

The formula for the odds ratio is:

$$OR = \frac{ad}{bc}$$

The formula for the *OR* designates the predictor's ratios of 1s to 0s within the positive outcome in the numerator, and the predictor's ratios of 1s to 0s within the negative outcome in the denominator. Note that the values must be coded accordingly. Table 36-1 displays the following notation to assist you in calculating the *OR*.

TABLE 36-1 STRUCTURE OF DATA FOR ODD RATIO CALCULATION		
	Yes (Presence)	No (Absence)
Yes (Presence)	*a*	*b*
No (Absence)	*c*	*d*

HAND CALCULATIONS

A retrospective associational study examined the medical utilization of homeless veterans receiving treatment in a Veterans Affairs health care system (LePage, Bradshaw, Cipher, Crawford, & Hooshyar, 2014). A sample of veterans seen in the Veterans Affairs health care system in 2010 ($N = 102{,}034$) was evaluated for homelessness at any point during the year, as well as chronic medical and psychiatric diseases, and medical utilization. The two variables in this example are dichotomous: homelessness in 2010 (yes/no) and having made at least one visit to the emergency department in 2010 (yes/no). The data are presented in Table 36-2. The null hypothesis is: *There is no association between homelessness and emergency department visits among veterans.*

TABLE 36-2 HOMELESSNESS AND ED VISITS		
	At least 1 ED Visit	No ED Visits
Homeless	807	1,398
Not homeless	15,198	84,631

The computations for the odds ratio are as follows:

Step 1: Fit the cell values into the *OR* formula:

$$OR = \frac{ad}{bc} = \frac{(807)(84{,}631)}{(1{,}398)(15{,}198)} = \frac{68{,}297{,}217}{21{,}246{,}804} = 3.21$$

$$OR = 3.21$$

Step 2: Compute the 95% confidence interval for the odds ratio. As demonstrated in Exercise 34, the confidence interval for any statistic is composed of three components: the statistic +/− *SE*(*t*). To compute a 95% confidence interval for the *OR*, you must first convert the *OR* into the natural logarithm of the *OR*. The natural logarithm of a number *X* is the power to which *e* would have to be raised to equal *X* (where *e* is approximately 2.718288). For example, the natural logarithm of *e* itself would be 1, because $e^1 = 2.718288$.

Convert the *OR* to the *ln(OR)*

$$ln(3.21) = 1.17$$

Step 3: Compute the standard error of $ln(OR)$:

$$SE_{ln(OR)} = \sqrt{\frac{1}{a} + \frac{1}{b} + \frac{1}{c} + \frac{1}{d}}$$

$$SE_{ln(OR)} = \sqrt{\frac{1}{807} + \frac{1}{1,398} + \frac{1}{15,198} + \frac{1}{84,631}}$$

$$SE_{ln(OR)} = \sqrt{.001239 + .000715 + .0000658 + .0000118}$$

$$SE_{ln(OR)} = 0.045$$

Step 4: Create the confidence interval (CI) still using the *ln(OR)*, with a *t* of 1.96:

$$95\% \ CI = ln(OR) +/- SE(t)$$

$$95\% \ CI = 1.17 +/- 0.045(1.96)$$

$$1.082 \text{ to } 1.258$$

Step 5: Convert the lower and upper limits of the CI back to the original *OR* unit:

$$e^{1.082} = 2.95$$

$$e^{1.258} = 3.52$$

This means that the interval of 2.95 to 3.52 estimates the population *OR* with 95% confidence (Kline, 2004; Pett, 2016). Moreover, because the CI does not include the number 1.0, the *OR* indicates a significant association between homelessness and emergency department visits.

Step 6: Interpret the directionality of the odds ratio
   An *OR* of $\cong$ 1.0 indicates that exposure (to homelessness) does not affect the odds of the outcome (ED visit).
   An *OR* of >1.0 indicates that exposure (to homelessness) is associated with a higher odds of the outcome (ED visit).
   An *OR* of <1.0 indicates that exposure (to homelessness) is associated with a lower odds of the outcome (ED visit).

The *OR* for the study was 3.21, indicating the odds of having made an emergency department visit among veterans who were homeless was higher than those who were not homeless. We can further note that homeless veterans were over three times as likely, or 221% more likely, to have made an emergency department visit (LePage et al., 2014). This value was computed by subtracting 1.0 from the *OR* 1.00 (3.21 − 1.00 = 2.21 × 100% = 221%). The difference between the obtained *OR* and 1.00 represents the extent of the lesser or greater likelihood of the event occurring.

SPSS COMPUTATIONS

The following screenshot is a replica of what your SPSS window will look like. The remaining data are viewable by scrolling down in the SPSS screen. The values in the data set must be coded as "1" or "0."

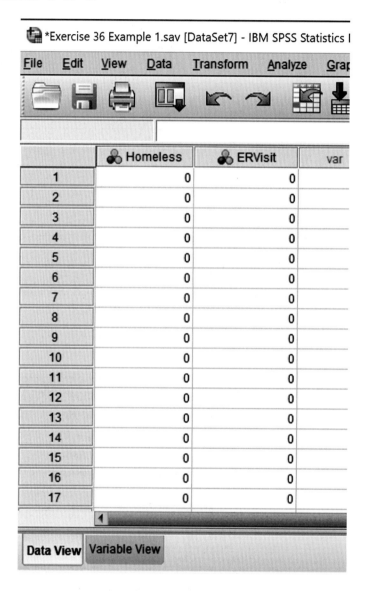

Step 1: From the "Analyze" menu, choose "Descriptive Statistics" and "Crosstabs." Move the two variables to the right, where either variable can be in the "Row" or "Column" space.

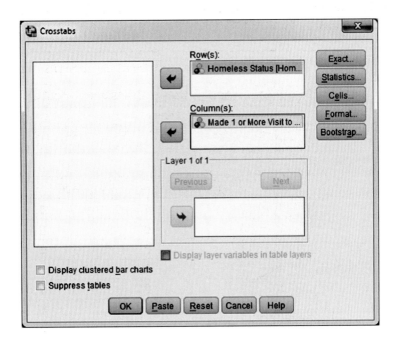

Step 2: Click "Statistics" and check the box next to "Risk." Click "Continue" and "OK."

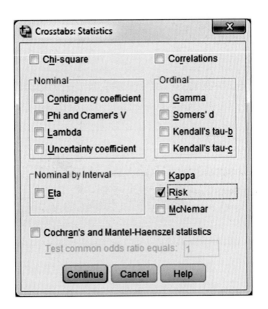

INTERPRETATION OF SPSS OUTPUT

The following tables are generated from SPSS. The first table contains the contingency table, similar to Table 36-2 presented previously. The order of the values in the contingency table is different than that of Table 36-2, but the actual values are the same. The second table contains the *OR* results.

Crosstabs

Homeless Status * Made 1 or More Visit to Emergency Department

Crosstabulation

Count

		Made 1 or More Visit to Emergency Department		Total
		No ER Visit	1 or More ER Visit	
Homeless Status	Not Homeless	84631	15198	99829
	Homeless	1398	807	2205
Total		86029	16005	102034

Risk Estimate

	Value	95% Confidence Interval	
		Lower	Upper
Odds Ratio for Homeless Status (Not Homeless / Homeless)	3.214	2.943	3.511
For cohort Made 1 or More Visit to Emergency Department = No ER Visit	1.337	1.295	1.380
For cohort Made 1 or More Visit to Emergency Department = 1 or More ER Visit	.416	.393	.440
N of Valid Cases	102034		

The 95% CI is 2.94 – 3.51

Observe that the *OR* value is 3.21

The last table contains the *OR* value in addition to the lower and upper limits of the 95% CI, respectively. The *OR* is located in the first row of the table. Note that there is no *p* value, because *OR*s are not traditionally reported accompanied by a *p* value; rather, the 95% CI is reported. The CI values calculated by SPSS are slightly different than the hand-calculated values of 2.95 and 3.52 due to rounding error.

FINAL INTERPRETATION IN AMERICAN PSYCHOLOGICAL ASSOCIATION (APA) FORMAT

The following interpretation is written as it might appear in a research article, formatted according to APA guidelines (APA, 2010). An *OR* was computed to assess the association between homelessness and emergency department use. Homeless veterans were significantly more likely to have made an emergency department visit in 2010 than the non-homeless veterans (36.6% versus 15.2%, respectively; *OR* = 3.21, 95% CI [2.94, 3.51].

STUDY QUESTIONS

1. What does an *OR* of 1.0 indicate?

2. Using the numbers in the contingency table, calculate the percentage of homeless veterans who made at least one visit to the emergency department.

3. Using the numbers in the contingency table, calculate the percentage of non-homeless veterans who made at least one visit to the emergency department.

4. Using the numbers in the contingency table, calculate the percentage of homeless veterans who did not make an emergency department visit.

5. A 95% CI was computed for an *OR* of 0.70. The lower and upper limits were 0.55 to 0.85, respectively. What do the results indicate?

6. A 95% CI was computed for an *OR* of 0.70. The lower and upper limits were 0.35 to 1.05, respectively. What do the results indicate?

7. A 95% CI was computed for an *OR* of 1.23. The lower and upper limits were 1.15 to 1.31, respectively. What do the results indicate?

8. What kind of design was used in the example? Was this design appropriate for conducting an *OR* analysis? Provide a rationale for your answers.

9. A researcher recodes the variable "more than one visit" from binary to a 4-category nominal variable: 1 = zero visits, 2 = 1–2 visits, 3 = 3–4 visits, 4 = more than 4 visits. The researcher wants to compare the homeless cohort to the non-homeless cohort on the newly recoded variable. What would be an appropriate statistical approach?

10. What result would have been obtained if the variables in the SPSS Crosstabs window had been switched, with ED Visit being placed in the "Row" and Homeless being placed in the "Column"?

Answers to Study Questions

1. An *OR* of 1.0 indicates no significant association between the two variables (Gordis, 2014).

2. There were 2,205 homeless veterans, 807 of which made at least one ED visit and 1,398 did not. Therefore, the percentage of homeless veterans who made at least one visit to the emergency department is calculated as $807 \div 2{,}205 = 0.366 \times 100\% = 36.6\%$.

3. There were 99,829 non-homeless veterans, 15,198 of which made at least one ED visit and 84,631 who did not. Therefore, the percentage of non-homeless veterans who made at least one visit to the emergency department is calculated as $15{,}198 \div 99{,}829 = 0.152 \times 100\% = 15.2\%$.

4. The percentage of homeless veterans who did not make an emergency department visit is calculated as $1{,}398 \div 2{,}205 = 0.634 \times 100\% = 63.4\%$.

5. An *OR* of 0.70 with 95% CI of 0.55 to 0.85 indicates a significant association between the two variables, because the CI does not contain 1.0. The probability of the event is 30% lower among the exposure/test group.

6. An *OR* of 0.70 with 95% CI of 0.35 to 1.05 indicates that there is no significant association between the two variables, because the CI contains 1.0.

7. An *OR* of 1.23 with 95% CI of 1.15 to 1.31 indicates a significant association between the two variables, because the CI does not contain 1.0. The probability of the event is 23% higher among the exposure/test group.

8. The study design in the example was a retrospective associational design, because the data were a retrospective examination of an associational research question. Moreover, both variables (homeless/non-homeless and visit/no visit) were nominal and binary. Therefore the research design was appropriate for an OR analysis (Gordis, 2014).

9. The appropriate statistical approach would no longer be an odds ratio, because one of the variables is not binary. Rather, the newly recoded variable is ordinal. To compare two groups on an ordinal variable, a Mann-Whitney U test would be appropriate (see Exercises 21 and 23; Pett, 2016).

10. Switching the variables in the SPSS Crosstabs window would have resulted in the exact same *OR* value and 95% CI values.

DATA FOR ADDITIONAL COMPUTATIONAL PRACTICE FOR QUESTIONS TO BE GRADED

This additional example uses the same data from the retrospective associational study by LePage and colleagues (2014). The two variables in this example are dichotomous: homelessness in 2010 (yes/no) and having used any illegal substance in 2010 (yes/no). The null hypothesis is: *There is no association between homelessness and illegal drug use among veterans.* These data are presented in Table 36-3 as a contingency table.

TABLE 36-3　HOMELESSNESS AND ILLEGAL SUBSTANCE USE		
	Illegal Drug Use	**No Illegal Drug Use**
Homeless	957	1,248
Not homeless	2,626	97,203

Questions to Be Graded

Name: _____ Class: _____

Date: _____

Answer the following questions with hand calculations using the data presented in Table 36-3 or the SPSS dataset called "Exercise 36 Example 2.sav" available on the Evolve website. Follow your instructor's directions to submit your answers to the following questions for grading. Your instructor may ask you to write your answers below and submit them as a hard copy for grading. Alternatively, your instructor may ask you to submit your answers online.

1. Are the data in Table 36-3 appropriate to compute an *OR*? Provide a rationale for your answer.

2. Compute the *OR*. Show your calculations.

3. Compute the 95% CI for the *OR*. Show your calculations.

4. Does the *OR* represent a significant association between homelessness and illegal drug use? Specify how you arrived at your answer.

5. Using the numbers in the contingency table, calculate the percentage of homeless veterans who used illegal substances.

6. Using the numbers in the contingency table, calculate the percentage of non-homeless veterans who used illegal substances.

7. Using the numbers in the contingency table, calculate the percentage of homeless veterans who did not use illegal substances.

8. Using the numbers in the contingency table, calculate the percentage of non-homeless veterans who did not use illegal substances.

9. Write your interpretation of the results as you would in an APA-formatted journal.

10. Was the sample size adequate to detect an association between the two variables in this example? Provide a rationale for your answer.

References

Aberson, C. L. (2019). *Applied power analysis for the behavioral sciences* (2nd ed.). New York: Routledge Taylor & Francis Group.

Aday, L., & Cornelius, L. J. (2006). *Designing and conducting health surveys* (3rd ed.). New York: John Wiley & Sons.

Aiken, L. S., & West, S. G. (1991). *Multiple regression: Testing and interpreting interactions*. Newbury Park, CA, and London: Sage.

Allison, P. D. (1999). *Multiple regression: A primer*. Thousand Oaks, CA: Pine Forge Press.

American Psychological Association (2010). *Publication manual of the American Psychological Association* (6th ed.). Washington, DC: American Psychological Association.

Aponte, J. (2010). Key elements of large survey data sets. *Nursing Economics, 28*(1), 27–36.

Armenta, B. E., Hartshorn, K. J., Whitbeck, L. B., Crawford, D. M., & Hoyt, D. R. (2014). A longitudinal examination of the measurement properties and predictive utility of the Center for Epidemiologic Studies Depression Scale among North American indigenous adolescents. *Psychological Assessment, 26*(4), 1347–1355.

Austin, P. C., & Steyerberg, E. W. (2012). Interpreting the concordance statistic of a logistic regression model: Relation to the variance and odds ratio of a continuous explanatory variable. *BMC Medical Research Methodology, 12*(82), 1–8.

Bannigan, K., & Watson, R. (2009). Reliability and validity in a nutshell. *Journal of Clinical Nursing, 18*(23), 3237–3243.

Bartlett, J. W., & Frost, C. (2008). Reliability, repeatability and reproducibility: Analysis of measurement errors in continuous variables. *Ultrasound Obstetric Gynecology, 31*(4), 466–475.

Benjamini, Y., & Hochberg, Y. (1995). Controlling the false discovery rate: A practical and powerful approach to multiple testing. *Journal of the Royal Statistical Society, 57*(1), 289–300.

Bhatta, S., Champion, J. D., Young, C. C., & Loika, E. A. (2018). Outcomes of depression screening among underserved adolescents accessing care through a school-based pediatric primary care clinic. *Journal of Adolescent Health, 62*(supp), S53-S54.

Bialocerkowski, A., Klupp, N., & Bragge, P. (2010). Research methodology series: How to read and critically appraise a reliability article. *International Journal of Therapy & Rehabilitation, 17*(3), 114–120.

Bond, G. R. (2004). Supported employment: Evidence for an evidence based practice. *Psychiatric Rehabilitation Journal, 27*(4), 345–359.

Boyko, E. J. (1994). Ruling out or ruling in disease with the most sensitive or specific diagnostic test: Short cut or wrong turn? *Medical Decision Making: An International Journal of the Society for Medical Decision Making, 14*(2), 175–179.

Bradley, K. L., Bagnell, A. L., & Brannen, C. L. (2010). Factorial validity of the Center for Epidemiological Studies Depression-10 in adolescents. *Issues in Mental Health Nursing, 31*(6), 408-412.

Breusch, T. S., & Pagan, A. R. (1979). A simple test for heteroscedasticity and random coefficient variation. *Econometrica: Journal of the Econometric Society, 47*(5), 1287-1294.

Brown, S. J. (2018). *Evidence-based nursing: The research-practice connection* (4th ed.). Burlington, MA: Jones & Bartlett.

Campo, M., Shiyko, M., & Lichtman, S. W. (2010). Sensitivity and specificity: A review of related statistics and current controversies in physical therapist education. *Journal of Physical Therapy Education, 24*(3), 69–78.

Centers for disease Control and Prevention, (CDC). U.S. Department of Health and Human services (2015). Body mass index. Retrieved July 13 from https://www.cdc.gov/healthyweight/assessing/bmi/.

Centers for Disease Control and Prevention (CDC). (2010). *National Center for Health Statistics: National Survey of Residential Care Facilities*. Atlanta, GA: CDC.

Charmaz, K. (2014). *Constructing grounded theory: A practical guide through qualitative analysis* (2nd ed.). Thousand Oaks, CA: Sage.

Cipher, D. J. (2019). Statistical decision tree for selecting an appropriate analysis technique. In S. K. Grove & J. R. Gray (Eds.), (2019). *Understanding nursing research: Building an evidence-based practice* (7th ed., p. 311). St. Louis, MO: Saunders.

Coddington, R. D. (1972). The significance of life events as etiologic factors in the diseases of children—II a study of a normal population. *Journal of Psychosomatic Research, 16*(3), 205-2013.

Cohen, J. (1962). The statistical power of abnormal–social psychological research: A review. *Journal of Abnormal Psychology, 65,* 145–153.

Cohen, J. (1988). *Statistical power analysis for the behavioral sciences* (2nd ed.). New York: Academic Press.

Cohen, J., & Cohen, P. (1983). *Applied multiple regression/correlation analysis for the behavioral sciences* (2nd ed.). Hillsdale, NJ: Erlbaum.

Consolidated Standards for Reporting Clinical Trials (CONSORT) Group. (2010). *Welcome to the CONSORT Website.* Retrieved October 20, 2018 from http://www.consort-statement.org.

Creswell, J. W., & Clark, V. L. P. (2018). *Designing and conducting: Mixed methods research* (3rd ed.). Thousand Oaks, CA: Sage.

Creswell, J. W., & Poth, C. N. (2018). *Qualitative inquiry & research design: Choosing among five approaches* (4th ed.). Thousand Oaks, CA: Sage.

Creswell, J. W. & Creswell, J. D. (2018). *Research design: Qualitative, quantitative and mixed methods approaches* (5th ed.). Thousand Oaks, CA: Sage.

Daniel, W. W. (2000). *Applied nonparametric statistics* (2nd ed.). Pacific Grove, CA: Duxbury Press.

de Winter, J. C. F., & Dodou, D. (2010). Five-point Likert items: *t*-test versus Mann-Whitney-Wilcoxon. *Practical Assessment, Research, and Evaluation, 15*(11), 1–16.

DeVon, H. A., Block, M. E., Moyle-Wright, P., Ernst, D. M., Hayden, S. J., Lazzara, D. J., et al. (2007). A psychometric toolbox for testing validity and reliability. *Journal of Nursing Scholarship, 39*(2), 155–164.

Dunbar, K. B., Agoston, A. T., Odze, R. D., Huo, X., Pham, T. H., Cipher, D. J., et al. (2016). Association of acute gastroesophageal reflux disease with esophageal histologic changes. *Journal of the American Medical Association, 315*(19), 2104–2112. doi:10.1001/jama.2016.5657.

Faul, F., Erdfelder, E., Buchner, A., & Lang, A. G. (2009). Statistical power analyses using GPower 3.1: Tests for correlation and regression analyses. *Behavior Research Methods, 41*(4), 1149–1160.

Flores, A., Burstein, E., Cipher, D. J., & Feagins, L. A. (2015). Obesity in inflammatory bowel disease: A marker of less severe disease. *Digestive Diseases and Sciences, 60*(8), 2436–2445.

Gaskin, C. J., & Happell, B. (2014). Power, effects, confidence, and significance: An investigation of statistical practices in nursing research. *International Journal of Nursing Studies, 51*(5), 795–806.

Gliner, J. A., Morgan, G. A., & Leech, N. L. (2009). *Research methods in applied settings* (2nd ed.). New York: Routledge.

Goetz, L., Howard, M., Cipher, D., & Revankar (2010). Occurrence of candiduria in a population of chronically catheterized patients with spinal-cord injury. *Spinal Cord, 48*(1), 51–54.

Goodwin, L. D. (2002). Changing conceptions of measurement validity: An update on the new standards. *Journal of Nursing Education, 41*(3), 100–106.

Gordis, L. (2014). *Epidemiology* (5th ed.). Philadelphia: Elsevier Saunders.

Gray, J. R., Grove, S. K., & Sutherland, S. (2017). *The practice of nursing research: Appraisal, synthesis, and generation of evidence* (8th ed.). St. Louis, MO: Saunders.

Grove, S. K., & Gray, J. R. (2019). *Understanding nursing research: Building an evidence-based practice* (7th ed.). St. Louis, MO: Saunders.

Hayat, M. J. (2013). Understanding sample size determination in nursing research. *Western Journal of Nursing Research, 35*(7), 943–956.

Heavey, E. (2019). *Statistics for nursing: A practical approach* (3rd ed.). Burlington, MA: Jones & Bartlett Learning.

Holmes Jr., L. (2018). *Applied biostatistical principles and concepts: Clinicians' guide to data analysis and interpretation.* New York: Routledge.

Hulley, S. B., Cummings, S. R., Browner, W. S., Grady, D. G., & Newman, T. B. (2013). *Designing clinical research* (4th ed.). Philadelphia: Lippincott Williams & Wilkins.

Hunt, C., Peters, L., & Rapee, R. M. (2012). Development of a measure of being bullied in youth. *Psychological Assessment, 24*(10), 156-165.

IBM Corp. (2017). IBM SPSS Statistics for Windows, Version 25.0. Armonk, NY: IBM Corp.

Kahveci, K. L., & Cipher, D. J. (2014). Acute care use originating from residential care facilities in the United States. Paper presented to the Annual Conference of the American Geriatrics Society. Orlando, FL.

Kandola, D., Banner, D., O'Keefe-McCarthy, S., & Jassal, D. (2014). Sampling methods in cardiovascular nursing research: An overview. *Canadian Journal of Cardiovascular Nursing, 24*(3), 15-18.

Kazdin, A. E. (2017). *Research design in clinical psychology* (5th ed.). Boston, MA: Pearson.

Kedika, R., Patel, M., Pena Sahdala, H. N., Mahgoub, A., Cipher, D. J., & Siddiqui, A. A. (2011). Long-term use of angiotensin converting enzyme inhibitors is associated with decreased incidence of advanced adenomatous colon polyps. *Journal of Clinical Gastroenterology, 45*(2), e12–e16.

King, A., & Eckersley, R. (2019). *Statistics for biomedical engineers and scientists: How to visulize and analyze data.* London Wall, London: Elsevier Academic Press.

Kim, M., & Mallory, C. (2017). *Statistics for evidence-based practice in nursing.* Burlington, MA: Jones & Bartlett Learning.

Kline, R. B. (2004). *Beyond significance testing.* Washington, DC: American Psychological Association.

Knapp, H. (2017). *Practical statistics for nursing using SPSS.* Thousand Oaks, CA: Sage.

Koo, T. K., & Li, M. Y. (2016). A guideline of selecting and reporting intraclass correlation coefficients for reliability research. *Journal of Chiropractic Medicine, 15*(2), 155-163.

Lee, Y. R., Tashjian, C. A., Brouse, S. D., Bedimo, R. J., Goetz, L. L., Cipher, D. J., & Duquaine, S. M. (2014). Antibiotic therapy and bacterial resistance in patients with spinal cord injury. *Federal Practitioner, 31*(3), 13-17.

Leedy, P. D., & Ormrod, J. E. (2019). Practical research: Planning and design (12th ed.). New York, NY: Pearson.

LePage, J. P., Bradshaw, L. D., Cipher, D. J., Crawford, A. M., & Hooshyar, D. (2014). The effects of homelessness on veterans' healthcare service use: An evaluation of independence from comorbidities. *Public Health, 128*(11), 985–992.

Levine, M. & Ensom, M. H. (2001). Post hoc power analysis: an idea whose time has passed? *Pharmacotherapy, 21*(4), 405–409.

Locke, B. Z., & Putnam, P. (2002). *Center for Epidemiologic Studies Depression Scale (CES-D Scale).* Bethesda, MD: National Institute of Mental Health.

Mancini, M. E., Ashwill, J., & Cipher, D. J. (2015). A comparative analysis of demographic and academic success characteristics of on-line and on-campus RN-to-BSN students. *Journal of Professional Nursing, 31*(1), 71–76.

Marsaglia, G., Tang, W. W., & Wang, J. (2003). Evaluating Kolmogorov's distribution. *Journal of Statistical Software, 8*(18),1–4.

Marshall, C., & Rossman, G. B. (2016). *Designing qualitative research* (6th ed.). Los Angeles, CA: Sage.

Melnyk, B. M., & Fineout-Overholt, E. (2019). *Evidence-based practice in nursing & healthcare: A guide to best practice* (4th ed.). Philadelphia: Lippincott Williams & Wilkins.

Moorhead, S., Swanson, E., Johnson, M., & Maas, M. L. (2018). Nursing Outcomes Classification (NOC): Measurement of health outcomes (6th ed.). St. Louis, MO: Elsevier.

National Heart, Lung, and Blood Institute (NHLBI). Classification of Overweight and Obesity by BMI, Waist Circumference, and Associated Disease Risks (2019). Retrieved from: https://www.nhlbi.nih.gov/health/educational/lose_wt/BMI/bmi_dis.htm

Ottomanelli, L., Goetz, L. L., Suris, A., McGeough, C., Sinnott, P. L., Toscano, R., Barnett, S. D., Cipher, D. J., Lind, L. M., Dixon, T. M., Holmes, S. A., Kerrigan, A. J., & Thomas, F. P. (2012). The effectiveness of supported employment for veterans with spinal cord injuries: Results from a randomized multi-site study. *Archives of Physical Medicine and Rehabilitation, 93*(5), 740-747.

Pett, M. A. (2016). *Nonparametric statistics for health care research: Statistics for small samples and unusual distributions* (2nd ed.). Thousand Oaks, CA: Sage.

Plichta, S. B., & Kelvin, E. (2013). *Munro's statistical methods for health care research* (6th ed.). Philadelphia: Lippincott Williams & Wilkins.

Polit, D. F., & Yang, F. M. (2016). *Measurement and the measurement of change: A primer for the health professionals.* Philadelphia: Wolters Kluwer.

Radloff, L. S. (1977). The CES-D scale: A self-report depression scale for research in the general population. *Applied Psychological Measures, 1*, 385–394.

Rasmussen, J. L. (1989). Analysis of Likert-scale data: A reinterpretation of Gregoire and Driver. *Psychological Bulletin, 105*, 167–170.

Ryan-Wenger, N. A. (2017). Precision, accuracy, and uncertainty of biophysical measurements for research and practice. In C. F. Waltz, O. L. Strickland, & E. R. Lenz (Eds.), *Measurement in nursing and health research* (5th ed., pp. 427–445). New York: Springer Publishing Company.

Shadish, W. R., Cook, T. D., & Campbell, D. T. (2002). *Experimental and quasi-experimental designs for generalized causal inference.* Chicago: Rand McNally.

Sharp, L. K., & Lipsky, M. S. (2002). Screening for depression across the lifespan: A review of measures for use in primacy care settings. *American Family Physician, 66*(6), 1001–1008.

Siddiqui, A. A., Sahdala, H. N. P., Nazario, H., Mahgoub, A., Patel, H., Cipher, D. J., & Spechler, S. J., et al. (2009). Obesity is associated with an increased prevalence of advanced adenomatous colon polyps in a male veteran population. *Digestive Disease and Sciences, 54*(7), 1560–1564.

Spurlock, D. R., & Hunt, L. A. (2008). A study of the usefulness of the HESI exit exam in predicting NCLEX-RN failure. *Journal of Nursing Education, 47*(4), 157–166.

Stevens, J. P. (2009). *Applied multivariate statistics for the social sciences* (5th ed.). London: Psychology Press.

Stevens, S. S. (1946). On the theory of scales of measurement. *Science, 103*(2684), 677–680.

Straus, S. E., Glasziou, P., Richardson, W. S., Rosenberg, W., & Haynes, R. B. (2011). *Evidence-based medicine: How to practice and teach EBM* (5th ed.). Edinburgh: Churchill Livingstone Elsevier.

Stone, K. S., & Frazier, S. K. (2017). Measurement of physiological variables using biomedical instrumentation. In C. F. Waltz, O. L. Strickland, & E. R. Lenz (Eds.), *Measurement in nursing and health research* (5th ed., pp. 379–425). New York: Springer.

Tabachnick, B. G., & Fidell, L. S. (2013). *Using multivariate statistics* (6th ed.). Needham Heights, MA: Allyn and Bacon.

Taylor, J., & Spurlock, D. (2018). Statistical power in nursing education research. *Journal of Nursing Education, 57*(5), 262–264.

Thompson, N. J., & Morris, R. D. (1994). Predicting injury risk in adolescent football players: The importance of psychological variables. *Journal of Pediatric Psychology, 19*(4), 415–429.

Thompson, S. K. (2002). *Sampling* (2nd ed.). New York: John Wiley & Sons.

Tran, S., Hooker, R. S., Cipher, D. J., & Reimold, A. (2009). Patterns of biologic use in inflammatory diseases: Older males. *Drugs and Aging, 26*(7), 607–615.

Velanovich, V. (2007) The development of the GERD-HRQL symptom severity instrument. *Diseases of the Esophagus, 20*, 130–134.

Viera, A. J., & Garrett, J. M. (2005). Understanding interobserver agreement: The kappa statistic. *Family Medicine, 37*(5), 360–363.

Villalonga-Olives, E., Forero, C. G., Erhart, M., Palaci-Vieira, J. A., Valderas, J. M., Herdman, M., ... Alonso, J. (2011). Relationship between life events and psychosomatic complainants during adolescence/youth: A structured equation model approach. *Journal of Adolescent Health, 49*(1), 199–205.

Waltz, C. F., Strickland, O. L., & Lenz, E. R. (2017). *Measurement in nursing and health research* (5th ed.). New York: Springer Publishing Company.

Weber, M. A., Schiffrin, E. L., White, W. B., Mann, S., Lindholm, L. H., Kenerson, J. G., ... Harrap, S. B. (2014). Clinical practice guidelines for the management of hypertension in the community: A statement by the American Society of Hypertension and the International Society of Hypertension. *Journal of Hypertension, 32*(1), 3–15.

White, H. (1980). A heteroskedasticity-consistent covariance matrix estimator and a direct test for heteroskedasticity. *Econometrica: Journal of the Econometric Society, 48*(4), 817–838.

Yates, F. (1934). Contingency tables involving small numbers and the χ^2 test. *Journal of Royal Statistical Society, 1*(2), 217–235.

Zar, J. H. (2010). *Biostatistical analysis* (5th ed.). Upper Saddle River, NJ: Pearson Prentice-Hall.

Appendix A
Critical Values for Student's *t* Distribution

Level of Significance (α), One-Tailed Test

	0.001	0.005	0.01	0.025	0.05	0.10

Level of Significance (α), Two-Tailed Test

Degrees of Freedom (*df*)	0.002	0.01	0.02	0.05	0.10	0.20
2	22.327	9.925	6.965	4.303	2.920	1.886
3	10.215	5.841	4.541	3.182	2.353	1.638
4	7.173	4.604	3.747	2.776	2.132	1.533
5	5.893	4.032	3.365	2.571	2.015	1.476
6	5.208	3.707	3.143	2.447	1.943	1.440
7	4.785	3.499	2.998	2.365	1.895	1.415
8	4.501	3.355	2.896	2.306	1.860	1.397
9	4.297	3.250	2.821	2.262	1.833	1.383
10	4.144	3.169	2.764	2.228	1.812	1.372
11	4.025	3.106	2.718	2.201	1.796	1.363
12	3.930	3.055	2.681	2.179	1.782	1.356
13	3.852	3.012	2.650	2.160	1.771	1.350
14	3.787	2.977	2.624	2.145	1.761	1.345
15	3.733	2.947	2.602	2.131	1.753	1.341
16	3.686	2.921	2.583	2.120	1.746	1.337
17	3.646	2.898	2.567	2.110	1.740	1.333
18	3.610	2.878	2.552	2.101	1.734	1.330
19	3.579	2.861	2.539	2.093	1.729	1.328
20	3.552	2.845	2.528	2.086	1.725	1.325
21	3.527	2.831	2.518	2.080	1.721	1.323
22	3.505	2.819	2.508	2.074	1.717	1.321
23	3.485	2.807	2.500	2.069	1.714	1.319
24	3.467	2.797	2.492	2.064	1.711	1.318
25	3.450	2.787	2.485	2.060	1.708	1.316
26	3.435	2.779	2.479	2.056	1.706	1.315
27	3.421	2.771	2.473	2.052	1.703	1.314
28	3.408	2.763	2.467	2.048	1.701	1.313
29	3.396	2.756	2.462	2.045	1.699	1.311
30	3.385	2.750	2.457	2.042	1.697	1.310
31	3.375	2.744	2.453	2.040	1.696	1.309

Level of Significance (α), Two-Tailed Test, cont'd

Degrees of Freedom (*df*)	0.002	0.01	0.02	0.05	0.10	0.20
32	3.365	2.738	2.449	2.037	1.694	1.309
33	3.356	2.733	2.445	2.035	1.692	1.308
34	3.348	2.728	2.441	2.032	1.691	1.307
35	3.340	2.724	2.438	2.030	1.690	1.306
36	3.333	2.719	2.434	2.028	1.688	1.306
37	3.326	2.715	2.431	2.026	1.687	1.305
38	3.319	2.712	2.429	2.024	1.686	1.304
39	3.313	2.708	2.426	2.023	1.685	1.304
40	3.307	2.704	2.423	2.021	1.684	1.303
45	3.281	2.690	2.412	2.014	1.679	1.301
50	3.261	2.678	2.403	2.009	1.676	1.299
55	3.245	2.668	2.396	2.004	1.673	1.297
60	3.232	2.660	2.390	2.000	1.671	1.296
65	3.220	2.654	2.385	1.997	1.669	1.295
70	3.211	2.648	2.381	1.994	1.667	1.294
75	3.202	2.643	2.377	1.992	1.665	1.293
80	3.195	2.639	2.374	1.990	1.664	1.292
85	3.189	2.635	2.371	1.988	1.663	1.292
90	3.183	2.632	2.368	1.987	1.662	1.291
95	3.178	2.629	2.366	1.985	1.661	1.291
100	3.174	2.626	2.364	1.984	1.660	1.290
200	3.131	2.601	2.345	1.972	1.653	1.286
300	3.118	2.592	2.339	1.968	1.650	1.284
∞	3.1	2.58	2.33	1.96	1.65	1.28

Appendix B
Critical Values of *r* for Pearson Product-Moment Correlation Coefficient

Level of Significance (α), One-Tailed Test

	0.05	0.025	0.01	0.005			0.05	0.025	0.01	0.005

Level of Significance (α), Two-Tailed Test

df = *n* − 2	0.10	0.05	0.02	0.01		*df* = *n* − 2	0.10	0.05	0.02	0.01
1	0.9877	0.9969	0.9995	0.9999		39	0.2605	0.3081	0.3621	0.3978
2	0.9000	0.9500	0.9800	0.9900		40	0.2573	0.3044	0.3578	0.3932
3	0.8054	0.8783	0.9343	0.9587		41	0.2542	0.3008	0.3536	0.3887
4	0.7293	0.8114	0.8822	0.9172		42	0.2512	0.2973	0.3496	0.3843
5	0.6694	0.7545	0.8329	0.8745		43	0.2483	0.2940	0.3458	0.3801
6	0.6215	0.7067	0.7887	0.8343		44	0.2455	0.2907	0.3420	0.3761
7	0.5822	0.6664	0.7498	0.7977		45	0.2429	0.2876	0.3384	0.3721
8	0.5493	0.6319	0.7155	0.7646		46	0.2403	0.2845	0.3348	0.3683
9	0.5214	0.6021	0.6851	0.7348		47	0.2377	0.2816	0.3314	0.3646
10	0.4973	0.5760	0.6581	0.7079		48	0.2353	0.2787	0.3281	0.3610
11	0.4762	0.5529	0.6339	0.6835		49	0.2329	0.2759	0.3249	0.3575
12	0.4575	0.5324	0.6120	0.6614		50	0.2306	0.2732	0.3218	0.3542
13	0.4409	0.5140	0.5923	0.6411		55	0.2201	0.2609	0.3074	0.3385
14	0.4259	0.4973	0.5742	0.6226		60	0.2108	0.2500	0.2948	0.3248
15	0.4124	0.4821	0.5577	0.6055		65	0.2027	0.2404	0.2837	0.3126
16	0.4000	0.4683	0.5426	0.5897		70	0.1954	0.2319	0.2737	0.3017
17	0.3887	0.4555	0.5285	0.5751		75	0.1888	0.2242	0.2647	0.2919
18	0.3783	0.4438	0.5155	0.5614		80	0.1829	0.2172	0.2565	0.2830
19	0.3687	0.4329	0.5034	0.5487		85	0.1775	0.2108	0.2491	0.2748
20	0.3598	0.4227	0.4921	0.5368		90	0.1726	0.2050	0.2422	0.2673
21	0.3515	0.4132	0.4815	0.5256		95	0.1680	0.1996	0.2359	0.2604
22	0.3438	0.4044	0.4716	0.5151		100	0.1638	0.1946	0.2301	0.2540
23	0.3365	0.3961	0.4622	0.5052		120	0.1496	0.1779	0.2104	0.2324
24	0.3297	0.3882	0.4534	0.4958		140	0.1386	0.1648	0.1951	0.2155
25	0.3233	0.3809	0.4451	0.4869		160	0.1297	0.1543	0.1827	0.2019
26	0.3172	0.3739	0.4372	0.4785		180	0.1223	0.1455	0.1723	0.1905
27	0.3115	0.3673	0.4297	0.4705		200	0.1161	0.1381	0.1636	0.1809
28	0.3061	0.3610	0.4226	0.4629		250	0.1039	0.1236	0.1465	0.1620
29	0.3009	0.3550	0.4158	0.4556		300	0.0948	0.1129	0.1338	0.1480
30	0.2960	0.3494	0.4093	0.4487		350	0.0878	0.1046	0.1240	0.1371
31	0.2913	0.3440	0.4031	0.4421		400	0.0822	0.0978	0.1160	0.1283
32	0.2869	0.3388	0.3973	0.4357		450	0.0775	0.0922	0.1094	0.1210
33	0.2826	0.3338	0.3916	0.4297		500	0.0735	0.0875	0.1038	0.1149
34	0.2785	0.3291	0.3862	0.4238		600	0.0671	0.0799	0.0948	0.1049
35	0.2746	0.3246	0.3810	0.4182		700	0.0621	0.0740	0.0878	0.0972
36	0.2709	0.3202	0.3760	0.4128		800	0.0581	0.0692	0.0821	0.0909
37	0.2673	0.3160	0.3712	0.4076		900	0.0548	0.0653	0.0774	0.0857
38	0.2638	0.3120	0.3665	0.4026		1000	0.0520	0.0619	0.0735	0.0813

df = Degrees of Freedom.

Appendix C
Critical Values of F for α = 0.05 and α = 0.01

Critical Values of F for α = 0.05

df Denominator	df Numerator																		
---	1	2	3	4	5	6	7	8	9	10	12	15	20	24	30	40	60	120	∞
1	161.4	199.5	215.7	224.6	230.2	234.0	236.8	238.9	240.5	241.9	243.9	245.9	248.0	249.1	250.1	251.1	252.2	253.3	254.3
2	18.51	19.00	19.16	19.25	19.30	19.33	19.35	19.37	19.38	19.40	19.41	19.43	19.45	19.45	19.46	19.47	19.48	19.49	19.50
3	10.13	9.55	9.28	9.12	9.01	8.94	8.89	8.85	8.81	8.79	8.74	8.70	8.66	8.64	8.62	8.59	8.57	8.55	8.53
4	7.71	6.94	6.59	6.39	6.26	6.16	6.09	6.04	6.00	5.96	5.91	5.86	5.80	5.77	5.75	5.72	5.69	5.66	5.63
5	6.61	5.79	5.41	5.19	5.05	4.95	4.88	4.82	4.77	4.74	4.68	4.62	4.56	4.53	4.50	4.46	4.43	4.40	4.36
6	5.99	5.14	4.76	4.53	4.39	4.28	4.21	4.15	4.10	4.06	4.00	3.94	3.87	3.84	3.81	3.77	3.74	3.70	3.67
7	5.59	4.74	4.35	4.12	3.97	3.87	3.79	3.73	3.68	3.64	3.57	3.51	3.44	3.41	3.38	3.34	3.30	3.27	3.23
8	5.32	4.46	4.07	3.84	3.69	3.58	3.50	3.44	3.39	3.35	3.28	3.22	3.15	3.12	3.08	3.04	3.01	2.97	2.93
9	5.12	4.26	3.86	3.63	3.48	3.37	3.29	3.23	3.18	3.14	3.07	3.01	2.94	2.90	2.86	2.83	2.79	2.75	2.71
10	4.96	4.10	3.71	3.48	3.33	3.22	3.14	3.07	3.02	2.98	2.91	2.85	2.77	2.74	2.70	2.66	2.62	2.58	2.54
11	4.84	3.98	3.59	3.36	3.20	3.09	3.01	2.95	2.90	2.85	2.79	2.72	2.65	2.61	2.57	2.53	2.49	2.45	2.40
12	4.75	3.89	3.49	3.26	3.11	3.00	2.91	2.85	2.80	2.75	2.69	2.62	2.54	2.51	2.47	2.43	2.38	2.34	2.30
13	4.67	3.81	3.41	3.18	3.03	2.92	2.83	2.77	2.71	2.67	2.60	2.53	2.46	2.42	2.38	2.34	2.30	2.25	2.21
14	4.60	3.74	3.34	3.11	2.96	2.85	2.76	2.70	2.65	2.60	2.53	2.46	2.39	2.35	2.31	2.27	2.22	2.18	2.13
15	4.54	3.68	3.29	3.06	2.90	2.79	2.71	2.64	2.59	2.54	2.48	2.40	2.33	2.29	2.25	2.20	2.16	2.11	2.07
16	4.49	3.63	3.24	3.01	2.85	2.74	2.66	2.59	2.54	2.49	2.42	2.35	2.28	2.24	2.19	2.15	2.11	2.06	2.01
17	4.45	3.59	3.20	2.96	2.81	2.70	2.61	2.55	2.49	2.45	2.38	2.31	2.23	2.19	2.15	2.10	2.06	2.01	1.96
18	4.41	3.55	3.16	2.93	2.77	2.66	2.58	2.51	2.46	2.41	2.34	2.27	2.19	2.15	2.11	2.06	2.02	1.97	1.92
19	4.38	3.52	3.13	2.90	2.74	2.63	2.54	2.48	2.42	2.38	2.31	2.23	2.16	2.11	2.07	2.03	1.98	1.93	1.88
20	4.35	3.49	3.10	2.87	2.71	2.60	2.51	2.45	2.39	2.35	2.28	2.20	2.12	2.08	2.04	1.99	1.95	1.90	1.84
21	4.32	3.47	3.07	2.84	2.68	2.57	2.49	2.42	2.37	2.32	2.25	2.18	2.10	2.05	2.01	1.96	1.92	1.87	1.81
22	4.30	3.44	3.05	2.82	2.66	2.55	2.46	2.40	2.34	2.30	2.23	2.15	2.07	2.03	1.98	1.94	1.89	1.84	1.78
23	4.28	3.42	3.03	2.80	2.64	2.53	2.44	2.37	2.32	2.27	2.20	2.13	2.05	2.01	1.96	1.91	1.86	1.81	1.76
24	4.26	3.40	3.01	2.78	2.62	2.51	2.42	2.36	2.30	2.25	2.18	2.11	2.03	1.98	1.94	1.89	1.84	1.79	1.73
25	4.24	3.39	2.99	2.76	2.60	2.49	2.40	2.34	2.28	2.24	2.16	2.09	2.01	1.96	1.92	1.87	1.82	1.77	1.71
26	4.23	3.37	2.98	2.74	2.59	2.47	2.39	2.32	2.27	2.22	2.15	2.07	1.99	1.95	1.90	1.85	1.80	1.75	1.69
27	4.21	3.35	2.96	2.73	2.57	2.46	2.37	2.31	2.25	2.20	2.13	2.06	1.97	1.93	1.88	1.84	1.79	1.73	1.67
28	4.20	3.34	2.95	2.71	2.56	2.45	2.36	2.29	2.24	2.19	2.12	2.04	1.96	1.91	1.87	1.82	1.77	1.71	1.65
29	4.18	3.33	2.93	2.70	2.55	2.43	2.35	2.28	2.22	2.18	2.10	2.03	1.94	1.90	1.85	1.81	1.75	1.70	1.64
30	4.17	3.32	2.92	2.69	2.53	2.42	2.33	2.27	2.21	2.16	2.09	2.01	1.93	1.89	1.84	1.79	1.74	1.68	1.62
40	4.08	3.23	2.84	2.61	2.45	2.34	2.25	2.18	2.12	2.08	2.00	1.92	1.84	1.79	1.74	1.69	1.64	1.58	1.51
60	4.00	3.15	2.76	2.53	2.37	2.25	2.17	2.10	2.04	1.99	1.92	1.84	1.75	1.70	1.65	1.59	1.53	1.47	1.39
120	3.92	3.07	2.68	2.45	2.29	2.17	2.09	2.02	1.96	1.91	1.83	1.75	1.66	1.61	1.55	1.50	1.43	1.35	1.25
∞	3.84	3.00	2.60	2.37	2.21	2.10	2.01	1.94	1.88	1.83	1.75	1.67	1.57	1.52	1.46	1.39	1.32	1.22	1.00

df = Degrees of Freedom.

Merrington, M., & Thompson, C. M. (1943). Tables of percentage points of the inverted beta (F) distribution. *Biometrika, 33*(1), 73–78.

Critical Values of *F* for α = 0.01

df Denominator	1	2	3	4	5	6	7	8	9	10	12	15	20	24	30	40	60	120	∞
1	4,052	4,999.5	5,403	5,625	5,764	5,859	5,928	5,982	6,022	6,056	6,106	6,157	6,209	6,235	6,261	6,287	6,313	6,339	6,366
2	98.50	99.00	99.17	99.25	99.30	99.33	99.36	99.37	99.39	99.40	99.42	99.43	99.45	99.46	99.47	99.47	99.48	99.49	99.50
3	34.12	30.82	29.46	28.71	28.24	27.91	27.67	27.49	27.35	27.23	27.05	26.87	26.69	26.60	26.50	26.41	26.32	26.22	26.13
4	21.20	18.00	16.69	15.98	15.52	15.21	14.98	14.80	14.66	14.55	14.37	14.20	14.02	13.93	13.84	13.75	13.65	13.56	13.46
5	16.26	13.27	12.06	11.39	10.97	10.67	10.46	10.29	10.16	10.05	9.89	9.72	9.55	9.47	9.38	9.29	9.20	9.11	9.02
6	13.75	10.92	9.78	9.15	8.75	8.47	8.26	8.10	7.98	7.87	7.72	7.56	7.40	7.31	7.23	7.14	7.06	6.97	6.88
7	12.25	9.55	8.45	7.85	7.46	7.19	6.99	6.84	6.72	6.62	6.47	6.31	6.16	6.07	5.99	5.91	5.82	5.74	5.65
8	11.26	8.65	7.59	7.01	6.63	6.37	6.18	6.03	5.91	5.81	5.67	5.52	5.36	5.28	5.20	5.12	5.03	4.95	4.86
9	10.56	8.02	6.99	6.42	6.06	5.80	5.61	5.47	5.35	5.26	5.11	4.96	4.81	4.73	4.65	4.57	4.48	4.40	4.31
10	10.04	7.56	6.55	5.99	5.64	5.39	5.20	5.06	4.94	4.85	4.71	4.56	4.41	4.33	4.25	4.17	4.08	4.00	3.91
11	9.65	7.21	6.22	5.67	5.32	5.07	4.89	4.74	4.63	4.54	4.40	4.25	4.10	4.02	3.94	3.86	3.78	3.69	3.60
12	9.33	6.93	5.95	5.41	5.06	4.82	4.64	4.50	4.39	4.30	4.16	4.01	3.86	3.78	3.70	3.62	3.54	3.45	3.36
13	9.07	6.70	5.74	5.21	4.86	4.62	4.44	4.30	4.19	4.10	3.96	3.82	3.66	3.59	3.51	3.43	3.34	3.25	3.17
14	8.86	6.51	5.56	5.04	4.69	4.46	4.28	4.14	4.03	3.94	3.80	3.66	3.51	3.43	3.35	3.27	3.18	3.09	3.00
15	8.68	6.36	5.42	4.89	4.56	4.32	4.14	4.00	3.89	3.80	3.67	3.52	3.37	3.29	3.21	3.13	3.05	2.96	2.87
16	8.53	6.23	5.29	4.77	4.44	4.20	4.03	3.89	3.78	3.69	3.55	3.41	3.26	3.18	3.10	3.02	2.93	2.84	2.75
17	8.40	6.11	5.18	4.67	4.34	4.10	3.93	3.79	3.68	3.59	3.46	3.31	3.16	3.08	3.00	2.92	2.83	2.75	2.65
18	8.29	6.01	5.09	4.58	4.25	4.01	3.84	3.71	3.60	3.51	3.37	3.23	3.08	3.00	2.92	2.84	2.75	2.66	2.5
19	8.18	5.93	5.01	4.50	4.17	3.94	3.77	3.63	3.52	3.43	3.30	3.15	3.00	2.92	2.84	2.76	2.67	2.58	2.4
20	8.10	5.85	4.94	4.43	4.10	3.87	3.70	3.56	3.46	3.37	3.23	3.09	2.94	2.86	2.78	2.69	2.61	2.52	2.42
21	8.02	5.78	4.87	4.37	4.04	3.81	3.64	3.51	3.40	3.31	3.17	3.03	2.88	2.80	2.72	2.64	2.55	2.46	2.36
22	7.95	5.72	4.82	4.31	3.99	3.76	3.59	3.45	3.35	3.26	3.12	2.98	2.83	2.75	2.67	2.58	2.50	2.40	2.31
23	7.88	5.66	4.76	4.26	3.94	3.71	3.54	3.41	3.30	3.21	3.07	2.93	2.78	2.70	2.62	2.54	2.45	2.35	2.26
24	7.82	5.61	4.72	4.22	3.90	3.67	3.50	3.36	3.26	3.17	3.03	2.89	2.74	2.66	2.58	2.49	2.40	2.31	2.21
25	7.77	5.57	4.68	4.18	3.85	3.63	3.46	3.32	3.22	3.13	2.99	2.85	2.70	2.62	2.54	2.45	2.36	2.27	2.17
26	7.72	5.53	4.64	4.14	3.82	3.59	3.42	3.29	3.19	3.09	2.96	2.81	2.66	2.58	2.50	2.42	2.33	2.23	2.13
27	7.68	5.49	4.60	4.11	3.78	3.56	3.39	3.26	3.15	3.06	2.93	2.78	2.63	2.55	2.47	2.38	2.29	2.20	2.10
28	7.64	5.45	4.57	4.07	3.75	3.53	3.36	3.23	3.12	3.03	2.90	2.75	2.60	2.52	2.44	2.35	2.26	2.17	2.06
29	7.60	5.42	4.54	4.04	3.73	3.50	3.33	3.20	3.09	3.00	2.87	2.73	2.57	2.49	2.41	2.33	2.23	2.14	2.03
30	7.56	5.39	4.51	4.02	3.70	3.47	3.30	3.17	3.07	2.98	2.84	2.70	2.55	2.47	2.39	2.30	2.21	2.11	2.01
40	7.31	5.18	4.31	3.83	3.51	3.29	3.12	2.99	2.89	2.80	2.66	2.52	2.37	2.29	2.20	2.11	2.02	1.92	1.80
60	7.08	4.98	4.13	3.65	3.34	3.12	2.95	2.82	2.72	2.63	2.50	2.35	2.20	2.12	2.03	1.94	1.84	1.73	1.60
120	6.85	4.79	3.95	3.48	3.17	2.96	2.79	2.66	2.56	2.47	2.34	2.19	2.03	1.95	1.86	1.76	1.66	1.53	1.38
∞	6.63	4.61	3.78	3.32	3.02	2.80	2.64	2.51	2.41	2.32	2.18	2.04	1.88	1.79	1.70	1.59	1.47	1.32	1.00

df = Degrees of Freedom.

From Merrington, M., and Thompson, C. M. (1943). Tables of percentage points of the inverted beta (*F*) distribution. *Biometrika, 33*(1), 73–78.

Appendix D
Critical Values of the χ^2 Distribution

df	Alpha (α) Level				
	0.10	0.05	0.025	0.01	0.001
1	2.7055	3.8415	5.0239	6.6349	10.8276
2	4.6052	5.9915	7.3778	9.2103	13.8155
3	6.2514	7.8147	9.3484	11.3449	16.2662
4	7.7794	9.4877	11.1433	13.2767	18.4668
5	9.2364	11.0705	12.8325	15.0863	20.5150
6	10.6446	12.5916	14.4494	16.8119	22.4577
7	12.0170	14.0671	16.0128	18.4753	24.3219
8	13.3616	15.5073	17.5345	20.0902	26.1245
9	14.6837	16.9190	19.0228	21.6660	27.8772
10	15.9872	18.3070	20.4832	23.2093	29.5883
11	17.2750	19.6751	21.9200	24.7250	31.2641
12	18.5493	21.0261	23.3367	26.2170	32.9095
13	19.8119	22.3620	24.7356	27.6882	34.5282
14	21.0641	23.6848	26.1189	29.1412	36.1233
15	22.3071	24.9958	27.4884	30.5779	37.6973
16	23.5418	26.2962	28.8454	31.9999	39.2524
17	24.7690	27.5871	30.1910	33.4087	40.7902
18	25.9894	28.8693	31.5264	34.8053	42.3124
19	27.2036	30.1435	32.8523	36.1909	43.8202
20	28.4120	31.4104	34.1696	37.5662	45.3147
21	29.6151	32.6706	35.4789	38.9322	46.7970
22	30.8133	33.9244	36.7807	40.2894	48.2679
23	32.0069	35.1725	38.0756	41.6384	49.7282
24	33.1962	36.4150	39.3641	42.9798	51.1786
25	34.3816	37.6525	40.6465	44.3141	52.6197
26	35.5632	38.8851	41.9232	45.6417	54.0520
27	36.7412	40.1133	43.1945	46.9629	55.4760
28	37.9159	41.3371	44.4608	48.2782	56.8923
29	39.0875	42.5570	45.7223	49.5879	58.3012
30	40.2560	43.7730	46.9792	50.8922	59.7031
31	41.4217	44.9853	48.2319	52.1914	61.0983
32	42.5847	46.1943	49.4804	53.4858	62.4872
33	43.7452	47.3999	50.7251	54.7755	63.8701
34	44.9032	48.6024	51.9660	56.0609	65.2472
35	46.0588	49.8018	53.2033	57.3421	66.6188
36	47.2122	50.9985	54.4373	58.6192	67.9852
37	48.3634	52.1923	55.6680	59.8925	69.3465
38	49.5126	53.3835	56.8955	61.1621	70.7029
39	50.6598	54.5722	58.1201	62.4281	72.0547
40	51.8051	55.7585	59.3417	63.6907	73.4020
41	52.9485	56.9424	60.5606	64.9501	74.7449
42	54.0902	58.1240	61.7768	66.2062	76.0838
43	55.2302	59.3035	62.9904	67.4593	77.4186
44	56.3685	60.4809	64.2015	68.7095	78.7495
45	57.5053	61.6562	65.4102	69.9568	80.0767

df = Degrees of Freedom.

Corty, E. (2007). *Using and interpreting statistics: A practical text for the health, behavioral, and social sciences.* St Louis, MO: Mosby.

Index

Page numbers followed by "*f*" indicate figures, and "*t*" indicate tables.